Biomedicine Review

A Review Manual, Test Prep and
Study Guide for Acupuncturists
and East Asian Medicine Practitioners

Second Edition

Catherine Follis, DC

Second Edition, July 2014
First Edition, October 2013

ISBN-13: 978-0991022519
ISBN-10: 0991022513

Disclaimer: This book attempts to be a review of materials learned in the educational setting at institutions teaching the practice of acupuncture. This book is for educational use only. This book does not render any medical advice, and is not meant to be used to diagnose, prescribe for, or treat any medical condition, illness or injury. The publisher and author of this book will not accept liability or responsibility for any damage or injury as a result of any actions performed by the reader using any information from this book. Please obtain proper health care instructions, medication and/or supplement advice, and treatment from a licensed health care provider. The materials in this review manual have been provided in the best attempt at being error free. If errors are present, the author and publisher cannot be held liable. Any errors or omissions, if present, will be attempted to be corrected in upcoming editions.

BIOMEDICINE REVIEW
A Review Manual, Test Prep and Study Guide for Acupuncturists and East Asian Medicine Practitioners

Table of Contents

CHAPTER 17: NUTRITION AND SUPPLEMENTS 275

INTRODUCTION: A GUIDE TO THIS MANUAL

Welcome to Biomedicine Review. Hopefully this book will be a good review and summary of many of the topics pertaining to Biomedicine that is taught in Acupuncture school. Here is an overall guide to this manual.

In Chapter 1, we discuss the importance of obtaining a proper health history that would be obtained by a Western Doctor. This health history information is also obtained by most health care providers! The health history intake and interview allow the health care provider to get a better understanding of the patient. Chapter 1 covers the different sections of the patient health history and reviews what types of information should be gathered in each section. In this chapter we also discuss the basic components of a Western Physical Examination: the vital signs and assessment techniques. Lastly, pain documentation methods and referred pain is covered.

In Chapters 2-14 of this review manual, each physiological system of the body (for example: muscular, digestive, urinary, cardiovascular, etc.) will be covered. In the beginning of the chapter for each system, a brief review of the anatomy and physiology of that system will be discussed. Being familiar with the anatomy and physiology of the body will help increase understanding of the structures examined during the physical exam and also the pathological changes that occur with different disease conditions. After reviewing the anatomy and physiology of each body system, this manual will then take a quick glance at the Western Physical Examination. This examination should be performed so that the health care provider can assess the health of each system in the body. Some of the more common abnormal findings that may be discovered during the examination process will be discussed. If a Western Doctor/physician might use advanced imaging tests to assist in diagnosis of a condition, commonly used imaging and diagnostic tests will be listed in each chapter for each system. Finally, at the end of these chapters, some of the pathologies that may occur in the body and affect each system will be listed. Pay particular attention to any "Red Flag Symptoms" listed for some of the pathologies. *Please note that the list of pathologies and abnormal findings may not be all-inclusive (there are LOTS of pathologies and abnormal exam findings), But, this manual will try to cover some of the more common ones.*

Just performing a physical examination may not offer all of the needed information for a physician to administer a proper diagnosis and/or treatment. In many cases additional laboratory tests may be ordered. These tests can include blood tests, urinalysis, and fecal studies. Screening examinations should be done on a regular basis. These examinations are usually preventative in nature and may be performed even when the patient is exhibiting no symptoms. A discussion on common laboratory tests and a timeline of when screening examinations should be performed is found in the Laboratory Studies and Screening Examination chapter (Chapter 15).

This manual will also discuss some of the main classes of pharmaceuticals and nutritional supplements which might be prescribed by a Western Doctor/physician. In the Pharmaceuticals Chapter (Chapter 16), each classification and category of drugs listed will have its mechanisms of action, uses, and side effects listed (as well as generic and trade names). In the Nutrition and Supplements Chapter (Chapter 17), common supplements taken by patients will be listed, including their proposed uses and side effects. Interactions between supplements and medications will also be discussed in both of these chapters.

Lastly, this book wraps up with the Safety Practices and Practice Management chapters. The Safety Practices chapter (Chapter 18) will offer a review on OSHA, a brief review on the universal precautions and clean needle technique, and CPR/first aid. The Practice Management chapter (Chapter 19) will discuss proper charting, HIPAA, referral guidelines, mandated reportable conditions, coding for treatments and procedures, malpractice and liability insurance, licensure and certification, and scope of practice. Concerning practice management, some of the topics covered here are set by individual states in their laws and regulations. So, be sure to check with the regulations in the specific state you may be practicing in. Washington State will be the "sample" state in this book, to give you an example of what some state laws and regulations will look like in regards to the practice of acupuncture.

At the end of each chapter, there are practice study and test questions pertaining to the information presented in each chapter. Check your knowledge of the materials in each chapter with these questions. The answers are also provided, so you can grade yourself as you complete the questions. In this manual, there are over 350 practice test questions for you to utilize as you work with this material.

This book is meant to be a review of the topics listed here and are hopefully topics you have already had some exposure to. Some of you may be using this book to help review for your certification exam. If you need more detail or more of a refresher, please refer to other resources to get more background information. Resources can include: your anatomy and physiology textbook, your CNT manual, materials from your First Aid/CPR class, HIV/AIDS and HIPAA trainings, materials from your classes (pathology, pharmacology, nutrition, etc.) or materials and practice management information you have learned in student clinic. If you are preparing for a certification examination and looking for more textbook recommendations, check out the bibliography that may be posted by the testing body. For example, the NCCAOM will list on their website (*www.nccaom.org*) an outline of the topics you will be tested on and a bibliography (which will list some textbooks which may contain some information that might be found on the exam). The outlines and bibliography provided by the certification body can be very helpful and help you strategize your studying. For example: on the content outline, it may list specific topics you will need to know (for example: knowing what a MRI is). So, obviously, if a topic or item is specifically mentioned in the study guide outline- learn it!! In other areas of the outline, it may give more of a general description of what you need to know (for example: knowing the anatomy and physiology of the body). Those areas may require more time and planning when studying, due to the limited guidance given to you by the outline. Review outlines also often times show what percentage of questions on the exam will come from the different topics listed on the outline. So, a topic which makes up 55% of the exam will have a lot more questions asked on it than a topic which is only worth 10% of the exam. While you want to study and master as much of the content on the exam outline as possible, knowing which section of the exam will be asked about more frequently may help you divide up the amount of time you spend studying on the different sections of the examination outline.

Whether you are a practicing acupuncturist who may be using this manual as a refresher and a review, or a student using this book to help support your certification examination studying efforts, I wish you all the best. I hope this manual may be of some value for you and ultimately for the care of the patients you will be able to serve and help.

CHAPTER 1: HISTORY TAKING AND THE PHYSICAL EXAMINATION

Here is a brief overview of what is involved in the physical examination performed by a Western doctor/physician (and many other health care providers, too!):

I. **History Taking/Interview**: A health care provider will obtain patient case history via an interview utilizing open ended questions, if possible. Some identifying *biographic information* (such as age, current address, phone number, email address, gender, marital status, occupation, insurance information) can be gained through the intake form. Topics covered should include:
    A. Chief Complaint and History of Present Illness
    B. Past Medical History
    C. Family History
    D. Personal History
    E. Social History
    F. Review of Systems (ask if patient has any issues with these systems)
        1. General Symptoms
        2. Diet
        3. Skin, Hair, Nails
        4. Head and Neck (EENT)
        5. Endocrine
        6. Chest and Lungs (Respiratory)
        7. Heart, Blood and Blood Vessels (Cardiovascular)
        8. Lymphatic and Lymph nodes
        9. Gastrointestinal (Digestive)
        10. Genitourinary
        11. Musculoskeletal
        12. Neurologic
        13. Psychiatric

II. **Examination**: After verbally discussing the above factors with the patient, the physical examination should begin. The four main examination procedures that should be done in the physical exam are:
    A. Inspection/Observation
    B. Palpation
    C. Percussion
    D. Auscultation
These four procedures should be done (if applicable) for each of the main systems listed above. Additional tests may be used as well for specific systems- for example: instrumentation, orthopedic tests, neurologic tests, etc.

History Taking and the Interview:

During the interview, the health care provider will obtain information about the patient's current health status and past history. This time also allows the health care provider to build rapport and trust with the patient. The health care provider should ensure that the environment is private during this process and the health care provider should work to make sure that the patient feels comfortable and welcome to share information. This could include:

- Making sure the patient is in a physically comfortable position during the interview (sitting, standing, whatever is most comfortable for them).
- The health care provider should use language that is warm, polite and non-offensive- encouraging the patient to offer more information about their condition.
- The health care provider should ensure that they are using body language that is open and welcoming (avoiding crossing their arms, looking bored, rolling their eyes as a response to patient statements, etc.)

Some information about the patient's condition and history can be obtained using an intake form, but a face-to face interview should always take place as well. The health care provider can use two main types of questions during the interview to obtain needed information:

- **Open-ended questions**- these questions allow the patient to answer the question in their own words. These questions usually cannot be answered with just a "yes" or "no". Open ended questions will offer the health care provider more information than using closed questions and should be used most often. For example:
  - *How did your injury happen?*
  - *Which foods seem to cause your digestive troubles?*
- **Closed questions**- these are very direct questions and can be answered with a "yes" or "no". Closed questions may help the health care provider focus the intake process so they can figure out the patient's main issues- but once an area of concern is established, then the health care provider will utilize open ended questions to provide more detailed information. For example:
  - *Are you having chest pain now?*
  - *Did you take your medication this morning?*
  - *Does anyone in your family have a history of diabetes?*

Let's now look at the main areas of information that will be obtained during the history taking interview.

Chief Complaint and History of Present Illness:

The chief complaint is the main reason the patient is seeking care today. Asking open ended questions will help gain information about the chief complaint:

- What is the main reason for seeking care today?
- What caused the symptoms (causative factors)? Where is the location of the symptoms?
- Has the patient has ever experienced these symptoms before?
- If symptoms are painful, have the patient rate the intensity of the pain using the Visual Analog Scale or Verbal Analog Scale
- Are symptoms constant or intermittent? What causes exacerbations and remissions/relief?
- Do the symptoms affect their lifestyle or daily activities?
- Have they seen another health care provider for these symptoms?

Past Medical History:

This is the time for the health care provider to get an idea of the health of the patient prior to this current condition. Questions the health care provider may ask pertaining to past medical history include:

- Have you been hospitalized before? If so, when, where and why?
- Any surgeries? If yes, when, where and why?
- What childhood illnesses did they experience? (For example: measles, mumps, chicken pox, polio, etc.),
- Have they suffered any major illness as an adult? (For example: tuberculosis, HIV, diabetes, hypertension, myocardial infarction, stroke, cancer, asthma, kidney or liver failure, etc.)
- Have they had any prior treatment for emotional, mood, psychiatric conditions? Any thoughts of suicide (past or present)? Any history of physical or emotional abuse (past or present)?
- Are they currently being treated for any medical problem (besides the chief complaint)? If yes, with whom (for example: PCP, naturopath, dietician, chiropractor, massage, PT, OT, counseling, acupuncture, medical specialists, dental care, etc.)?
- Have they experienced a serious physical injury in their lifetime?
- What medications are they taking? What is the dosage and frequency? This will include ALL medications, including prescription, over-the-counter, herbal, homeopathic, nutritional and dietary supplements.
- Does the patient have any allergies? If so, to what (food, medication, environmental factors, supplement or herbal)? What are the symptoms of the typical allergic reaction they experience and what treatments do they employ if they are having an allergic reaction?
- Have they had a transfusion before?
- Note if any of the past medical history of the patient would be a risk factor for future health conditions.

Family History:

Obtaining a family history is important. Family history may reveal a link and higher risk for some diseases and conditions.

- Have any other blood relatives experienced the patient's chief complaint?
- Determine ethnicity of patient and their family
- Ask about the health of family members. Are parents and siblings still alive? If not, what was the cause of death, and at what age?
- Did any close relatives suffer from any major medical illness or conditions? Ask for family history of: heart disease, high blood pressure, cancer, tuberculosis, stroke, epilepsy, diabetes, kidney disease, glaucoma, thyroid disease, autoimmune diseases, arthritis, blood diseases, asthma, allergies, addictions or any other familial (hereditary) diseases.
- Ask of age and health of spouse and any children.
- Note if any of the family history could be a risk factor for future health conditions (ex: history of breast cancer in parent and siblings increases risk of breast cancer in the patient)

Personal and Social History:

In this section, the health care provider is gaining information on the patient's personal past history and their current activities of daily living. If any of these things are impacted by their current medical condition, that information should be noted. Information to be obtained should include:

- Ask the patient about their home environment as a youth (divorced parents, married parents, raised by single parent, socioeconomic class)
- Ask the patient about current home environment (who are they living with)
- What does the patient do for a living? Do they enjoy their job? What goes on at work in a typical day (what do they do, how many hours worked per day)? Are they in a physically dangerous or challenging job? Are they exposed to toxic substances while at work?
- Does the patient serve in the military? If yes, how long and where?
- Do they follow a religion? Do their religious beliefs affect their diet, dress, or other health practices?
- How much sleep does the patient get at night? How is their quality of sleep at night?
- Does the patient exercise? If so, ask patient to describe their exercise program.
- What hobbies and interests does the patient have?
- What are sources of stress in the patient's life? What stress relieving activities do they perform?
- Does the patient smoke cigarettes? If yes, how many per day?
- Does the patient smoke or consume marijuana? If yes, how much per day?
- Does the patient drink alcohol? If yes, how much per day? Or, the health care provider may instead choose to utilize the *CAGE assessment* for alcohol abuse. The CAGE assessment is a simple assessment- the provider asks the patient these four questions:
  - Have you ever felt the need to **Cut Down** on your drinking?
  - Do you feel **Annoyed** by people complaining about your drinking?
  - Do you ever feel **Guilty** about your drinking?
  - Do you ever drink an **Eye-opener** in the morning to relieve shakes?

  Two or more "yes" responses suggest the patient may have a problem with alcohol abuse. *(Ewing, John A. "Detecting Alcoholism: The CAGE Questionnaire" JAMA 252: 1905-1907, 1984)*
- Does the patient use illicit drugs? If yes, what type and how often?
- Does the patient consume caffeine (coffee, tea, energy drinks)? If yes, how much per day?
- Have the patient describe their typical diet. Do they avoid any foods? If so, why?
- Ask about their sexual history. Do they have any concerns? What is their number of partners? Any history of sexually transmitted diseases?

Review of Systems:

In this section, the health care provider takes a quick glance at all of the systems of the body to determine if more follow up is needed. Depending on the patient and their health, for some systems the health care provider may only take a few seconds to ask about, whereas other systems may have a few minutes or more devoted to them if a patient indicates a problem or issue (more follow up questions can then be done to get more information.)

✓ *General symptoms*
- Is the patient experiencing fever, malaise, fatigue, chills, night sweats?
- What is the height and weight of the patient? Have they noticed any significant weight loss or weight gain in the last year?

✓ *Diet*
- If not already discussed in the "habits" section of the Personal History:
  - Ask about the patient's appetite, food likes and dislikes, and dietary restrictions
- Ask if the patient takes vitamin or other supplementation.

- Ask the patient about caffeine, alcohol, and water intake.
- Any food allergies or intolerances should be noted. If an allergy or intolerance is mentioned, the health care provider should note what sort of reaction they experience, and what sort of treatment/medication they use in the event of an allergic response.
- A diet journal could be requested from the patient.

✓ *Skin, Hair, or Nails-*
- Does the patient suffer from rashes, allergic reactions, eruptions, pigmentation or texture change on their skin?
- Does the patient notice excessive sweating, hair and nail growth?
- Does the patient notice excessive hair loss, nail weakness or discoloring?

✓ *Head and Neck-*
- General:
  - Does the patient suffer from headaches? If yes, what is the location, frequency, length of episodes and any known triggers of their headaches?
  - Does the patient experience dizziness? Loss of consciousness?
  - Has the patient ever had a head injury?
- Eyes:
  - When was their last eye examination? Have they noticed any change in their vision? Any history of eye trauma?
  - Does the patient wear glasses or contacts? If so, what is their uncorrected vision? Have they had any corrective vision surgery?
  - Does the patient have glaucoma, color blindness, or cataracts?
  - Does the patient suffer from blurred vision, double vision, or excessive tearing? Does light bother their eyes? Do they have trouble seeing at night?
  - Does anyone in their family have a history of familial eye diseases? (congenital glaucoma, retinal degeneration, macular degeneration, strabismus, amblyopia, astigmatism)
- Ears:
  - Has the patient ever had ear surgery? If so, why and when?
  - Does the patient have poor hearing or notice a change in their sense of hearing? Do they wear a hearing aid?
  - Does the patient experience a loss of balance (vertigo) or ringing in the ears (tinnitus)?
  - Does the patient experience ear pain, swelling or discharge?
- Nose:
  - Has the patient ever experienced nasal surgery? If so, where and why?
  - Does the patient feel their ability to smell is impaired?
  - Have they ever experienced sinus infections or nosebleeds? If so, how frequently?
  - Does the patient have nasal problems which cause breathing difficulties, frequent sneezing, or nasal discharge?
- Teeth and Mouth:
  - When was the last time the patient went to the dentist?
  - Does the patient experience mouth sores? Bleeding gums?
  - Does the patient have a loss of the sense of taste?
  - Does the patient have a toothache? Any other pain in the mouth?
  - Does the patient wear dentures?
  - Does the patient have difficulty swallowing food or liquids?
- Neck:
  - Does the patient have pain, swelling or stiffness in the neck?
  - If yes, for how long? What makes it feel better? What makes it feel worse?

✓ **Endocrine System-**
- Does the patient notice any enlargement around their thyroid?
- Has the patient experienced any unexplained weight change?
- Is the patient experiencing heat or cold intolerance, increased thirst, increased hunger, changes in facial or body hair, increased hat and glove size?
- Does the patient take any hormone medications?

- For Males (these questions could also be asked in the Genitourinary section):
  - What was their age at the onset of puberty?
  - Are they experiencing any difficulty with libido, erections, emissions, infertility?
  - Are they experiencing any testicular pain? What is the frequency of their testicular self-exams? Have they had their prostate examined and/or screening tests done? (Note, younger males may have not had this performed yet)
  - Does the patient notice pain or lumps in the breast tissue, or a change in contour?

- For Females (these questions could also be asked in the Genitourinary section):
  - What was their age of onset for menses?
  - What is the patient's cycle length? Have the patient describe their menses (duration and amount of flow, is there any pain during menses, any clotting?)
  - When was the patient's last gynecological exam? When was their last Pap smear? Have they ever had an abnormal Pap? If yes, what follow up was done?
  - If applicable, what was the patient's age at menopause?
  - Is the patient experiencing any difficulty with libido or infertility?
  - Is the patient currently pregnant? Have they been pregnant before? If yes, how many pregnancies? Any miscarriages? Any abortions?
  - How many children does the patient have? How was the delivery of each child? (Length of labor, type of delivery, any complications?)
  - Does the patient use birth control? If yes, what type?
  - Does the patient perform monthly breast self-examinations?
  - If applicable, when was their last mammogram and what were the results?
  - Does the patient notice any breast pain, tenderness, lumps, change in breast contour, or discharge from nipples?

✓ **Chest and Lungs (Respiratory System):**
- Does the patient experience pain with breathing, dyspnea (difficulty breathing), shortness of breath, a persistent cough, or wheezing?
- Does the patient have shortness of breath during exercise or when lying down?
- Does the patient have a productive cough? If so, do they cough up blood?
- Any respiratory sensitivity to airborne particles (smoke, pollen, etc.)? Any sensitivity of breathing with exercise or breathing cold/hot air temperatures? If yes, document what sort of reaction they have from exposure, any treatments for exposure should be noted as well.
- Does the patient have a history of emphysema, pneumonia, asthma or frequent respiratory infections?
- Has the patient ever had a positive TB skin test? Have they ever had a chest x-ray? If yes, when and what were the results?

✓ **Heart, Blood, Blood Vessels (Cardiovascular System):**
- Does the patient experience palpitations, an irregular heartbeat, a fast heartbeat, chest pain or distress? If yes, document any causes, timing, duration, exacerbating and relieving factors.
- Does the patient have hypertension (high blood pressure)? If yes, what treatments and/or dietary changes are they doing?
- Does the patient have a history of angina?
- Has the patient had a myocardial infarction (heart attack)? If yes, when?

- Has the patient had any prior cardiovascular tests (ECG, blood tests, stress tests, etc.)? If yes, when and what were the results?
- Does the patient have a history of anemia? If yes, what type?
- Does the patient have a tendency to bruise or bleed easily? Do they have a history of abnormal blood clotting?
- Does the patient have varicose veins, swollen ankles, or intermittent pain in their legs?

✓ **Lymphatic System and Lymph Nodes:**
- Is there any enlargement or tenderness in the armpit region, groin region, or along the neck?
- Does the patient have prior history of cancer in the lymph nodes?

✓ **Gastrointestinal (Digestive) System:**
- Has the patient experienced any gastrointestinal symptoms such as: nausea, vomiting, loss of appetite, abdominal pain, frequent belching or passing of gas?
- Has the patient recently gained or lost weight?
- How often does the patient have a bowel movement? What is the color, odor, consistency of the stools? Has there been any change in their elimination pattern? Does the patient use laxatives?
- Does the patient have a history of ulcers or hemorrhoids?
- Does the patient have hepatitis, jaundice, any other liver or gallbladder disease?
- Any history of colon cancer or colon polyps?

✓ **Genitourinary System:**
- What color is the patient's urine? Is it clear or cloudy? Is there any odor associated with it? Have they ever seen blood in their urine?
- Is there any pain or burning with urination, incontinence, urgency, decreased flow or dribbling?
- Does the patient get up during the night to urinate? If yes, how many times?
- Is the patient experiencing suprapubic pain or flank pain?
- Has the patient ever had a UTI? If yes, how many?
- Has the patient ever been treated for kidney stones? If yes, when?
- Any history of STD's?

✓ **Musculoskeletal System:**
- Is there any difficulty with sitting, standing, walking?
- Does the patient have pain in any muscles or joints? If yes, where?
- Does the patient have any history of arthritis, gout, back injuries, or muscle weakness?

✓ **Neurologic System-**
- Has the patient ever had a seizure?
- Does the patient have a tremor?
- Any history of tremors, twitching, weakness or paralysis, abnormalities of sensation in any part of their body?
- Is there any concern with loss of memory or mental confusion?

✓ **Psychiatric-**
- Does the patient ever experience mood swings?
- Does the patient ever feel anxious, depressed, unable to cope, or unable to concentrate?
- Is the patient currently experiencing sleep disturbances?
- Is the patient feeling unusually stressed?
- Is the patient experiencing suicidal thoughts?
- Does the patient seem to comprehend the interview, are they responding to questions in a reasonable manner?

Pain Patterns and Documenting Pain Levels:

Often, pain or discomfort is what brings a patient to a health care provider's office. Being able to appropriately analyze and document pain symptoms is important.

Referred Pain

Referred pain is where an underlying organ is having dysfunction, but the area of pain where the patient reports discomfort may be removed from the location of the underlying pathology.

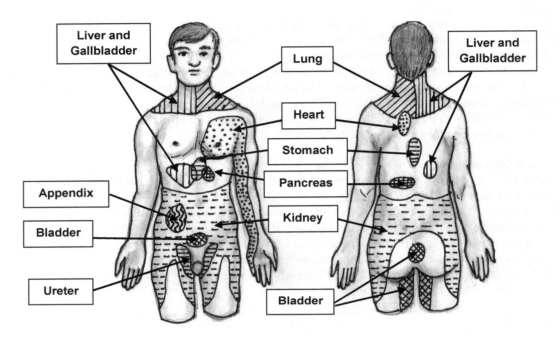

Localized Pain

Localized pain is pain that is felt near the area of dysfunction. Patient is usually asked to describe the pain. Common descriptive terms are: ache, burning, throbbing, cramping, stabbing, sharp, dull, hot, zinging, and pinching. These terms may be used in combination (ex: dull ache, sharp stabbing pain, etc.).

It should also be noted if this pain is:
- ➢ Constant
- ➢ Intermittent
- ➢ Acute
- ➢ Chronic

During the course of a physical exam, the patient should be told to let the examiner know if any portions of the exam are changing the levels of pain that they are currently experiencing (increasing pain or decreasing the pain) and if the quality of pain changes (example: pain changes from aching to stabbing when examiner lifts patient arm).

Pain Intensity Scales:

Pain intensity scales are used as a way for a patient to report their subjective pain level. These scales can be used to rate a patient's pain level on an overall daily basis, or can be used to rate pain during a specific activity or event. These scale results should be kept in the patient's chart, or can be incorporated into the "S" Subjective section of a SOAP chart. These scales can also be used to rate a patient's sense of wellness or rate activity of a particular body system (example: rating digestive activity).

There are two common pain intensity scales used by health care providers: the **Verbal (Numerical) Analog Scale** and the **Visual Analog Scale.**

Verbal (Numerical) Analog Scale: From a scale of 0-10, patient *verbally* tells practitioner what their pain level is.

> ➢ 0= no pain, 10= most severe pain.

> ➢ It should be noted in the chart if a patient is currently talking pain reducing medication. The health care provider should try to get a verbally reported pain level from the patient for when they are NOT under the influence of the medication, and then another verbal analog score for the patient when they are under the influence.

Visual Analog Scale: Here, the patient uses a slide rule to indicate their pain level, or marks an area on a visual scale chart to indicate their pain level. There may or may not be any numbers located on the chart indicating pain levels. Below are examples of charting methods in which the patient writes an "X" on the line below to mark their level of pain.

For example:

On the scale below, mark your pain levels today:

◄───►

No pain   **Excruciating**

Or

On the scale below, mark your pain levels today:

No pain   **Moderate Pain**   **Unbearable Pain**

◄───►

0   1   2   3   4   5   6   7   8   9   10

The Examination:

Vital Signs:

One of the things included in a physical examination will be an assessment of the vital signs. Some health care providers will take the vital signs before they proceed with the rest of the examination. Often times on a visit to the Western Doctor/physician, the vital signs will be recorded by the nurse or a medical assistant before the doctor enters the room. Other physicians and health care providers will take the different vital signs when they are assessing the appropriate system (for example, they will note the respiratory rate when examining the respiratory system).

The vital signs are:

✓ **Body Temperature**: Normal Ranges- 96.7-100.5 degrees Fahrenheit (depending on the route used for measurement).
  - Oral temperature is normally 97.7-99.5 degrees Fahrenheit.
  - Axillary (armpit): 96.7-98.5 degrees Fahrenheit
  - Rectal: 98.7-100.5 degrees Fahrenheit
  - Tympanic: 98.2-100 degrees Fahrenheit
  - Temporal: 98.2- 100.1 degrees Fahrenheit

✓ **Pulse**: Normal Ranges- 60-100 pulses per minute. Palpate a superficial artery (often the lateral portion of the wrist or alongside the trachea), and count the number, rate, rhythm, and amplitude of the pulsations.

✓ **Respirations-** Normal rate- 16-20 breaths per minute. Pay attention to the rate and depth of the breathing. Look for any use of accessory muscles when breathing (for example- the neck muscles). Note any abnormal sounds while breathing.

✓ **Blood Pressure-** Equipment used: *sphygmomanometer* (the cuff and bulb) and *stethoscope*, and the sounds heard while taking a blood pressure are called *Korotkoff's sounds*.
  - Optimal blood pressure is Systolic 100-119 mmHg and Diastolic 60-79 mmHg.
  - Prehypertension is Systolic 120-139 mmHg or Diastolic 80-89 mmHg
  - Stage 1 Hypertension is Systolic 140-159 mmHg or a Diastolic of 90-99 mmHg
  - Stage 2 Hypertension is Systolic greater than 160 mmHg or Diastolic greater than 100 mmHg.
  - Hypertensive Crisis is Systolic greater than 180 or Diastolic greater than 120 mmHg

✓ Some texts will also include **height** and **weight** as part of the vital signs. Even if these are not considered a "vital sign", they should be obtained during an initial visit.

Assessment Techniques:

When proceeding to examine the individual systems of the body (respiratory, gastrointestinal, etc.), four main techniques are usually performed. Not all techniques will be performed on every body part (for example- no deep palpation or auscultation on the eyeball).

- *Inspection/Observation*- Inspect each body system using vision (primarily) but also smell & hearing. Observe, color, size, location, movement, texture, symmetry, odors, and sounds in the area of the body being assessed. When possible, compare structures bilaterally and note any differences from one side to the other. For example: during a breathing assessment- watch the motion of the chest bilaterally, note odors on the breath (fruity), and listen for any wheezing/gurgling.

- *Palpation*- A few pointers with palpation- Try to keep your fingernails short and hands warm. Palpate suspected tender areas last. Begin palpation with wide surfaces of finger pads, and gradually isolate with finger tips if needed. Begin with light palpation (depressing skin ½" to ¾"), then if no tenderness proceed to deep palpation (if needed) to assess deeper internal organs. Assess for texture (rough, smooth, hard, etc.), moisture (wet or dry), temperature, motion (is the area vibrating, twitching, or still), pain or tenderness.

- *Percussion*- Involves the health care provider tapping their fingers or hands quickly and sharply against parts of the patient's body while listening to the sound produced and noting any tenderness. Percussion is used to determine size, shape, location and tenderness of certain organs. It can also be used to assess organ density (is the organ solid, fluid filled, or filled with gas).

- *Auscultation*- Using a stethoscope and listening for various heart, breath, and bowel sounds

Practice Study and Test Questions:

1) What is considered biographic data?
    A) Age
    B) Gender
    C) Current address
    D) All of the above

2) Which of the following questions is an example of an open ended question?
    A) How do your symptoms affect your daily living activities?
    B) Do you have neck pain now?
    C) Have you taken your medication today?
    D) Does it hurt when you urinate?

3) In what section of the health history should the following information be placed: "The patient's mother has had breast cancer"
    A) Past Medical History
    B) Family History
    C) Social History
    D) Musculoskeletal System History

4) The patient's exercise frequency and routine should be documented under:
    A) Biographic Data
    B) Family History
    C) Past Medical History
    D) Personal and Social History

5) The patient reports they are experiencing palpitations. What portion of the review of systems would discover this information?
    A) Heart, Blood, Blood Vessels (cardiovascular)
    B) Neurologic
    C) Genitourinary
    D) Gastrointestinal (Digestive)

6) The patient reports they are experiencing an enlarged, painless lump in their armpit. What portion of the review of systems would discover this information?
    A) Gastrointestinal (Digestive)
    B) Neurologic
    C) Lymphatic and Lymph Node
    D) Chest and Lungs (Respiratory)

7) Pain in the pancreas can refer to
    A) Left Shoulder
    B) Left side of the mid-low back
    C) Lower left abdomen
    D) Inner thighs

8) Normal temperature, taken orally, is within the range of
    A) 96.7-98.5 degrees Fahrenheit
    B) 98.2-100 degrees Fahrenheit
    C) 98.7-100.5 degrees Fahrenheit
    D) 97.7-99.5 degrees Fahrenheit

9) An examination technique in which the physician taps their fingers on the chest of the patient, is called
    A) Percussion
    B) Deep palpation
    C) Auscultation
    D) Light palpation

10) A sphygmomanometer is used
    A) to measure temperature rectally
    B) to assist in palpation of the abdomen
    C) when taking a blood pressure
    D) when percussing the chest

11) Normal respiratory rate is between
    A) 10-15 breaths per minute
    B) 30-35 breaths per minute
    C) 60-100 breaths per minute
    D) 16-20 breaths per minute

12) The appendix may refer pain to the
    A) lower left abdominal region
    B) right shoulder
    C) down the left arm
    D) lower right abdominal region

13) A patient's chief complaint is cramping in the abdominal region. What question would be helpful in learning more about the chief complaint and would be noted in the chief complaint/history of present illness section of the health history?
    A) What makes the abdominal cramping feel worse?
    B) What is the age of your spouse?
    C) Does your family have a history of glaucoma?
    D) Does the patient have a history of a tremor?

14) A patient states *verbally* that their pain is an 8/10. This would be recorded using the
    A) Verbal Analog Scale
    B) Visual Analog Scale
    C) Vital Analog Scale
    D) None of the above

15) Pre-hypertension is defined as
    A) Systolic greater than 180 mmHg and Diastolic greater than 120 mmHg
    B) Systolic 100-119 mmHg and Diastolic 70-89 mmHg
    C) Systolic 160 mmHg and Diastolic 100 mmHg
    D) Systolic 120-139 mmHg and Diastolic 80-89 mmHg

16) Inspection/Observation of a body system uses the following senses
    A) Vision
    B) Smell
    C) Hearing
    D) All of the above

17) Auscultation is performed using
    A) light pressure with the fingertips
    B) a sphygmomanometer
    C) a stethoscope
    D) All of the above

18) The kidney can refer pain to
    A) in the left chest and left arm
    B) in the upper central back region
    C) the low back and into the thighs
    D) upper left abdominal area

19) Asking the patient if they are exposed to any toxic substances while at work would most likely be done during which part of the health history interview?
    A) Past Medical History
    B) Personal and Social History
    C) Family History
    D) Genitourinary System

20) Should a patient be asked during the health history interview if they have ever experienced mood swings, anxiety, depression, or difficulty concentrating?
    A) Never, mental health issues should not be covered in the health history interview
    B) Perhaps, if the health care provider has time
    C) Yes

21) A patient rates their pain as a 5/10 on a verbal analog scale. This information should be reported in which section of the chart note?
- A) Subjective
- B) Objective
- C) Assessment
- D) Plan

22) Information pertaining to the patient's last eye examination should be recorded in which section of the Review of Systems?
- A) Head and Neck
- B) Genitourinary
- C) Endocrine
- D) Chest and Lungs

23) Your patient is a military veteran. His service should be noted in which portion of the health history interview?
- A) Family History
- B) Endocrine System
- C) Personal and Social History
- D) Musculoskeletal System

24) Hypertensive crisis is defined as
- A) 115/79
- B) 140/90
- C) 160/100
- D) a blood pressure greater than 180/120

25) A tympanic temperature reading is taken
- A) in the mouth
- B) on the surface of the forehead
- C) in the ear
- D) in the rectum

Answers: 1) D 2) A 3) B 4) D 5) A 6) C 7) B 8) D 9) A 10) C 11) D 12) D 13) A 14) A 15) D 16) D 17) C 18) C 19) B 20) C 21) A 22) A 23) C 24) D 25) C

CHAPTER 2: ORIENTATION TO THE HUMAN BODY-AN INTRODUCTION TO ANATOMY AND PHYSIOLOGY

These notes are not meant to be an all-inclusive anatomy and physiology course. They are just a review of some of the main points. Please refer to your materials/textbook from your A&P course for more details

The Sciences of Anatomy and Physiology:

Anatomy: The study of the internal and external structures of the body and the physical relationship of these structures. Basically anatomy is the study of "parts"- where the body parts are located, sizes, shapes, colors of the parts. **Macroscopic (Gross Anatomy):** the study of BIG parts- parts you can see with the unaided eye. [Examples: *surface anatomy, regional anatomy* or *systemic anatomy, etc.*] **Microscopic Anatomy:** the study of parts too small to be seen without use of a microscope. There are two main types of anatomy we study with a microscope- cytology and histology. *Cytology* is the study of individual cells and the structures that compose them. And, *histology* is the study of tissues (a tissue is a group of cells).

Physiology: How organisms perform their vital functions- in other words WHAT do the parts do? Examples of types of physiological studies: *cell physiology, systemic physiology* and *pathological physiology.*

Levels of Organization:

The human body can be organized into SIX levels of organization, starting with the smallest microscopic building blocks and eventually combining and forming the most complex level (which is us, as a human being).

    1. *Chemical Level-* atoms, molecules, elements, compounds. This is the basis of all matter- everything around us and in us.

    2. *Cellular Level-* the cell is the smallest unit of life. Chemicals, molecules, compounds combine to form cells. Only living organisms contain cells.

    3. *Tissue Level-* a tissue is a group of similar cells all working together to accomplish a specific function

    4. *Organ Level-* two or more tissues working together will combine to form an organ. Organs can usually perform more than one function.

    5. *Organ System-* two or more organs working together form an organ system. Organ systems can usually handle complex bodily processes. There are 11 organ systems:

        a. Integumentary System
        b. Skeletal System
        c. Muscular System
        d. Nervous System
        e. Endocrine System
        f. Cardiovascular System (sometimes called Circulatory System)
        g. Lymphatic System
        h. Respiratory System
        i. Digestive System
        k. Urinary System
        l. Reproductive System

    6. *Organism Level-* Composed of all 11 organ systems working together to form a complete human being.

Homeostasis:

Homeostasis is the existence of a stable, constant, internal environment. Our body works hard to maintain homeostasis. Homeostatic balance is a crucial concept in maintaining health, wellness, and life. If we are unable to maintain homeostasis, this can lead to illness- even death. Our body uses the Nervous System and Endocrine System to regulate homeostasis. There are three main parts involved in homeostasis regulation:

1) Receptor- these are neuron sensors located throughout our body that constantly take measurements on what is happening in us and around us. There are many different types of receptors in our body specializing in measuring different types of stimuli.

2) Control Center- (aka Integration Center) - this is where we process the measurements that were detected by the receptor. This is usually our brain.

3) Effector- this is the bodily response of a cell or organ to try to move the body back into homeostatic balance. The control center gives the effector instructions on what it should do.

The effector response will be in either one of two forms: Negative Feedback or Positive Feedback.

- **Negative Feedback:** This feedback response negates (or stops) whatever pattern the original stimulus was causing. In most cases in our body (over 90% of the time) negative feedback is a GOOD thing and is the primary way that we maintain homeostasis. For example, if body temperature is rising, negative feedback will stop the temperature from increasing further and work to lower the temperature back down into the normal range for a healthy body.

- **Positive feedback:** This feedback enhances, increases, or exaggerates whatever pattern or activity is occurring. This type of feedback is used whenever a potentially dangerous or stressful process must be finished quickly. There are a few situations when positive feedback is healthy- the blood clotting mechanism and the process of childbirth are two examples. Unfortunately, positive feedback can also be dangerous- this process allows the body to potentially get out of control. We can see this in cases of illness or trauma where the body is no longer able to maintain a stable internal environment.

The Anatomy and Physiology of a Cell (Cytology):

A cell is the smallest unit of life. It is composed of three main parts:
1. Plasma (Cell) Membrane
2. Cytoplasm
3. Nucleus

Let's review these three components of a cell.

Plasma (Cell) Membrane:

The cell membrane is the outer covering of the cell. It can also be called the *plasma membrane* or the *plasmalemma*. It functions to: act as a physical protective barrier, regulate exchange of materials with the environment, detect changes in the extracellular fluid, offer structural support, and serve as the location where cells can attach to one another.

The cell membrane is composed of Lipids, Proteins, and Carbohydrates. **Lipids- (fats)** make up the majority of our cell membrane. The cell membrane is sometimes called a *phospholipid bilayer*, due to the fact that it is made out of two layers of phospholipid molecules. **Proteins** function to: anchor/attach cells together, identify cells, act as enzymes, serve as receptors, and transport materials across the membrane. **Carbohydrates** can be quite large, and create an additional outer covering of the cell called the *glycocalyx*.

The Cytoplasm

Cytoplasm is defined as the material located between the cell membrane and the membrane surrounding the nucleus inside the cell. Two main components of the cytoplasm are the *cytosol* and the *organelles*.

Cytosol (intracellular fluid) - composed of mostly water with dissolved nutrients, ions, proteins, and waste products. The cell membrane keeps this fluid separate from the extracellular fluid (the fluid outside the cell). Cytosol contains more potassium than extracellular fluid; extracellular fluid contains more sodium than cytosol. Cytosol contains more proteins than extracellular fluid, and cytosol will also contain carbohydrates and lipids for cell usage.

Organelles- are structures suspended within the cytosol that perform most of the cell functions. Here are some of the main organelles in the cell:
- **Cytoskeleton-** the cell skeleton. Made of proteins (microfilaments, intermediate filaments, microtubules).
- **Microvilli-** Fingerlike projections of the cell membrane which increase the surface area of the cell.
- **Centrioles-** The centrioles are found within the centrosome and are associated with the movement of DNA during cell division.
- **Cilia-** long slender extensions of the cell membrane- found especially in the respiratory and reproductive systems.
- **Ribosomes-** perform protein synthesis in the cell.
- **Proteasomes-** contain protein digesting enzymes (proteases) and break down damaged or denatured proteins in the cytoplasm.
- **Endoplasmic Reticulum-** There are two types of Endoplasmic Reticulum. Smooth Endoplasmic Reticulum has no ribosomes attached to it and specializes in synthesizing phospholipids, cholesterol, steroid hormones, glycerides, and glycogen. Rough Endoplasmic Reticulum has ribosomes attached to it; therefore, it assists in protein modification.
- **Golgi Apparatus-** consists of five or six flattened discs. Its functions are: modification and packaging of secretions to be released from the cell, renewing the cell membrane, and packaging enzymes for use inside the cell.
- **Lysosomes-** Are vesicles filled with digestive enzymes and are used to clean the cell and remove larger unwanted materials, damaged organelles, bacteria and inactive cell structures.
- **Peroxisomes-** break down fatty acids and other organic compounds. As they digest materials, they produce hydrogen peroxide- a potentially dangerous free radical (which is then further broken down into oxygen and water).
- **Mitochondria-** An organelle surrounded by a double membrane. It is filled with numerous folds called *cristae* and mitochondrial DNA. Metabolic reactions in the matrix convert carbohydrates (especially glucose) into the high energy compound / fuel called **ATP (Adenosine Triphosphate)**. The production of ATP involves glucose being broken down into pyruvic acid in the cytosol. The pyruvic acid enters the mitochondria and is processed through the **Tricarboxylic Acid Cycle (TCA cycle)** - also known as the ***Krebs Cycle***. The TCA cycle will break down the remainder of the pyruvic acid, *ONLY* if oxygen is present. Pyruvic acid will ultimately be broken down into carbon dioxide, water and dozens of molecules of ATP.

The Nucleus

The nucleus is the largest organelle in the cell. It is the control center of the entire cell. The nucleus is surrounded by a *nuclear envelope*- a membrane that keeps the nucleus separate from the rest of the cytoplasm. In order for the nucleus to be able to communicate with other parts of the cell, there are *nuclear pores* (small holes) in the nuclear envelope. Most cells are uninucleate (having only one nucleus).

The nucleus contains **nucleoplasm** (fluid) and a **nuclear matrix** for support and structure. It also contains **nucleoli,** which synthesize ribosomal RNA and the ribosomal subunits. Lastly, the nucleus contains

chromosomes, which are made up of strands of DNA attached to histones (proteins). There are 46 chromosomes (23 pairs of chromosomes) in the nuclei of somatic cells

DNA contains the instructions for proper protein synthesis in the cell. DNA tells the cell how to build its components, repair itself, adapt to changes in the environment, and regulates all of the activities of cell metabolism. DNA is composed of a pattern of four repeating nitrogenous bases linked together in a long strand. The four nitrogenous bases are: *Adenine (A), Thymine (T), Cytosine (C)* and *Guanine (G).*

Most cells can divide and form new cells. **Mitosis** is the term used to describe the division of the nucleus of a somatic body cell into two brand new cells. A cell spends most of its life in a phase called *interphase.* Interphase is the time in which the cell is performing its regular body functions. Towards the end of interphase, the cell will get ready to divide into two new cells. During the last portion of interphase, the nucleus will create a second set of chromosomes (called DNA replication). When mitosis occurs, there are four steps involved. *Prophase* is the first step of mitosis, and is the time in which the nuclear envelope dissolves, exposing the DNA and chromosomes. *Metaphase* is the second phase, and is where the chromosomes line up along the middle of the cell. *Anaphase* is the third step and is when the chromosomes separate. One full set of chromosomes gets pulled to one end (pole) of the cell, while the second set of chromosomes is pulled to the opposite end (pole) of the cell. *Telophase* is the last step of mitosis and is when the nuclear envelope reforms around both sets of chromosomes. And, the cell then divides down the middle, creating two brand new cells.

The Anatomy and Physiology of Tissues (Histology)

As a group of cells work together, that larger structure is called a **tissue.** The study of tissues is called **histology.** There are four basic types of tissues: *epithelial, connective, muscular,* and *nervous* tissues.

Epithelial Tissues:

Epithelial tissues perform four basic functions: provide physical protection, control permeability, provide sensation and produce specialized secretions. Epithelial tissues consist of tightly packed cells. When naming the various types of epithelial tissues, scientists looked at the thickness of the epithelial tissues. If the cells in the epithelial tissue are one layer thick, the tissue is called a *simple epithelium*. If the tissue is more than one cell layer thick, it is called a *stratified epithelium*. The thicker stratified types of epithelium are going to offer more physical protection than the simple epithelium.

Classifications of Epithelial Tissue:
1. **Squamous Epithelium**- squamous cells are thin, flat and irregular in shape. *Simple Squamous Epithelium*- most delicate type of epithelium. Used in areas where absorption or diffusion takes place. *Stratified Squamous Epithelium*- located where mechanical stress is severe. The many layers of cells provide good protection from physical or chemical damage. The epidermis of the skin is a good example.
2. **Cuboidal Epithelium**- cuboidal cells resemble square boxes. *Simple Cuboidal Epithelium*- lines portions of the kidney tubules and glands. *Stratified Cuboidal Epithelium*- relatively rare, found in portions of the sweat glands and mammary glands
3. **Columnar Epithelium**- columnar shaped cells appear rectangular- taller than the cuboidal cells. *Simple Columnar Epithelium*- occurs where absorption takes place, and can also be used in areas where protection is needed. *Pseudostratified Ciliated Columnar Epithelium*- columnar epithelium that has its surface covered with cilia. This is commonly found in the respiratory system. *Stratified Columnar Epithelium*- relatively rare, some are found lining portions of the pharynx, epiglottis, and anus.
4. **Glandular Epithelia:** these cells are designed to produce secretions. Collections of these epithelial cells form glands. There are two kinds of glands. *Endocrine Glands* release their secretion into interstitial fluid, blood or lymph for transport throughout the body to their target tissue (ex: hormone producing glands like the pituitary and thyroid). *Exocrine glands* release their secretions into ducts, which then carry the secretions directly to their destination (ex: sweat glands and salivary glands).

Connective Tissue:

Connective tissues, in many cases, work closely with epithelial tissue. Connective tissues have three basic components: *specialized cells*, *extracellular protein fibers*, and *ground substance* (a fluid, which combines with the extracellular proteins to make a substance called extracellular matrix).

The functions of connective tissue are: providing a framework for the body; transporting fluids and dissolved materials; protecting delicate organs; supporting, surrounding and connecting other types of tissue; storing energy reserves (fats); and defending the body from microorganisms.
Classifications of Connective Tissues:
1. **Loose Connective Tissues**- these are packing materials of the body- they fill in spaces, cushion, and stabilize other tissues and organs. Some examples: *Areolar Tissue*- very open tissue, with lots of ground substance and little fibers (for example, in subcutaneous tissue). *Adipose Tissue*- contains lots of adipocytes, which store fat. *Reticular Tissue*- fibrous mesh found in the liver, spleen, and lymph nodes.
2. **Dense Connective Tissue**- often called *collagenous tissues*. Some examples: *Dense Regular Connective Tissue*- collagen fibers run parallel to each other. Tendons, ligaments, and aponeurosis are great examples of dense regular connective tissue. *Dense Irregular Connective Tissue*- collagen fibers form an interwoven mesh network. These tissues strengthen and support areas that are under stress. *Elastic Tissue*- dominated by elastic fibers. Examples are the elastic ligaments that support the spine
3. **Blood**- A type of fluid connective tissue.
4. **Lymph**- A type of fluid connective tissue.
5. **Cartilage**- A type of supporting connective tissue. Cartilage matrix is a firm gel. Chondrocytes (cartilage cells) live in the matrix. There are a few types of cartilage: *Hyaline Cartilage*- most common type. A very tough, somewhat flexible cartilage. Found in the ribs and also composes the articular cartilage. *Elastic Cartilage*- contains elastic fibers, so it is resilient and flexible. Forms the auricle (flap of the outer ear), tip of the nose, and epiglottis. *Fibrocartilage*- matrix has little ground substance, but a lot of interwoven collagen fibers. Found in the intervertebral discs and the menisci of the knee.
6. **Bone**- the matrix of bone is roughly 2/3 calcium salts- which is what gives bones their very hard and solid consistency. The remainder of the matrix is mostly collagen and living bone cells (osteocytes, osteoblasts and osteoclasts).

Muscular Tissue

Muscular tissue will provide movement in our body. There are three main types of muscle in the body. We will discuss them in more detail when we cover the muscular system, but here is a brief overview.

1. **Skeletal Muscle**- attaches onto the bones (skeleton) of the body. Skeletal muscle cells are relatively large, long and slender. Therefore they can sometimes be called "muscle fibers". Due to being so long in length, skeletal muscle cells are *multinucleated* (contain many nuclei). Skeletal muscle cells are *striated* (having a striped appearance) when looked at under a microscope. Skeletal muscle cells are under *voluntary* control from the nervous system.

2. **Cardiac Muscle**- located only in the heart. Cardiocytes (cardiac muscle cells) are smaller than skeletal muscle cells and have only one nucleus. Cardiac muscle cells have a very limited ability to repair themselves. Cardiac muscle cells, like skeletal muscle are *striated*. Cardiac cells have a unique connection between one another called *Intercalated Discs*. These cells are under *involuntary* control.

3. **Smooth Muscle**- located inside of our organs and blood vessels. These muscle cells are small and are capable of division- therefore can heal after injury. Smooth muscle is *non-striated* and is under *involuntary* control of the nervous system. Digestive system contains a lot of smooth muscle.

Neural Tissue:

Neural Tissue is also known as nerve tissue or nervous tissue. Its function is to transmit electrical messages throughout the body. We will discuss this tissue more in the nervous system. There are two main types of cells in neural tissue.

Neurons- these cells actually transmit the electrical messages, and can be very long in length. Neurons contain three main parts: *Cell Body, Dendrites,* and the *Axon.*

Neuroglia (or **glial cells**) - these cells support, repair, protect, and supply nutrients to the neurons.

Directional Terminology from the Anatomical Position:

Anatomical Position: The patient is standing upright, looking straight ahead, arms at the side with the *palms facing forward.*
Prone Position: The patient is lying on the treatment table *face down (on their stomach).*
Supine Position: The patient is lying on the treatment table *face up (on their back)*
Lateral Recumbant Position: The patient is side-lying

Anterior or **Ventral**	The front (belly) side of the body
Posterior or **Dorsal**	The back side of the body
Superior	Closer to the head or a higher position in the body
Inferior	Closer to the feet or a lower position in the body
Cranial or **Cephalic**	Head Region
Caudal	Region near the buttocks
Medial	Closer to the body midline or center
Lateral	Further away from the body midline
Distal	A structure or part further away from the trunk of the body (used when describing locations in the arms or legs)
Proximal	A structure or part closer to the trunk of the body (used when describing locations in the arms or legs)
Superficial	A structure closer to the body surface
Deep	A structure farther inside the body away from the surface
Oculus/Ocular	Eye region
Bucca or **Buccal**	Cheek Region
Nares or **Nasal**	Nose region
Oris or **Oral**	Mouth Region
Axilla	Armpit Region
Brachium	Upper arm, between the shoulder and elbow
Olecranon	Posterior (back) side of the elbow
Antecubitis	Anterior (front) side of elbow
Antebrachium	Also known as the forearm, between the elbow and wrist
Carpus	Wrist Region
Manus	Hand area
Pollex	Thumb area
Digitis or **Phalanges**	Region around the fingers or toes
Upper limb	Clinical term for the entire arm
Cervicis or **Cervical**	Neck Region
Thoracis or **thorax**	Chest region
Mamma or **mammary**	Breast area
Abdomis	Abdominal (belly) area
Umbilical	The area around the Naval (Belly-button)
Inguinal	Area around the groin

Lumbus or **Loin**	Low back area
Gluteal	Buttock region
Femoral	Thigh Area
Patellar	Knee-cap area
Popliteal	Posterior surface (back) of knee
Cruris	Lower leg area, between knee and foot
Sural	Calf area
Tarsus or **tarsal**	Ankle area
Calcaneal	Heel of foot
Pes or **Pedal**	Foot region
Hallux	Big toe region
Plantar or **planta**	Bottom of foot area
Lower limb	Clinical term for entire leg

Practice Study and Test Questions:

1) The existence of a stable, constant internal environment is called
    A) Homeostasis
    B) Positive feedback
    C) Physiology
    D) Anatomy

2) Which organelle produces ATP in a cell?
    A) Ribosome
    B) Centriole
    C) Mitochondria
    D) Peroxisome

3) Which word is used to describe the armpit region?
    A) carpus
    B) axilla
    C) ocular
    D) inguinal

4) Which of the following is NOT a type of connective tissue?
    A) blood
    B) bone
    C) muscle
    D) tendons

5) The patient is standing upright, looking straight ahead, arms at the side with the palms facing forward. What position is the patient in?
    A) Supine
    B) Anatomical Position
    C) Prone
    D) Lateral recumbant

6) Which type of muscle is located in the digestive organs?
    A) Cardiac
    B) Smooth
    C) Skeletal

7) The patient is lying face down on the treatment table. What position is the patient in?
A) Supine
B) Lateral recumbant
C) Prone
D) Anatomical Position

8) What is the directional term which means "farther away from the midline of the body"?
A) Lateral
B) Medial
C) Superior
D) Caudal

9) A nucleus of a cell contains how many pairs of chromosomes?
A) 23
B) 12
C) 40
D) 31

10) Which of the following is NOT a nitrogenous base found in DNA?
A) Uracil
B) Guanine
C) Cytosine
D) Adenine

11) The epidermis of the skin is an example of
A) stratified columnar epithelium
B) simple cuboidal epithelium
C) simple squamous epithelium
D) stratified squamous epithelium

12) The brachium is the area of the body
A) in the palm of the hand
B) between the elbow and wrist
C) between the shoulder and elbow
D) between the hip and knee

13) Most cells are
A) binucleate
B) uninucleate
C) anucleate
D) multinucleate

14) Which organelle performs protein synthesis in a cell?
A) Mitochondria
B) Golgi Apparatus
C) Ribosome
D) Lysosome

15) The study of the internal and external structures of the body is called
A) Anatomy
B) Physiology
C) Geology
D) Phrenology

Answers: 1)A 2)C 3)B 4)C 5)B 6)B 7)C 8)A 9)A 10)A 11)D 12)C 13)B 14)C 15)A

CHAPTER 3: THE INTEGUMENTARY SYSTEM

The functions of your integumentary system are: protection, excretion, maintenance of body temperature, synthesis of Vitamin D3 (cholecalciferol), storage of nutrients and sensory reception

The skin has two main layers to it. The superficial layer is called the *epidermis*. Under the epidermis, lies the *dermis*. Deep to the dermis (although not usually considered a layer of the skin) is the *hypodermis/ subcutaneous layer*.

The Epidermis-

Consists of stratified squamous epithelium, and is avascular (no blood supply). The layers of cells in the epidermis closest to the basal lamina (the base of the epithelium) are alive, very active, and constantly dividing. These layers can draw nutrients from the blood supply in the deeper part of the skin, the dermis. As the layers get pushed further away from the basal lamina (out toward the surface of the epidermis) the cells run out of nutrients and die. Therefore, the cells that you touch when you are touching the surface of your skin are dead. These dead cells will gradually fall off and will be replaced by cells being pushed up from deeper regions of the epidermis.

Keratinocytes are the most abundant cell in the epidermis, and make up the multiple layers of cells in the epidermis. These cells produce *keratin,* which is a tough fibrous protein used to give the skin strength and making it "water-resistant". Also located in the epidermis are *melanocytes* (produce pigment), *Merkel cells* (nerve endings), *Langerhans cells* (immune system cells), and dendritic cells. The epidermis is arranged in five sub-layers (strata) in areas of *thick skin* (palms of hand, soles of feet), or there are four sub-layers in the *thin skin* (which covers the rest of our body). The layers of the epidermis are as follows, moving from the basal lamina (deepest region of the epidermis) out towards the surface of the skin:

1. **Stratum Germinativum** (aka **Stratum Basale**) - It is the innermost layer of the epidermis. The main types of cell in this layer are the *basal cells* (aka germinative cells). These are stem cells, which continuously divide to produce new keratinocytes. *Merkel Cells* are found here and are sensitive to touch. Cells in the stratum germinativum and spinosum produce Vitamin D.
2. **Stratum Spinosum** (which means "spiny layer"). It is superficial to the stratum germinativum and is composed of usually 8-10 layers of keratinocytes. Cell division still may occur here. This layer contains *Langerhans Cells*- used in the immune system
3. **Stratum Granulosum** (which means "grainy layer"). Is located superficial to stratum spinosum and consists of 3-5 layers of keratinocytes. Cell division usually has stopped, and keratinocytes begin to flatten
4. **Stratum Lucidum**- also called the "clear layer". Is located on top of the stratum granulosum, and found only in areas of "thick skin" (the palms of the hand and soles of the feet).
5. **Stratum Corneum**- The exposed surface of skin. It is 15-30 layers thick (of dead keratinocytes), and this layer has undergone *keratinization*. It takes 15-30 days for a cell to move from the stratum germinativum to the stratum corneum. And, then the dead cell usually remains on the surface of the stratum corneum for about 2 weeks before it is sloughed off.

Skin color is caused by the following pigments in the skin. <u>Carotene</u>- a yellow-orange pigment, found often in the stratum corneum. Carotene can also be found in vegetables, such as carrots and squashes. <u>Melanin</u>- is a pigment that can range from yellow, red, brown, and/or black. Melanin is produced by *melanocytes* located in the stratum germinativum. Melanin is used to provide *UV protection*. <u>Oxygenated Hemoglobin</u>- found in the red blood cells, and gives skin a pink to red hue. The amount of this coloration can vary from moment to moment. Some abnormal skin colors can indicate diseases and be used in diagnosis by a medical doctor, for example: *jaundice, cyanosis, deep bronze color (excess MSH or Addison's disease),* and *vitiligo*.

The Dermis

The dermis lies underneath the epidermis, and on top of the subcutaneous layer. It has two main layers: *the papillary layer* (the more superficial region of the dermis, located directly underneath the epidermis), and *the reticular layer* (the deeper and thicker layer). The dermis contains blood vessels, collagen fibers, elastic fibers, hair follicles, sweat glands, oil glands, nerve endings and lymphatic vessels.

The Hypodermis/ Subcutaneous Layer

The subcutaneous layer is also known as the hypodermis. While not technically a part of the integument, this is the fascial layer that attaches the skin (dermis and epidermis) onto the underlying structures (like muscle, organs, etc.). The subcutaneous layer is composed of adipose tissue (fat), and areolar connective tissue. Large arteries and veins travel in the upper portion of the subcutaneous layer, and large quantities of blood can be found in the veins located there. The fat in this layer is used as a shock absorber, energy reserve, and as a layer of insulation.

Accessory Structures

Hair Follicles and Hair- Hair is located everywhere *except* on the palms of the hand, sides of the fingers and toes, the lips, sides and soles of the feet, and some parts of the external genitalia. Hair offers protection from UV exposure, cushions body surfaces from impact, acts as insulation, assists with filtering entrances to the nose and ears, protects the surface of the eye (eyelashes), and they can act as sensory receptors. Assisting these functions are two structures: the *root hair plexus* (the nerve plexus of sensory nerves that surround the base of the hair), and *arrector pili* (muscles that attach to the sheath that surrounds the hair follicles- when we are cold, these muscles contract and give us goose bumps).

The hair begins in the dermis at the *hair bulb* (the base of the hair follicle), then the *hair root* extends up from the hair bulb through the dermis halfway to the surface of the skin. The hair root then becomes the *hair shaft*, which is the portion of the hair that we see extending off of the surface of the skin. The superficial layer of the hair bulb, called the *hair matrix*, is responsible for forming the hair. Dividing cells in the center of the hair matrix will form the inner core, or *medulla* of the hair. Cells slightly farther from the center of the matrix will make the intermediate layer of the hair, called the *cortex*. Cells in the outer edges of the matrix will make the outer surface of the hair called the *cuticle*. Hair is composed of strands of keratin (a protein produced by the keratinocytes). Differences in hair color are due to different pigment shades produced by the melanocytes in the hair papilla.

Sebaceous (Oil) Glands: These are glands which release their secretions into hair follicles. The liquid secretion, called **sebum,** will follow that hair follicle and hair shaft towards the surface of the skin. Sebum's functions are: lubrication, moisturizing/conditioning, and it can act as an antibacterial substance. On non-hairy parts of the body (face, back, chest, nipples), there are *sebaceous follicles* which release sebum directly to the surface of the skin. In the developing fetus, the sebaceous glands become very active, and form a protective superficial coating on the skin called the *vernix caseosa*.

Sudoriferous (Sweat) Glands: There are two types of sweat glands. *Apocrine Sweat Glands* are found in the armpits, the nipple area, and in the groin. These apocrine glands secrete their products into the hair follicles. This secretion is sticky, cloudy, and potentially odorous when exposed to bacteria on the skin surface. These glands begin production at puberty. *Merocrine (Eccrine) Sweat Glands* are the most numerous of the sweat glands- located all over the body. There are 2-5 million eccrine sweat glands, with the palms and soles containing the highest numbers. The main functions of sweat are: cooling the skin surface temperature, excretion, and protection. Mammary glands (milk producing glands in the breast) and ceruminous glands (wax producing glands in the ear) are modified sweat glands.

Nails are found on tips of fingers and toes. The visible section of the nail is called the *nail body*, which covers the area of the epidermis called the *nail bed*. The free edge of the nail extends off the tip of the finger and covers the *hyponychium*, an area of thickened stratum corneum. The nail is produced at the *nail root*, and a portion of the nail root will extend over the top of the exposed nail- called the *eponychium* (also called the cuticle). The majority of the nail bed has good blood circulation, giving it a pink color. Near the root, the blood vessels may become obscured, which leaves a pale half-moon area called the *lunula*. The nail is composed of tightly packed dead cells filled with hard keratin.

Physical Examination of the Integumentary System:

Skin Examination:

1. Inspect/Observe the color of the skin (all over the body)
   - Look for areas of bruising, cyanosis, pallor, jaundice, erythema, hypopigmented and hyperpigmented areas
2. Inspect/Observe any rash, lesions or markings. Note location, pattern and if there is any bleeding or discharge found. See skin rash chart on next page for more details
3. If any freckles/moles are found: the **"ABCDE"** guidelines are used to document any potentially abnormal findings:
   - **A**= Asymmetry. Asymmetrical lesions have a higher risk of malignancy
   - **B**= Border. An irregular border could indicate malignancy
   - **C**= Color. The mark should be only one color and the color should match other markings in the body. Blue or black lesions should be especially noted
   - **D**= Diameter. Larger than 6 mm increases risk of malignancy
   - **E**= Evolving. Moles that are changing in shape, color, or size increase risk of malignancy
4. Palpate the skin for texture, turgor and moisture levels
5. Palpate the skin for temperature (palpate areas of the body bilaterally to compare temperature)

Hair Examination:

1. Inspect/observe hair. Note distribution, quantity and color
2. Palpate hair for texture

Nail Examination:

1. Inspect/observe nails. Note color, shape, contour, angle of nail base
2. Palpate the nail. Check for secure attachment.
3. Check peripheral circulation:
   - Press on the nail bed and release. Note how long it takes for the color to return. Normal result: Color should return within 3 seconds.

SKIN PATHOLOGIES WITH RASH-LIKE SYMPTOMS

Disease Name	Cause	Incubation period after exposure	Is rash localized or widespread?	Description of rash and other symptoms
Chicken Pox (Varicella)	Varicella zoster virus (a type of herpesvirus)	10-21 days. 14-16 days on average	Widespread	Adults may have 1-2 days of fever before rash. Children usually have the rash appear first. The rash begins first on the head, then spreads to the trunk, then to the arms and legs. The majority of lesions are on the trunk. Lesions are 1-4 mm in diameter and have a blister-like appearance. Blisters are itchy and are filled with a clear fluid. The area around the base of the blister is usually reddened. Other symptoms in a child may include fatigue, pruritis (itching) and a temperature (up to 102°) for 2-3 days. Symptoms may be more severe in an adult. Usually no scarring remains after rash resolves. Contagious.
Shingles (Herpes zoster)	Varicella zoster virus	First exposure to varicella zoster virus causes chicken pox (see above). Recurrent episodes (that can happen decades after the primary exposure) result in shingles.	Localized, usually following the dermatome of a sensory nerve	Lesion outbreak is usually unilateral (only on one side of the body) and usually involving only one dermatome level. Most common areas of outbreak are on face or trunk. Often, 2-4 days prior to the rash, there can be pain and paresthesia in the area. The pain can continue while the rash is present. The rash has blistering lesions, with a reddened inflamed area underneath. The blisters usually scab over in 7-10 days and completely heal within a few weeks without any scarring.
Measles (Rubeola)	Rubeola virus (a type of paramyxovirus)	From exposure to fever is 10-12 days From exposure to rash is approximately 14 days	Widespread	First symptoms are a fever, which lasts 2-4 days on average. The fever can climb up to 103-105°F. After the fever, a cough and runny nose may develop. Then *Koplik spots* (bluish white spots) will form in the mucosa of the mouth. Koplik spots form 1-2 days before the body rash. The rash will then begin on the forehead and then spreads down the face. From the face it spreads to the neck, down to the trunk, into the arms, and lastly onto the legs and then feet. The rash is itchy, and is made up of splotchy patches of red or reddish-brown tiny bumps. Usually no blisters are present. The rash lasts 5-6 days and will then eventually fade in the order that it appeared. Contagious.

SKIN PATHOLOGIES WITH RASH-LIKE SYMPTOMS (CONTINUED)

Disease Name	Cause	Incubation period after exposure	Is rash localized or widespread?	Description of rash and other symptoms
Small pox	Variola major (90% of cases); Variola minor (10% of cases)	7-17 days; (with an average of 12-14 days)	Widespread	First symptoms (prodrome): are fever (101-104°F), headache, fatigue, and body ache- lasts 2-4 days. Then the rash begins. It first starts as small red spots in the mouth and on the tongue. These spots can blister and then break open and then spread into the throat. A rash next begins on the face, then extremities, then trunk and can become widespread within 24 hours. The rash becomes blistered over the next 3-4 days. The blisters are filled with a thick, cloudy, pus-like fluid. The blisters have a depression (dimple) in the middle (a key clinical sign) and are hard and round when touched. After about five days, the blisters crust and scab. The scabs will fall off and leave pitted scars- usually 3 weeks after rash onset. It is only *after* all the scabs have fallen off that the person is no longer contagious.
Herpes simplex	Herpes Simplex Virus Type I (aka oral herpes) Herpes Simplex Virus Type II (aka genital herpes)	2-7 days	Localized HSV-I usually around the mouth- "cold sore" HSV-II usually in genital region	A blister or many small blisters appear near the lips (vermillion border) or genital region. The blisters break and the remaining sores are often painful and tender. A person is infectious for 7-12 days and can spread the infection to others. These lesions recur in about 60-80% of infected patients. Recurrent episodes are usually milder and shorter.
Lyme Disease	Borrelia Burgdorferi (usually spread via tick bite)	3-30 days (average 7 days)	Localized	Rash begins as a reddened area at the base of the tick bite. The rash expands outward from the initial area giving a "bulls-eye" appearance. This expanding rash is called erythema migrans (EM). The rash may be inflamed and warm to the touch, but usually is not itchy. The infection can linger in the body for weeks, months or years after the rash fades. Prolonged symptoms can include Bell's Palsy, headaches, pain and swelling in joints, heart palpitations, or shooting pain. Not usually spread via human-human contact- usually spread via tick bite.

SKIN PATHOLOGIES WITH RASH-LIKE SYMPTOMS (CONTINUED)

Disease Name	Cause	Incubation period after exposure	Is rash localized or widespread	Description of rash and other symptoms
Impetigo	Group A Streptococci Or Staphylococcus Aureus	7-10 days after exposure to Streptococcus 4-10 days after exposure to Staphylococcus	Localized	Can occur anywhere in the body. Usual areas of outbreak are around the nose, mouth, hands or arms. Red bumps appear on the skin, which release a yellowish pus-like secretion. This secretion will often dry and create a crust that sticks to the skin. The rash lasts 2-3 weeks. This is highly contagious.
Hand-Foot-and-Mouth Disease (HMFD)	Coxsackievirus or Enterovirus	3-6 days	Localized to hands, mouth, and feet	Symptoms begin with fatigue, sore throat and a fever (101-103°F). A day or two later a rash with blisters may appear in the mouth and on the hands, feet, and sometimes the gluteal region. The rash and blisters last for approximately one week. Most common in children under age 5. Can be spread to others through contact with fecal material.
Candidiasis	Candida (most commonly candida albicans)		Localized	Candidiasis can occur in many areas of the body. It can occur in the vagina (causing a white, cottage cheese-like discharge). It can occur in the mouth as thrush (causing thick white patches on the tongue). It can also occur as a rash on the skin (called intertrigo). In intertrigo, the rash may be present in warm, moist areas of the body, such as: armpits, groin, under breast tissue and in the folds of skin of the obese. The skin appears red and can be tender.
Athlete's foot	Tinea pedis (other tinea infections can arise on other parts of the body)		Localized	This rash is usually localized to the feet and is commonly located between the toes, but can also be seen on the bottom and/or sides of the foot. The skin can be reddened, flaky, itchy, and/or painful.
Rosacea	Unkown- Possible genetic or environmental	N/A	Localized	Redness on the face- usually over the nose and cheeks. The area may feel warm and inflamed. In the area of reddened skin, there may also be pus filled acne-like pimples. Most common in women (age 30-60), with lighter colored complexions. The rash may come and go. Triggers can include spicy foods, alcohol, temperature extremes, sunlight, stress, or some types of medications.

SKIN PATHOLOGIES WITH RASH-LIKE SYMPTOMS (CONTINUED)

Disease Name	Cause	Incubation period after exposure	Is rash localized or widespread	Description of rash and other symptoms
Psoriasis	Not fully understood It is an immune system problem- an autoimmune disease		Localized	Rash looks like red patches of skin covered with dry silvery scales. The skin may become cracked and bleed. The area may itch and be tender/painful. Often seen on extensor surfaces of the body. The rash may come and go. Triggers can include cold weather, stress, trauma to the skin, other infections, smoking, alcohol intake, and some medications.
Systemic Lupus Erythematosus (SLE or Lupus)	Autoimmune disease			Rash appears on sun-exposed areas of the face, ears, neck, arms and legs. The rash can be scaly, red and cause the skin to thicken. The rash is not usually painful or itchy. A "malar rash" is a butterfly shaped rash that appears over the cheeks and the bridge of the nose. The rash is very photosensitive and will worsen with sun exposure. Lupus can also affect joints (arthritis), brain, lungs, blood vessels and the pericardium.
Atopic dermatitis (Eczema)	Unknown- Possibly genetic, and/or immune system malfunction	N/A	Localized	A patchy-looking rash often found on hands, feet, on the anterior surface of the elbow, in the popliteal region (behind the knee), ankles, wrist, face, neck and upper chest. Not all of these areas will be affected at one time. The rash may be red to a brownish gray color and can be itchy. Small raised bumps may be present, and these bumps may leak exudate (which can create a crust on the skin). The skin can also get scaly, dry and cracked. If the patient scratches the rash, due to the itching, the skin can get infected. Symptoms can come and go and can be worsened by things like dry skin, stress, changes in temperature, soaps/detergents, foods, wool or certain types of fabrics, or cigarette smoke.

Abnormal Examination Findings of the Skin, Hair, and Nails

Abnormal findings, if necessary, should be referred to patients PCP or a dermatologist

Skin:

Abnormal colors: abnormal coloration of the skin could indicate:
- *Bronzing/Brown-* caused by increased melanin. This can be due to sun exposure, pregnancy, Addison's disease
- *Blue* (cyanosis) - caused by deoxygenation of blood. This can be due to environment (anxiety, cold temperature), heart or lung disease, abnormal hemoglobin in the blood
- *Red* (erythema) - caused by increased visibility of oxyhemoglobin and/or increased blood flow to an area. Can be due to inflammation, fever, blushing, allergic reaction
- *Yellow* (jaundice) - caused by increased bilirubin (from bile) or carotenemia in the blood. This can be due to liver disease, hemolysis of blood cells, or increased carotene intake from yellow/orange fruits and veggies
- *Pale/Pallor-* could be due to decreased melanin or decreased oxyhemoglobin as a result of albinism, vitiligo, shock, syncope, anemia, nephritic syndrome

Pruritus- Is an unpleasant itching sensation. It is a very common skin disorder and can be caused by many things, such as: contact with something that irritates the skin, drug use, emotional upset, heat ("heat rash").

Spider Angioma- a central red spot with many thin arms extending off of it (like a spider or a sun with many rays). If only one is present, it may be benign. More than 5 could indicate liver failure or cirrhosis. Pregnant women may develop these due to increased estrogen levels. These spots will blanch (lighten in color) when pressure is applied.

Café-au-lait spots- flat light brown patches on skin surface, usually appearing during the first few years of life (but may occur later). These spots are larger than freckles, and usually a more irregular shape than most birthmarks. More than six spots on the body could be a sign of neurofibromatosis

Port-wine hemangiomas- (aka *port wine stains*). Purple colored and usually present at birth

Chloasma- increased skin pigmentation over the nose and cheeks. Commonly seen during pregnancy

Keloid- is an excessive overgrowth of scar tissue. Can be found in an area of skin damage or can arise spontaneously. They are more common in African Americans.

Scaling- excessive layers of keratinized cells on top of skin surface

Crusting- dried residue of pus, serum or blood found on surface of the skin.

Anhydrosis- no sweating

Hyperhidrosis- excessive sweating

Furuncle- inflammation of a hair follicle, may be filled with pus

Comedo- a plugged opening of a sebaceous gland (oil gland), often called a "blackhead"

Wheal- an area on the skin that is inflamed, and may also be slightly raised. May itch and will feel warm to the touch. Hives can sometimes present as this.

Acrochordon- aka *"skin tag"*- This is a non-cancerous overgrowth of skin. We have an increased risk of developing them as we age. More common in people who are overweight, have diabetes or are pregnant.

Petichiae- a small lesion (usually less than 3 mm), which is often red or purple. This is usually from a broken blood vessel. This lesion does not blanch when pressure is applied.

Purpura- a lesion slightly larger than petichiae (usually 3-10 mm), and is often red or purple. This is usually a result of a broken blood vessel. This lesion does not blanch when pressure is applied.

Ecchymosis- (sometimes called a *"bruise"*)- a lesion larger than purpura (usually greater than 10 mm/ 1 cm), and is often red or purple. This is usually a result of a broken blood vessel. This lesion does not blanch when pressure is applied.

Birthmarks- generally flat and can range in color from tan to red to brown. Can be found all over the body

Freckles- are small flat lesions, which are usually red-brown or brown in color. Primarily on face, arms and back. May fade or darken due to sun exposure.

Moles- flat or slightly elevated. These spots are usually evenly pigmented, tan to dark brown. Found on all areas of the body.

Cool skin could indicate circulation disorder, shock, and hypothyroidism

Localized increased warmth can indicate infection, inflammation, or an area that has been burned.

Turgor test: Gently squeeze/pinch the skin on the forearm. Upon letting go, if the skin quickly returns to its original shape, the patient has normal turgor. If the skin maintains a tented appearance or takes longer than 30 seconds to return to its original shape, the patient has poor turgor. This could be due to dehydration or edema.

Hair:

Alopecia- diffuse hair loss. Can be a result of a few different scenarios:
- Hair loss with thin, shiny, atrophic skin; weak pulses; and cool extremities could be a result of *arterial insufficiency*
- Hair loss with translucent and charred skin could be the result of a *burn*
- Hair loss, including the outer third of the eyebrows, thin coarse hair on the face, sluggishness, and weight gain could be the result of *hypothyroidism*

True (frank) baldness - is a genetically determined and sex-influenced condition.
Male pattern baldness is caused by follicular response to DHT (a hormone- dihydrotestosterone)

Hirsutism- is excessive hairiness in women on body and face. Can be a result of drug therapies, endocrine disorders (Cushing's syndrome, acromegaly, PCOS- polycystic ovary syndrome)

Nails:

Digital Clubbing- appears as a thickened nail that is curved at the end. The nail angle will be greater than 180 degrees. Can be caused by different pathologies
- Digital clubbing with dyspnea, pursed lip breathing, barrel chest, peripheral cyanosis, are signs of *emphysema*
- Digital clubbing with wheezing, dyspnea, neck vein distention, palpitations, and edema, are signs of *heart failure*
- Digital clubbing with hemoptysis, dyspnea, wheezing, chest pain, weight loss, and fever are signs of *lung and pleural cancer*

Yellow nails could be due to smoking or jaundice

Leukonychia- white spot on the nail, usually as a result of trauma

Beau's lines- transverse grooves in the nail that run parallel to the lunula. Can be a sign of acute illness, malnutrition, and anemia

Koilonychia- Thin spoon shaped nails, with lateral edges that turn upwards. This is often caused by hypochromic anemia (iron deficiency anemia). Can also be caused by Raynaud's disease, chronic diseases, or malnutrition

Pitting in nails- are little pits or divots visible on the nail surface. Often seen in patients with psoriasis

Onycholysis- this is a separation of the nail from the nail bed. Can be caused by psoriasis, hyperthyroidism, contact dermatitis or minor trauma to someone with long fingernails,

Advanced Imaging and Diagnostic Tests of the Skin

Biopsy- Removal of tissue samples from affected area. Tissue samples are then analyzed, usually under a microscope for abnormalities. Physicians take biopsies of areas that look abnormal and use them to detect cancer, precancerous cells, infections, and other conditions. For some biopsies, the doctor inserts a needle into the skin and draws out a sample; in other cases, tissue is removed during a surgical procedure or scraped away with the edge of a scalpel. The tissue or secretions gathered from lesions can be cultured to detect the presence of bacteria, or can be assessed for other abnormal growth (cancer, etc.).

Scratch Test (for Allergies) - This test checks for a skin reaction to common allergy-provoking substances, such as foods, molds, dust, plants, or animal proteins. If the skin reacts to a substance, chances are that the individual is allergic to it. In adults, the test is done on the forearm; in children it's done on the upper back. Some people are tested for as many as a few dozen at one visit. Individual drops of fluid (containing allergens of the allergy provoking substances) are dripped in rows across the skin. The doctor uses a needle to make small light scratches in the skin under each drop, to help the skin absorb the fluid. The doctor notes where each drop of fluid was placed, either by keeping a chart or by writing a code on the area of skin being tested. The patient will need to stay still long enough (usually about 20 minutes) to give the skin time to react. At the end of the waiting time, the doctor will examine each needle scratch for redness or swelling.

Pathologies of the Integumentary System

For additional infectious diseases that may affect this system, please refer to the Communicable/Infectious Disease chart in Chapter 10.

Abscess- is an accumulation of pus, usually caused by a bacterial infection. Symptoms may be local swelling, redness, heat, pain in the area. Purulent (pus) discharge may leak out of the area.

Acne – an active infection (by the bacteria *P. acnes)* of blocked sebaceous glands. This causes *open comedos* *("blackheads")* or *closed comedos ("whiteheads")*. Topical antibiotics, vitamin-A derivatives, or peeling agents may reduce scarring from acne. The prescription drug *Accutane* reduces oil gland activity on a long term basis, and is often used to treat acne.

Alopecia- an autoimmune or genetic disease in which there is hair loss on the scalp (or elsewhere on the body). It can occur in men or women. In males, it can cause male pattern hair loss. In females it can cause a thinning of hair throughout the head. The drug *Rogaine* or corticosteroids may be used for treatment.

Athlete's Foot- is a fungal infection (*tinea pedis*). <u>*Red Flag symptoms*</u>*: dry, itchy cracked skin on the feet. Can commonly be seen on the skin in-between the toes, on the soles, or top of the foot. Deep cracks in the skin can lead to bleeding.* If this fungal infection is on other areas of the body, it goes by different names: on the head (*tinea capitis*), on the trunk "ringworm" (*tinea corporis*), on the groin "jock itch" (*tinea cruris*), and in the nails (*tinea ungulum*).

Burn – tissue damage and cell death caused by intense heat, electricity, UV radiation, or certain chemicals (like acids). Severe burns are very prone to infection, reduce the skin's ability to thermoregulate, and can cause dehydration (and a resulting electrolyte imbalance), which can lead to *circulatory shock* (inadequate blood circulation).

Burns are classified according to severity as:
- **First-degree or partial thickness** – damage to the epidermis only and redness (erythema) is present.
- **Second-degree burn** affects the epidermis and the upper part of dermis, with blistering, pain and redness possibly occurring.
- **Third-degree or full thickness burns** usually involve entire thickness of skin. In this most severe burn, there may be less pain and discomfort, due to complete damage to nerves in the area. Extensive third degree burns cannot heal themselves, so often skin grafts must be used to cover the area of damage.

Candidiasis- is a fungal infection of the skin caused by the *Candida* species (most commonly *Candida albicans*). If it occurs in the mouth/tongue it can be called *thrush*. If it occurs in the vagina, it can be called *vaginitis*. Candida can also be a cause of some diaper rashes in babies. Other areas that are prone to candida infections are areas that are moist and warm (armpits, groin, under the breast, in excess skin rolls of the obese).

Cellulitis- is a bacterial infection of the skin (usually *Streptococcus* or *Staphylococcus* bacteria). This infection can gradually spread through the hypodermis and dermis of the skin. The skin will become red and swollen, and the area will gradually spread and enlarge. Usually cellulitis develops in an area where there has been some sort of wound to the skin.

Chicken Pox- (also called **Varicella**) - a contagious viral illness caused by the *varicella-zoster virus (*a member of the herpes family). Symptoms include fever and headache. A rash then begins- with small itchy fluid filled blisters forming on the body. The rash begins on the face or trunk and then can spread to other areas. These blisters are filled with a clear fluid which contains live virus. The blisters will eventually dry and scab- usually leaving no scar. Usually the person recovers with no complications. The same virus which causes chicken pox causes shingles.

Cold sores ("fever blisters") – small, fluid-filled blisters that itch and sting, usually caused by an infection by the *herpes simplex virus type 1 (HSV-1)*. They usually occur around the mouth, and can be activated by emotional stress, fever, or UV radiation.

Contact dermatitis – is a type of dermatitis with symptoms of itching, redness, and swelling of the skin, progressing to blistering. It is caused by skin exposure to chemicals that provoke allergic responses in sensitive individuals. *Pruritis* is the clinical term for an irritating, itching sensation of the skin.

Decubitus ulcers (bedsores) – an *ulcer* is an area where the skin tissue degenerates and dies (necrosis) due to a lack of blood flow. Bedsores occur when the weight of the body puts prolonged pressure on skin that lies over bony areas, restricting the blood supply. This, in turn, weakens and damages the skin- creating ulcerations. Often seen in people who are bedridden, or in people who are mobile but have circulatory issues.

Eczema- (also called **atopic dermatitis***). Can be triggered by temperature changes, fungi, chemical irritants (detergents, etc.), and stress. Hereditary factors and environmental factors (or both) can predispose an individual to this condition. Symptoms can include itchy skin, red bumps on the skin which can crust when scratched, red or brown dry areas on the skin, or cracked skin.

Folliculitis – a local inflammation of sebaceous glands or hair follicles. Usually caused by *Staphylococcus aureus*. A *furuncle* ("boil") can result if the duct of the gland becomes blocked.

Hansen's disease (leprosy): caused by a bacterium. The bacterium destroys cutaneous nerve endings which are sensitive to pain, touch, heat, and cold. Damage to the distal tissues occur; due to the fact the individual no longer feels pain in the area.

Hirsutism- excessive hair growth on women that occurs in patterns usually seen in males (for example: on the chin, upper lip). Can be a result of drug therapies, endocrine disorders (Cushing's syndrome, acromegaly)

Herpes- A viral infection. *Herpes simplex virus type 1 (HSV-1)* is the usual cause of cold sores. *Herpes simplex virus type 2 (HSV-2)* is the usual cause of genital herpes. In both cases, painful, blistering lesions can appear on the skin. Live virus is found in the fluid of these lesions and can be transmitted to others. HSV-2 is one of the most common sexually transmitted diseases in the US. The virus lives in the spinal nerves and will cause periodic outbreaks of the lesions.

Hyperkeratosis- (aka: calluses and corns). Excessive keratin production. Calluses are flatter patches of hyperkeratization, while corns are a more localized build-up of keratin. Commonly seen on the hands and feet.

Impetigo- a skin infection caused by the *Staphylococcus* or *Streptococcus* bacteria. <u>*Red Flag symptoms*</u>: *Red spots form on the skin, which turn into blistering pustules followed by a yellow crust. Can be itchy.* Can be seen in infants and children, and is easily spread in close contact (daycare, etc.).   Impetigo is an infection on the surface of the skin, while cellulitis is a bacterial infection involving the deeper portions of the skin (dermis and hypodermis).

Keloid- a thickened mass of scar tissue, often with a shiny epidermal covering. Most commonly seen in the upper back, chest, shoulders, and earlobes. This can occur in an area of prior injury, or occasionally, spontaneously.

Lice- *Pediculus humanus* are the lice found on the body and scalp. Bites can cause redness and itching. The lice are small, but can be seen with the eye. Eggs are laid at the base of hairs near the skin. *Phthirus pubis* is the pubic louse or "crabs". <u>*Red Flag symptoms of head lice*</u>: *small whitish flecks on the shaft of the hair, near the scalp; seeing lice crawling in the hair; tickling sensation on head; and itching.* <u>*Red Flag symptoms of pubic lice*</u>: *itching in genital area, tickling sensation, and seeing the darker and larger lice crawling on the skin and hair.*

Lyme Disease- a condition caused by an infection with *Borrelia Burgdorferi*. This bacterium is spread via the deer tick. After the tick bites a human, often a red rash (described as a "bull's eye") forms in the area of the bite. This expanding rash is called *erythema migrans (EM)*. In addition, the person may initially feel flu-like symptoms (fatigue, fever, body aches, stiff neck, and headache). After a few weeks (if left untreated), arthritis may set in- causing painful, swollen joints. Treatment is antibiotic therapy.

Mastitis- Infection of the breast tissue. Often seen in the first few weeks of breast-feeding. The nipples can become cracked and raw, allowing easy infection by *the Staphylococcus Aureus* bacteria.

Measles (also known as **Rubeola)** - caused by the *Rubeola virus*. Highly contagious. Symptoms can include *Koplik spots* (bluish-white spots in the mouth), followed by a red itchy rash all over the body. Fever, runny nose and a cough are also usually present. It can also cause ear infections, pneumonia, encephalitis, or death (in rare cases). The MMR vaccine (measles, mumps, rubella) is available for this disease.

Mumps- a contagious disease caused by the *Mumps virus*. Symptoms are fever, headache, muscle aches and fatigue. The salivary glands will then swell (called *parotitis*). Possible complications are inflammation of the testicles (*orchitis*) or ovaries (*oophoritis*), which can lead to sterility. Inflammation of the brain (*encephalitis*) or meningitis can occur.

Psoriasis – chronic condition characterized by reddened epidermal lesions covered with dry, silvery scales. Stem cells in the stratum germinativum show increased activity, causing hyperkeratosis in areas of the skin. Normally, in an individual, stem cells will divide once every 20 days. In an individual with psoriasis, they can divide every day and a half. Commonly affects areas of skin on the scalp, elbows, palms, soles, groin, or nails. When it is severe, it can be disfiguring and debilitating. While the cause is unknown, attacks are often triggered by trauma, infection, hormonal changes, or stress.

Raynaud's phenomenon (Raynaud's disease) - most commonly affects women. A vigorous sympathetic nervous system response causes excessive constriction of small arteries in the hands, feet, ears, and nose. Often triggered by exposure to the cold. Skin in the area changes color as blood flow is disrupted. First it becomes pale, and then turns blue. Eventually the skin will turn red once blood flow returns.

Rosacea- A chronic inflammatory skin disorder. Usually affects adults. Symptoms are flushing, papules, and pustules seen on face. Etiology is unknown. The symptoms may come and go. Triggers can include certain foods or beverages, very hot or cold weather, sun exposure, stress, strong emotions, and some medications.

Scabies- a parasitic infection of *Sarcoptes scaibei*. Highly contagious. The mite burrows under the skin and lays its eggs. <u>Red Flag symptoms</u>- *Intense itching; redness can be seen in the area of infection, and often burrows can be seen under the skin.* Areas commonly infected are between fingers, wrists and groin.

Seborrheic Dermatitis- inflammation around normally active sebaceous glands. This causes the area to become red and swollen. Thick crusting or scaling of the skin may be seen. Glands in the scalp are often the most affected ("dandruff" in adults, "cradle cap" in infants).

Shingles- caused by the virus that causes chicken pox- the *Herpes varicella zoster* virus. The virus lives in the dorsal root of the spinal nerves. During an outbreak, the virus will travel along the nerve pathway (from the root of the spinal nerve out to the surface of the skin). Blistering lesions follow a pattern along sensory nerve dermatomes. There can be intense pain also associated with the lesions.

Small Pox- infection caused by the *Variola major* and *Variola minor* viruses. After a two week incubation period, symptoms arise- such as: fever, headache, fatigue. A flat, red rash then appears, first on face and arms, then spreading to trunk. The rash first appears red and then forms blistering lesions (the blisters often have a dimpled appearance). The fluid in the blisters first is clear and then turns to pus. The blisters eventually dry and scab, and will leave deep permanent pitted scars. Blisters can also form in the nose, mouth and throat. Blindness and death can occur

Skin Cancers- There are many types of skin cancer. Here are a few examples

- **Basal cell carcinoma** – the skin cancer that is the least malignant and most common. *Red Flag symptoms- shiny, dome-shaped lesions that later develop a central ulcer with pearly beaded edge. It occurs most often in sun-exposed areas the face.* It rarely *metastasizes* (spreads).
- **Squamous cell carcinoma** – a type of skin cancer. *Red Flag Symptoms: lesions that are characterized as scaly, reddened papules (small, rounded elevations).* It is also capable of metastasis, and appears most often on the scalp, ears, dorsal surfaces of the hands, and lower lip.
- **Malignant melanoma** – cancer of the melanocytes, usually caused by too much sun exposure. It is one of the least common skin cancers, but is the most deadly—it metastasizes rapidly, which lowers the survival rate- especially if it is not caught early. *Red Flag Symptoms: lesions appear as spreading brown or black patches, can arise spontaneously or develop from a mole or pigmented spot. Physicians often used the ABCDE rule when looking at pigmented spots: A=Asymmetry, B=Border, C=Color, D=Diameter (6 mm) and E= if the lesion is evolving (changing) over time.*

Systemic Lupus Erythematosus (SLE) – "Lupus" Symptoms: butterfly shaped rash over the nose and cheeks. Affects women nine times as often as men. Immune system antigen recognition breaks down and the immune system produces autoantibodies. Autoantibodies attack normal healthy body cells instead of invading pathogens. This is a widespread autoimmune disease causing vast amounts of damage to tissues like the clotting factors, RBC's, platelets, and lymphocytes. In addition to the skin rash, kidney damage, arthritis, anemia, vascular inflammation and CNS deficits can result. Treatment: administering drugs to depress the immune system and/or corticosteroids.

Urticaria (also called *"wheals"* or *"hives"*) - an extensive allergic reaction to a food, drug, an insect bite, infection, stress, or some other stimulus.

Vitiligo- destruction of melanocytes in areas of skin. The patches of skin in these regions will lose pigmentation and appear very white.

Warts- caused by the *Human papilloma* virus (HPV). Rough, elevated bumps on the skin. Common on hands and feet. These growths form in the epidermis, can be present for weeks, months, and much longer.

Xerosis- (aka "dry skin") is a common complaint of the elderly and those who live in arid climates. The outer layers of the skin start to deteriorate and become scaly.

Practice Study and Test Questions:

1) When checking peripheral circulation, how long should it take for color to return to the nail bed after pressure is applied?

    A) Within 3 seconds
    B) Within 5 second
    C) Within 10 seconds
    D) Within 30 seconds

2) Cyanosis can indicate

    A) increased blood flow to an area
    B) increased melanin production
    C) deoxygenation of the blood
    D) increased bile in the blood from a liver problem

3) Diffuse hair loss is a symptom of
   A) impetigo
   B) cellulitis
   C) malignant melanoma
   D) alopecia

4) Dry, itchy cracked skin on the feet or in-between the toes can be a sign of
   A) cellulitis
   B) decubitus ulcer
   C) tinea pedis (athlete's foot)
   D) keloid

5) A butterfly shaped rash over the nose and cheeks may be a sign of
   A) xerosis
   B) Systemic Lupus Erythematosus
   C) vitiligo
   D) seborrheic dermatitis

6) Intense itching, redness, and the appearance of burrows under the skin can be signs of
   A) scabies
   B) impetigo
   C) cellulitis
   D) folliculitis

7) Red lesions on the skin which may blister and then be covered by a yellow crust are signs of
   A) hirsutism
   B) contact dermatitis
   C) Raynaud's
   D) impetigo

8) Excessive hairiness on a woman's body and/or face is called
   A) alopecia
   B) hirsutism
   C) acrochordon
   D) varicella

9) White flecks on the shaft of hair near the scalp and itching on the head may be signs of
   A) pubic lice
   B) head lice
   C) scabies
   D) rosacea

10) The pigment producing cell in the epidermis is called a
   A) melanocyte
   B) keratinocyte
   C) carotenocyte
   D) epidermocyte

11) Increased pigmentation over the nose and cheeks is called
   A) pruritus
   B) spider angioma
   C) chloasma
   D) ecchymosis

12) Digital clubbing can be a result of
      A) Emphysema
      B) Heart Failure
      C) Lung Cancer
      D) All of the above

13) Which type of burn involves the epidermis and the upper part of the dermis?
      A) first degree burn
      B) second degree burn
      C) third degree burn
      D) fourth degree burn

14) Pitting in the nails can be seen in patients who have
      A) Hansen's Disease
      B) Candidiasis
      C) Psoriasis
      D) Lupus

15) Excessive sweating is called
      A) anhydrosis
      B) petichiae
      C) comedo
      D) hyperhidrosis

16) A red "bull's eye" rash may be a sign of
      A) Lyme disease
      B) psoriasis
      C) herpes simplex
      D) chicken pox

17) The ABCDE guidelines performed in the physical examination are used to assess for
      A) cardiac arrhythmias
      B) malignant melanoma
      C) psoriasis
      D) MRSA

18) Hair follicles, oil glands, sweat glands, nerve endings, and blood vessels are all found in which layer of the skin?
      A) epidermis
      B) hypodermis
      C) subcutaneous layer
      D) dermis

Answers: 1) A 2) C 3) D 4) C 5) B 6) A 7) D 8) B 9) B 10) A 11) C 12) D 13) B 14) C 15) D 16) A 17) B 18) D

CHAPTER 4: THE SKELETAL SYSTEM

The skeletal system is made up of approximately 206 bones. The functions of this system include protection, support, storage of minerals and lipids, blood cell production (called *hematopoiesis*), and leverage for movement.

Bones can be classified according to their shapes.
- **Long Bones**- examples: humerus, femur, phalanges, radius, ulna, tibia, fibula
- **Flat Bones**- examples: skull bones, facial bones, ribs, sternum
- **Irregular bones**- examples: vertebra, coxal
- **Short and Sesamoid bones**- examples: Short bones= carpals, tarsals; Sesamoid= patella

The long bones are composed of the following parts. The *diaphysis* is the shaft portion of the bone. It is composed of dense *compact bone*. There is a hollow tube running down through the middle of the diaphysis, called the *medullary cavity*. The medullary cavity is filled with adipose tissue, called *yellow marrow*. The yellow marrow is used for shock absorption within the bone (and is composed of adipose material). The outside of the diaphysis is covered with a thin membranous covering called the *periosteum*. The periosteum serves as an attachment point for tendons and ligaments. The ends of long bones are called the *epiphyses*. The epiphyses are composed of *spongy bone*. The perforated holes in the spongy bone are filled with hematopoietic tissue called *red bone marrow*. The red bone marrow is the hematopoietic tissue (blood forming tissue). The outside of the epiphyses are covered with *articular cartilage*, a smooth surface which assists in joint functioning. Located at the junction between the diaphysis and epiphyses is the *metaphysis*. In a growing child, the metaphysis was the location of the epiphyseal (growth) plates.

Flat bones are formed slightly differently. The flat bones look somewhat like an Oreo cookie. Compact bone forms the outer surfaces of flat bones (much like the two cookie wafers on an Oreo). The inside of the flat bones are filled with spongy bone.

Surface Features of Bones:

This is terminology which describes bumps and grooves on the surface of bones. Some of these structures are able to be palpated, and we use them as landmarks when looking for structures, point locations, etc.
- Elevations and projections: For example- *process, ramus*
- Processes formed where tendons and ligaments attach: Examples*: trochanter, tuberosity, tubercle, crest, line,* and *spine*
- Processes used in articulation with adjacent bones: Examples: *head, neck, condyle, trochlea,* and *facet*
- Depressions: For example- *fossa* and *sulcus*
- Openings: Examples: *foramen, canal, fissure, sinus,* and *antrum*

Bone Histology:

Bones are composed of bone matrix and bone cells.

Bone Matrix: The matrix of bone is composed of **calcium phosphate** (accounts for 2/3 the weight of bone) and calcium hydroxide. These two substances combine to form *hydroxyapatite crystals* and *calcium carbonate*. The other main component of bone is **collagen fibers**, which accounts for roughly 1/3 of the weight of the bone. The collagen allows the bones to have some flexibility (to prevent shattering), and also provide a framework for the hydroxyapatite crystals to attach to. Bone matrix is often laid out in layers called *lamellae*.

Bone Cells: Bone cells only account for about 2% of the mass of the bone, but play very important roles. There are 4 main bone cells:

1. **Osteocytes-** mature bone cells that account for the majority of the bone cells. Osteocytes live in a pocket (called a *lacuna*) surrounded by bone matrix. Osteocytes maintain and monitor the protein and mineral content of the matrix, and can assist in the repair of bone (by becoming an osteoblast or osteoprogenitor cell).
2. **Osteoblasts** ("bone builders") - produce new bone matrix (a process called *osteogenesis*). They make and release *osteoid*, a material filled with protein and other organic components. Calcium salts then get deposited into the osteoid.
3. **Osteoprogenitor cells-** These are stem cells which divide to maintain the population of osteoblasts. These cells are very important in the healing of fractures.
4. **Osteoclasts** ("bone destroyers") - these are descendants of monocytes (white blood cells) and are responsible for removing bone matrix. These cells contain acids and enzymes which can dissolve and break down the matrix. This resorption process is called *osteolysis*.

There are two forms of Osseous Tissue- **compact bone** and **spongy bone**. Compact bone is dense, solid bone. It is found as a protective outer covering of spongy bone, and in located in areas of bone which are under high levels of physical stress (such as the diaphysis of long bones). It is composed of *osteons*- concentric *lamellae* (rings of bone tissue) surrounding a *central (Haversian) canal*. Other passageways, known as *perforating canals* (also called the canals of Volkmann) run perpendicular to the bone surface and penetrate deeper into the bone towards the marrow cavity. The central (Haversian) canals and perforating canals carry blood vessels and nerves through the interior of the bone.

Spongy bone is also strong, but is composed of more of a light-weight material than compact bone. Lamellae in spongy bone are not laid out in concentric rings like in compact bone. Instead, the matrix will form plates of strong bone material called *trabeculae*. These trabeculae branch and form a honeycomb looking structure. Often, filling the open spaces between the trabeculae in spongy bone will be the red bone marrow.

Bone Development and Growth:

The bony skeleton begins to form in an embryo about six weeks after fertilization. The bones of an embryo at this age are actually made out of cartilage or fibrous membranes, not bone tissue. During the time in the womb, the embryo/fetus' bones will begin to ossify (transform from cartilage/membranous tissue into bone tissue). The bones will continue to grow, develop, and calcify after birth up until about age 25. Two terms are important to understand here. **Ossification** is the term which means bone formation. **Calcification** is the deposition of calcium in body tissues.

There are two major forms of ossification- Endochondral and Intramembranous:

1) **Endochondral Ossification:** When our skeleton is developing, most bones (for example, all of our long bones) develop in this way. Bones in the embryo begin as tiny structures made out of hyaline cartilage. The conversion of these cartilage models of our bones into osseous (bone) tissue is called endochondral ossification. In endochondral ossification, chondrocytes (cartilage cells) in the center of the diaphysis will die, and blood vessels will penetrate into this area. Osteoblasts will begin to form in this area and become *the primary center of ossification*. Cartilage in the primary center of ossification will be converted into bone tissue by the osteoblasts. Then, chondrocytes in the center of each epiphysis will die and be replaced by osteoblasts. These become the *secondary ossification centers*. This will lead to ossification occurring in the epiphysis of the bones. The very tip of the epiphysis does not ossify; the hyaline cartilage will remain as a protective cap over the top of the epiphysis. We call this the *articular cartilage*, and it acts as a shock absorber and as a smooth surface inside of our joints where bone meets bone. In between the epiphysis and diaphysis (in the area of the metaphysis), there will also be a layer of cartilage called the *epiphyseal cartilage* (or *epiphyseal/growth plate*). When the epiphyseal cartilage grows, it causes the ends of the bone to be pushed farther apart, and the bone will lengthen. Osteoblasts from the diaphysis

gradually turn that new cartilage to bone. When the epiphyseal cartilage is completely converted to bone, growth of the bone in length will stop.

2) **Intramembranous Ossification**: This type of ossification is done in the flat bones of the skull, mandible, and clavicle. In an embryo, these bones start off as flat sheets of fibrous connective tissue membranes. These membranes have osteoblasts invading throughout, gradually turning the membranes into bone. There are no ossification centers in intramembranous ossification.

The Constant Changes in our Bones:

Bone matrix is constantly being broken down and re-made to ensure continuous strength and durability. This process is called **bone remodeling**. In young adults, one fifth of the skeleton is broken down and replaced each year. There are many factors that can affect the strength of our bones. *Regular, general exercise* encourages the osteoblasts to stay active and keep our bones strong. *Hormones* can also affect our bones. Growth hormone, thyroxine, estrogen, androgens, and calcitonin all work to increase osteoblast activity and/or increase calcium availability. Parathyroid hormone works to stimulate osteoclasts and therefore increases calcium levels in the blood. *Nutrition* can also be another factor in ensuring longevity of our bones. In addition to calcium, adequate levels of phosphorous, Vitamin D, Vitamin C, Vitamin A, and Vitamin B12 are all needed for proper bone development and maintenance.

The ability of bone to replace itself is especially important when repairing a fracture. Fracture repair is accomplished in a few steps. After injury, a large blood clot, or *fracture hematoma*, will form to stop the loss of blood, and will create a fibrous mesh in the injury site. The hematoma will be replaced by cartilaginous tissue. Osteoblasts will move into the area and transform the cartilaginous tissue into an area of thickened bony tissue, called a bony callus. For the next few months, up to over a year, osteoclasts and osteoblasts will continue to remodel the fracture area. The thickened callus will gradually be carved back down to a more normal shape, and compact bone will replace the spongy bone, if needed.

In a medical setting, bone fractures may be classified by four "either/or" classifications:
1. Position of bone ends after fracture:
    - **Nondisplaced**— fractured ends retain normal position/alignment
    - **Displaced**— fractured ends are out of normal alignment with each other
2. Completeness of the break
    - **Complete**— broken all the way through
    - **Incomplete**— not broken all the way through
3. Orientation of the break to the long axis of the bone:
    - **Linear**— parallel to long axis of the bone
    - **Transverse**— perpendicular to long axis of the bone
4. Whether or not the bone ends penetrate the skin:
    - **Compound (open)**— bone ends penetrate the skin
    - **Simple (closed)**— bone ends do not penetrate the skin

For example, a radiology report could read: "Radiology study shows a simple nondisplaced fracture of the right humerus. It is a complete transverse fracture in the mid-diaphyseal region. "

Anatomical Location of Bones in the Body

The bones of the body can be arranged according to their location. The skeleton can be divided into two main regions: the **axial skeleton** and the **appendicular skeleton**. The axial skeleton contains all of the bones of the cranial region, facial region, vertebral column and thoracic cage. The appendicular skeleton is composed of the pectoral girdle, bones of the upper extremity, pelvic girdle and lower extremity. (*Number in parenthesis indicates total number of that bone in the body. Often if "2" is indicated, that means there is one on the left side of the body and one on the right.)

Cranial Bones:
- Frontal bone
- Parietal bones (2- left and right)
- Occipital bone
- Temporal bones (2- left and right)
- Sphenoid bone
- Ethmoid bone

Facial Bones:
- Mandible
- Maxillary bones (maxillae) (2)
- Zygomatic bones (2)
- Nasal bones (2)
- Lacrimal bones (2)
- Palatine bones (2)
- Vomer
- Inferior nasal conchae (2)

Vertebral Column:
- Cervical Spine Vertebrae (7)
- Thoracic Spine Vertebrae (12)
- Lumbar Spine Vertebrae (5)
- Sacrum
- Coccyx

Thoracic Cage (Also includes the 12 thoracic vertebra):
- Ribs (12 pairs)
- Sternum

Pectoral Girdle:
- Clavicles (2)
- Scapula (2)

Upper Extremity:
- Humerus (2)
- Radius (2)
- Ulna (2)
- Carpals (Scaphoid, lunate, triquetrum, pisiform, trapezium, trapezoid, capitate, hamate- each hand will contain these 8 bones)
- Metacarpals (10 total- 5 per hand)
- Phalanges (Proximal, middle, distal) (28 total- 14 per hand)

Pelvic Girdle:
- Coxal Bones (2)

Lower Extremity:
- Femur (2)
- Tibia (2)
- Fibula (2)
- Patella (2)
- Tarsals (Calcaneus, talus, navicular, cuboid, medial cuneiform, intermediate cuneiform, lateral cuneiform- each foot will contain these 7 bones)
- Metatarsals (10 total- 5 per foot)
- Phalanges (Proximal, middle, distal) (28 total- 14 per foot)

Physical Examination of the Skeletal System

Due to the tight-knit working nature of the skeletal and muscular system, the physical examination of the muscular and skeletal system is combined in the Musculoskeletal Examination. This examination and abnormal findings are found at the end of the Muscular System chapter.

Pathologies of the Skeletal System

For additional infectious diseases that may affect this system, please refer to the Communicable/Infectious Disease Chart in Chapter 10.

Achondroplasia: results from abnormal epiphyseal activity. A child's epiphyseal cartilages grow abnormally slowly in this condition, leading to short, stocky limbs. The trunk will grow to normal size, and internal neural and organ development is normal, the limbs are just very short in these individuals. This is usually caused by an abnormality on chromosome #4.

Ankylosing Spondylitis: a condition which causes vertebra or other spinal areas to fuse together. Most commonly affects the sacroiliac joints, the lumbar vertebra and sacrum, the hips and shoulder. The cause isn't completely understood, but people with the HLA-B27 gene have a much higher risk of developing it. The joints will be come stiff as the fuse together, and pain can also accompany the loss of motion. Men are more likely to develop this than women.

Arthritis: is defined as synovial joint inflammation. There are many types of arthritis. Arthritis always involves damage to the articular cartilage- however the cause of the damage will vary with the many different types of arthritis. Here are a few of the more common types of arthritis:

- **Gouty arthritis (gout)** – excessive uric acid from the blood crystallizes and is deposited in the soft tissues of joints, causing sharp pain. It affects mostly men, and most commonly appears in the joint at the base of the big toe.
- **Osteoarthritis (OA)** – also known as *degenerative arthritis*, or *degenerative joint disease (DJD)*. It is a chronic, progressive, degenerative condition that eventually destroys the articular cartilage within synovial joints, replacing it with osseous growths called **osteophytes/bone spurs**. This "wear-and-tear arthritis" mostly affects people over the age of 60, causing pain, stiffness, and decreased range of motion in the affected joints. In the U.S. population, 25% of women and 15% of men over the age of 60 have this condition. The joint degeneration may be visible on an x-ray.
- **Rheumatoid arthritis (RA)** – a chronic inflammation of the synovial membrane of joints that leads to a thickening and eventual bony fusion (**ankylosis**) of joint tissues. It one of many types of *autoimmune diseases*, which are disorders that cause the body's immune system to try to destroy its own tissues. RA typically affects the joints of the extremities, and like most autoimmune diseases, it is characterized by periodic flare-ups and remissions, and affects more women than men.

Bone cancer- cancer of the bone. If the cancer originates in the bone tissue it is called primary bone cancer. If it has spread from another body part to the bones it is called a metastatic cancer. Most cancer in the bone is metastatic cancer (often coming from the lung, breast or prostate). There are different types of primary bone cancer, some examples are: *osteosarcoma* (usually in knee or arm), *chondrosarcoma* (commonly in pelvis, upper leg and shoulder), and *Ewing Sarcomas* (usually in spine, pelvis, arms or legs). <u>*Red Flag symptoms*</u>: *pain in bone and possible swelling in the area.* Bone scan, X-ray, CT, MRI, and PET scans can be used for diagnosis. Biopsy can be done to confirm presence. Treatment may involve surgery, radiation and/or chemotherapy.

Bunion (Hallux valgus) - a deformity at the base of the big toe. The big toe will deviate laterally. This usually has gradual onset. Pain can be at the area of the bunion along with redness and swelling. Wearing high heels, tight fitting shoes, and genetics can all be risk factors. X-ray may be done to visualize the joint.

Bursitis – an inflammation of the bursae, which are fluid-filled "pillows" that decrease friction in some synovial joints. Bursitis is most often caused by joint overuse or direct physical trauma to a bursa sac. Symptoms: Painful joint, and joint may be visibly swollen/red on inspection. Common in shoulder, elbow and hip joint. Treatment could include: NSAIDs, needle aspiration to remove fluid, corticosteroid injections.

Frozen Shoulder (Adhesive capsulitis) - pain and stiffness in the shoulder joint. Range of motion can be increasingly compromised. Symptoms start gradually, and can last weeks, months, even a year. NSAIDs and stretching exercises are often prescribed. Shoulder range of motion orthopedic tests are used for diagnosis.

Glenohumeral Dislocation- (also called **shoulder dislocation**) Occurs when the head of the humerus is forced out of the glenoid cavity. This may also result in labrum tears and/or tears of glenohumeral ligaments. Most common dislocation of the shoulder is the Anterior-Inferior dislocation.

Herniated disc (disc herniation) – the shock-absorbing *intervertebral discs* are located between the vertebrae, and are composed of mostly fibrocartilage (called the *annulus fibrosis*) with water-filled, jelly-like centers (called the *nucleus pulposus*). If the discs lose water and the spinal ligaments stiffen and weaken (both of which tend to happen as we get older), the nucleus pulposus may bulge out through the annulus fibrosus and possibly press on the spinal cord or spinal nerve roots, causing pain and numbness.

Hyperostosis: the excessive formation of bone. (In a way, this is the opposite of osteopenia). In hyperostosis, the osteoclasts slow down and stop working. This causes bone resorption to stop. The osteoblasts continue laying down new bone matrix, while the osteoclasts are unable to clear old bone matrix out of the tissue. In children, this can lead to abnormal growth and development of bones.

Kyphosis (aka: "round-back" "hunchback"). The thoracic curvature is greatly exaggerated. This can be a result of osteoporosis, where the vertebral bodies of the spine develop compression fractures. The compression of the vertebra can cause the curvature of the spine to change.

Lordosis (aka: "swayback") the lordotic curvature of the lumbar spine is exaggerated. This causes the buttocks and the abdomen to protrude abnormally.

Lyme Disease- a condition caused by an infection with *Borrelia Burgdorferi*. This bacterium is spread via the deer tick. After the tick bites a human, often a red rash (described as a "bull's eye") forms in the area of the bite. In addition, the person may initially feel flu-like symptoms (fatigue, fever, body aches, stiff neck, and headache). After a few weeks (if left untreated), arthritis may set in- causing painful, swollen joints. Treatment is antibiotic therapy. Diagnosis is done by blood tests, symptoms, and history of a tick bite.

Marfan's Syndrome- a connective tissue disorder where excess amounts of cartilage is deposited in the epiphyseal cartilages. An individual with Marfan's Syndrome usually is very tall and has very slender, long limbs. The changes seen in bone growth are usually not harmful. This disease can be life threatening because it also affects the connective tissue in the cardiovascular system, which can cause potentially deadly disorders with the heart and arteries. This is usually caused by a genetic defect on chromosome #15.

Myositis Ossificans: abnormal deposition of bone in and around muscles. A muscle trauma can lead to calcification within the muscle tissue. In other very severe cases, the cause is unknown. In these severe cases, the muscles of the neck, back, and upper limb are gradually replaced by bone.

Osteogenesis imperfecta: Collagen fiber and bone formation is decreased in this condition. Osteoblast activity is abnormal, and in severe cases the bones are very fragile. Fibroblast activity is also abnormal, which can lead to weakened ("loose") tendons and ligaments around the joint. This is an inherited connective tissue disorder.

Osteomalacia- the bones appear normal (they grow to normal size and proportions), but the bones are weak and flexible due to poor mineralization.

Osteomyelitis- is a painful and destructive bone infection, generally caused by bacteria. Most common in people over the age of 50. Often develops after surgery or trauma to the bone. Surgery to remove the damaged bone may need to be done, as well as antibiotic therapy (usually through an IV). A bone biopsy is the best test for diagnosis and allows the physician to see which bacteria is involved (so that the physician can choose the appropriate antibiotic for treatment).

Osteophyte (also called **bone spurs**) - these are bony projections and outgrowths which occur on the surface of bone. Often are seen in areas where there is a lot of impact or activity. Can be seen commonly on vertebra of the spine, on the calcaneus (heel), the knee, hip, shoulder or fingers. Some osteophytes can cause pain or reduce range of motion; others do not cause any symptoms. Can be diagnosed on an x-ray.

Osteoporosis – a loss in bone density and mass leading to porous, light, and brittle bones that are prone to fractures. It's caused by calcium resorption outpacing calcium deposit in bones, which tends to increase as people (especially women) get older. Contributing factors include a decrease in sex hormones (such as estrogen, which inhibits osteoclast activity), a diet lacking adequate calcium and vitamin D, and insufficient weight-bearing exercise. DEXA (Dual X-ray absorptiometry) is the best diagnostic test to check for osteoporosis. X-ray may also show bone density loss. Prescription drugs in the bisphosphonate category (such as *Fosamax*), reduce osteoclast activity. A mild loss of bone mass and density can be called *osteopenia*.

Paget's Disease (aka *Osteitis Deformans*): Can be caused by heredity or environmental factors (including possible a viral infection). This condition has areas of increased osteoclastic activity, leading to localized areas of osteoporosis. Meanwhile, in other areas of the skeletal system, osteoblast activity will increase leading to abnormal excessive bone matrix deposit (for example: thickening and enlarging bones in the skull). The combination of both of these abnormal activities leads to a progressively deforming skeleton. Bisphosphonate treatment (*Fosamax*) may help with this condition.

Rickets – a disease of children in which bones fail to calcify and become soft, causing misshapen bones, especially the weight-bearing ones. It's usually due to inadequate dietary calcium or vitamin D during ossification.

Scoliosis: abnormal lateral curvature of the spine. This lateral deviation can occur in one or more of the moveable vertebra. This is the most common spinal curvature disorder. This can be caused by developmental disorders, infections of the spine, or muscular paralysis. In most cases, the cause is unknown.

Scurvy- a condition involving weak, brittle bones due to a lack of Vitamin C. Vitamin C is also needed for the proper health of other tissue which contains collagen (skin, connective tissues), so other symptoms may also accompany scurvy, including life threatening ones.

Shin Splints- pain, tenderness, and possibly swelling along the tibia. Can be caused by running on hard surfaces for long periods of time, running with improper footwear, or participating in sports which have a lot of sudden starting and stopping (basketball, for example).

Spina Bifida: This is the most common neural tube defect and will begin in the third week of embryonic development. This condition occurs as the vertebrae are forming around the neural tube. In this condition, the spinal cord grows in an abnormal shape, and the vertebral arches are unable to form around the spinal cord. The vertebra now does not offer protection to the spinal cord, and the meninges (outer membrane covering the spinal cord) bulge outwards. Most common in the thoracic, lumbar, or sacral regions. Heredity and maternal diet play a role. It is now recommended that a pregnant woman take 400 – 800 micrograms of folic acid a day. In mild cases, the open gap in the vertebra can be corrected surgically. In severe cases, the brain or spinal cord may not develop properly and death may occur.

Spinal Stenosis- a narrowing of the vertebral spinal canal (which houses the spinal cord) or of the intervertebral foramina (the area where the spinal nerves exit the spinal cord). This can increase pressure on the spinal cord or spinal nerves, causing numbness in areas of the body and/or muscle weakness.

Spondylolisthesis- is where one vertebra slips forward on the vertebra below it. Most commonly at L5/S1 (lowest lumbar vertebra and sacrum). Spondylolisthesis can be rated depending on how much the vertebra has slipped out of place. Grade 1 (is the mildest amount of slippage) through Grade 5 (most severe- is also called *spondyloptosis*). The grade of spondylolisthesis will determine the treatment. Treatment can range from nothing (for very, very mild cases), limiting exercise or activities of daily living, NSAIDs to relieve pain symptoms, chiropractic care, physical therapy or surgery. Commonly diagnosed with an x-ray.

Sprain – the ligaments and joint capsule that reinforce a joint are stretched or torn, causing inflammation. Healing is slow due to the poor blood supply to the dense (fibrous) connective tissue. A **dislocation** (or luxation) occurs when the sprain is so severe that the bones are forced out of their normal positions. A partial dislocation is called a **subluxation**.

Temporomandibular Joint Disorder (TMJD) - disorder of the temporomandibular joint (TMJ). Symptoms can be jaw clicking/popping, pain on chewing or palpation of the TMJ, decreased jaw movement, headaches and/or neck pain. TMJD can be a result of teeth clenching/grinding, whiplash, anxiety, or osteoarthritis of the joint.

Unhappy Triad- a knee injury in which the anterior cruciate ligament (ACL), medial collateral ligament (MCL) and medial meniscus are torn. Usually caused by a blow to the outside of the knee. Usually diagnosed with a MRI

Practice Study and Test Questions:

1) The radius is an example of a
    A) flat bone
    B) long bone
    C) short bone
    D) sesamoid bone

2) Osteosarcoma, Ewing's sarcoma, and chondrosarcoma are examples of
    A) bone cancer
    B) arthritis
    C) fractures
    D) skin cancer

3) Hematopoietic tissue in the bone is the
    A) periosteum
    B) yellow bone marrow
    C) red bone marrow
    D) metaphysis

4) An autoimmune disease in which the synovial membrane of the joints is damaged is called
    A) rheumatoid arthritis
    B) spina bifida
    C) hyperostosis
    D) Paget's disease

5) Bone strength and bone density can be influenced by
      A) nutrition
      B) regular exercise
      C) hormones
      D) all of the above

6) The pathology in which one vertebra slips forward on the vertebra below it is called
      A) rosacea
      B) osteogenesis imperfecta
      C) Marfan's Syndrome
      D) spondylolisthesis

7) Chronic progressive destruction of the articular cartilage within joints (seen in patients usually over the age of 60) is called
      A) gouty arthritis
      B) achondroplasia
      C) osteoarthritis
      D) TMJD

8) Bisphosphonate treatment may help with
      A) Paget's disease
      B) Myositis Ossificans
      C) Osteoporosis
      D) Both A and C

9) Which of the following conditions may be treated with antibiotics?
      A) Lyme disease
      B) rickets
      C) adhesive capsulitis
      D) osteomalacia

10) Pain, tenderness, and possibly swelling along the tibia may be signs of
      A) unhappy triad
      B) spondylolisthesis
      C) lordosis
      D) shin splints

11) Which part of the disc may bulge and compress spinal cord or spinal nerves in a herniated disc?
      A) nucleus pulposus
      B) annulus fibrosis
      C) periosteum
      D) inferior facet

12) Upon inspection/observation of a patient in the standing positions, it is noted that their abdomen and buttocks are protruding abnormally. This could be a sign of
      A) osteomyelitis
      B) kyphosis
      C) lordosis
      D) gouty arthritis

13) The cell which produces new bone matrix and is needed for proper growth and development of bones is the
    A) osteoprogenitor cells
    B) osteocytes
    C) osteoclasts
    D) osteoblasts

14) Folic acid supplementation for a pregnant mom is recommended to try to prevent
    A) spina bifida
    B) Paget's disease
    C) Marfan's syndrome
    D) osteogenesis imperfecta

15) The best test for diagnosing osteoporosis is
    A) PET scan
    B) CT scan
    C) MRI
    D) DEXA- dual x-ray absorptiometry

16) An injury in which the ACL, MCL and medial meniscus is torn is called
    A) Unhappy triad
    B) Subluxation
    C) Myositis ossificans
    D) bursitis

17) A bone biopsy is the best diagnostic tool for
    A) osteopenia
    B) osteomyelitis
    C) rickets
    D) Marfan's syndrome

18) The most common type of shoulder dislocation is
    A) anterior-superior
    B) posterior-inferior
    C) anterior-inferior
    D) posterior-superior

19) Which of the following conditions are caused by a genetic chromosomal defect?
    A) Marfan's syndrome
    B) Achondroplasia
    C) scurvy
    D) Both A and B

20) A deficiency of calcium and/or vitamin D in children can cause
    A) rickets
    B) myositis ossificans
    C) osteomyelitis
    D) scurvy

Answers: 1) B 2) A 3) C 4) A 5) D 6) D 7) C 8) D 9) A 10) D 11) A 12) C 13) D 14) A 15) D 16) A 17) B 18) C 19) D 20) A

CHAPTER 5: THE MUSCULAR SYSTEM

There are **3 types of muscular tissue** found in the body, and each has a specialized structure and corresponding function ...

1. **Skeletal muscle tissue** – Is located on the skeleton of the body, or attached to the skin of the face. It appears *striated* (striped) under a microscope, and is under *voluntary* (conscious) control by the nervous system. Striations are formed because of the presence of sarcomeres. Skeletal muscle usually contains more than one nucleus per cell (multinucleated). Skeletal muscle will be the main focus of this chapter.

2. **Smooth muscle tissue** – is found in the walls of hollow *visceral* (internal) organs- especially in the digestive and urinary tracts, blood vessels, reproductive tract, and respiratory passages. It is uninucleate, has *no striations* (therefore, has no sarcomeres), and is *involuntary* (not under conscious control). It produces *peristalsis* (movement by squeezing), *dilation* (widening), and *constriction* (narrowing). Since smooth muscle fibers do not contain organized sarcomeres, the thick filaments are just scattered in the sarcoplasm. This allows smooth muscle to exhibit much better *plasticity* than skeletal muscle. This means that smooth muscle tissues can still contract well when they are stretched, while skeletal muscle does not.

3. **Cardiac muscle tissue** – is found only in the heart and is *striated* and *involuntary*. Cardiac muscle cells (also called cardiocytes) are smaller than skeletal muscle cells and are connected to one another by specialized sites called **intercalated discs**. Usually cardiac muscle cells contain only one nucleus and rely on aerobic metabolism (oxygen) to get the energy they need to contract. Because of this need for oxygen, cardiac muscle cells have many mitochondria and myoglobin (used to store oxygen).

From here on out in this chapter, we will focus on Skeletal Muscle.

Skeletal Muscle Anatomy and Physiology:

Skeletal muscle has a variety of functions. It produces movement, maintains posture, maintains body position, supports soft tissue, maintains body temperature, and will guard entrances and exits of the body.

Skeletal muscle is composed of densely packed muscle cells, which are called *muscle fibers* or *myofibers*. There are also blood vessels, nerve fibers, and three layers of connective tissue coverings in a muscle. The *endomysium* is the connective tissue covering which surrounds each muscle fiber or myofibers. The *perimysium* is the connective tissue layer which bundles several myofibers into *fascicles* (groups/bundles of muscle fibers). The *epimysium* covers the outside of the entire muscle (which is many fascicles grouped together).

Microscopic Anatomy of Skeletal Muscle:

Skeletal muscle cells are also called *muscle fibers* or *myofibers*. These muscle cells are large and multinucleated (containing many nuclei). The cell membrane of a muscle cell is called the *sarcolemma*, and it surrounds the cytoplasm of a muscle cell (called the *sarcoplasm*). *T-Tubules (Transverse tubules)* are passageways which run perpendicular to the muscle fibers and penetrate deep inside the muscle. They serve as a communication passageway to allow nerve action potentials (nerve messages) to travel deep within the muscle.

If we use our microscope and take a journey deep inside a muscle cell, we will see many **myofibrils** which run the length of the entire muscle cell. Each skeletal muscle cell contains hundreds to thousands of myofibrils. T-tubules will wrap around the myofibrils, and allow communication between them. Where T-tubules wrap around the myofibrils, a membrane is formed that covers the external surface of the myofibril. This membrane is called the *sarcoplasmic reticulum*. As the sarcoplasmic reticulum nears the T-tubule, expanded chambers form, which are called the *terminal cisternae*. The sarcoplasmic reticulum and terminal cisternae are storage areas for Ca^{+2} (Calcium ions). If a nerve message travels through the T-tubule, it triggers the terminal cisternae to release the stored calcium ions. Calcium ions will play an important part in skeletal muscle contraction- which we will discuss in a few moments.

Inside of each myofibril, are many bundles of **myofilaments**. Myofilaments are microscopic pieces of protein, and there are many of these proteins in each myofibril. It is these myofilaments which allow our muscle to contract, or shorten. There are two types of myofilaments which overlap one another in our myofibrils:

1. **Thin Filament**: The thin filament is composed mostly of a protein called *actin*. In the thin filament, there are also strands of tropomyosin and troponin (called the "troponin-tropomyosin complex"). *Tropomyosin* is used to cover "binding sites" on the thin filament- this prevents unwanted muscle contraction. *Troponin* is a substance that attaches onto tropomyosin to hold it in position, and is sensitive to calcium ions. The troponin-tropomyosin complex is crucial in allowing muscle contractions to occur. You can think of troponin and tropomyosin as "bodyguards" for the thin filament. They prevent unwanted contact from the thick filament. They will only allow contact between the thick and thin filament to occur if calcium is present- and this then leads to contraction.

2. **Thick Filament**: Composed mostly of a bundle of *myosin* protein molecules twisted around a titan core. Each myosin molecule has an elongated *tail* and a wider *head*. The head of the thick filament will attach onto the binding site of the thin filament. This forms cross bridges with the thin filament, which is a crucial step during muscle contraction.

Actin and Myosin are arranged into repeating little bundles called *sarcomeres*. Each myofibril will contain approximately 10,000 sarcomeres. At each end of the muscle cell, the actin and myosin are attached to the inside of the sarcolemma (the cell membrane). When viewing a sarcomere under a microscope, each sarcomere has a darker colored band (A band) and a lighter colored band (I band). This alternating pattern of darker colored bands and lighter colored bands cause skeletal muscle to have a striated appearance when viewing it under the microscope.

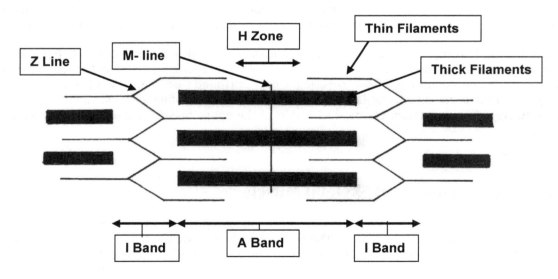

- **A Band**: darker colored and located in the center of the sarcomere. Each A band is the length of the thick filament, and has three subdivisions:
    1. *M Line*- the central portion of each thick filament is connected to adjacent thick filaments by proteins that run in the M-line. The M-line stabilizes the thick filaments.
    2. *H Zone*- (or *H band*) is a lighter region on either side of the M-line. Contains all thick filaments, no thin filaments.
    3. The *Zone of Overlap*- thin filaments will overlap thick filaments here.
- **I Band**: lighter colored region, which is found on either side of the A band. The I band only contains thin filaments (actin). At the end of the sarcomere, a *Z line* is present- this is the boundary between adjacent sarcomeres.

Sliding Filament Model and Skeletal Muscle Contraction:

The steps involved in muscle contraction are called the **Sliding Filament Model.** To summarize, muscle contraction occurs when the thin filament slides and overlaps the thick filament. During muscle contraction, the thin and thick filament do not change size, they just overlap one another. Before the thick and thin filaments can begin moving, two criteria must be met.
1. ***Energy/Fuel***: Adenosine Triphosphate/ATP (the fuel used by all body cells) must be present.
2. ***Nervous System Stimulation***: A message (*action potential*) from the nervous system must be transmitted to the muscle, telling it to contract. A *motor neuron* carries messages from the brain out to the muscle cells. This general area where this communication between neuron and muscle cell occurs is called the *neuromuscular junction*. The motor neuron has an enlarged end, called the synaptic terminal. The synaptic terminal will come near to, but not touch, the motor end plate of the muscle fiber. The space between the synaptic terminal of the neuron and the motor end plate of the muscle fiber is called the *synaptic cleft*. In order to get the action potential (nerve message) from the neuron to the muscle fiber, it must cross over the synaptic cleft. As the action potential travels down the length of the neuron and reaches the synaptic terminal, the synaptic terminal will release a chemical messenger which is able to cross the synaptic cleft. This chemical messenger is called a *neurotransmitter*, and the specific type of neurotransmitter used in skeletal muscle contraction is called *acetylcholine (ACh)*. One motor neuron will stimulate a certain number of muscle fibers within a muscle- this is called a *motor unit.* The more motor units stimulated within a muscle, the stronger the contraction.

Let us assume that both of these criteria are present, and now we will see how muscle contraction occurs:
1. Acetylcholine (Ach) is released by the motor neuron.
2. After crossing the synaptic cleft, ACh binds to receptors on the sarcolemma (cell membrane) of the muscle cell. This transmits the message (action potential) to the muscle cell.
3. T-tubules spread the action potential throughout the muscle fiber.
4. The sarcoplasmic reticulum and terminal cisternae release stored calcium ions.
5. The calcium ions will travel to the thin filament, stimulating troponin.
6. Troponin will move tropomyosin off of the binding sites on the thin filament (actin), thereby exposing the binding site.
7. The thick filament (myosin), energized by ATP, swings and locks onto the thin filament at the binding site, forming a cross bridge.
8. The thick filament pulls the thin filament during the power stroke. The filaments begin to overlap one another (shortening the length of the muscle and causing muscle contraction).
9. More ATP will bind to the myosin head, allowing it to detach from the binding site.
10. If ACh, calcium ions, and ATP are still present, more myosin heads will bind and pull the thin filament again, increasing the contraction further.

When the muscle relaxes, acetylcholine is broken down by acetylcholinesterase. This ends the action potential. The sarcoplasmic reticulum and terminal cisternae reabsorb the calcium ions. After the calcium is removed, tropomyosin moves back into its initial position, covering the binding sites of the thin filament. And, finally, the thin filament passively slides back to its initial position, and the muscle relaxes and returns to its original length.

Skeletal muscle fibers follow the *All or None Principle*. This principal states that individual muscle fibers will contract to their fullest extent possible or not at all. The whole muscle, however, is capable of partial contractions. Skeletal muscle contractions can vary according to the frequency in which they are stimulated. A **twitch** is a single stimulus-contraction-relaxation sequence in a muscle fiber. **Complete tetanus** is when repeated stimulation of the muscle occurs before the relaxation phase begins. Peak muscle tension builds quickly. This occurs in virtually all muscle contractions.

There are two main types of skeletal muscle contractions. During an **isotonic contraction**, muscle tension increases and muscle length changes (and movement of joints are visible). In an isotonic *concentric* contraction, the muscle tension (strength) exceeds the resistance (the weight of the object being moved) and the muscle shortens (ex: lifting a weight during a bicep curl). During an isotonic e*ccentric* contraction, the muscle tension is less than the resistance and the muscle lengthens. This is a controlled lengthening of the muscle (for example: lowering the weight during a bicep curl). In an **isometric contraction**, the muscle length does not change during the contraction (for example: pushing as hard as you can against a brick wall.) The speed of contraction will increase as resistance decreases. Therefore, you can lift a lighter object faster than a heavy object.

Energy Use and Muscular Activity:

Muscle cells use a massive amount of energy (adenosine triphosphate- ATP) to maintain contractions. To sustain the need for ATP during activity, there are four main ways a muscle can make ATP.

1. **Stored ATP**- a muscle cell can store a small amount of ATP. This usually can fuel 4-6 seconds of muscular activity
2. **Phosphorylation "Recharging" of ADP with CP**- When ATP is used for fuel, it is broken down into ADP+P (Adenosine Diphosphate + Phosphate). This ADP can be recycled and re-used when combined with CP (Creatine Phosphate). Creatine Phosphate donates its phosphate group and adds it to ADP. This "re-charges" the ADP back into ATP again for re-use. The muscle stores enough CP to recycle ADP back into ATP for another 15 seconds.
3. **Glycolysis**- In the cytoplasm of the cell, glucose can be broken down into 2 pyruvate molecules and 2 ATP. This does not require oxygen.
4. **The Krebs (Citric Acid Cycle) and Oxidative Phosphorylation**- The pyruvate formed by glycolysis will move from the cytoplasm into the mitochondria of the cell. In the mitochondria, pyruvate is converted into Acetyl CoA, NADH and carbon dioxide. The Acetyl CoA will then run through the Krebs (Citric Acid) Cycle. As it is broken down by enzymes, it forms one ATP, carbon dioxide, NADH and $FADH_2$ molecules. In the presence of oxygen (called Oxidative Phosphorylation), NADH and $FADH_2$ will be processed via the electron transport chain to form even more ATP. When using the Krebs Cycle and then Oxidative Phosphorylation (requiring oxygen being present)- one molecule of glucose will produce 36-38 ATP.

Muscle fatigue will occur with strenuous activity. This can be caused by a number of factors, such as: depletion of metabolic reserves in the muscle, decrease of pH in muscle fibers or the blood, physical damage to the muscle, and increased lactic acid in the muscle (after exercise lactic acid can be recycled back into pyruvic acid by the liver, or removed from the body in our urine). After exercise, our muscles will go into a recovery phase, where they clean and replenish themselves. *Oxygen Debt* is the amount of oxygen needed for this cleaning and replenishment process.

Muscle Performance:

Performance is measured in terms of power and endurance. Two main factors can affect the performance capabilities of a muscle:

1. Types of Muscle Fibers
    *   **Fast Twitch Fibers**- large sized muscle fibers, with densely packed myofibrils, but few mitochondria. These fibers are great at quick and powerful contractions, but have poor endurance. These fibers can also be called *white muscle fibers* or *Type II-A fibers.*
    *   **Slow Twitch Fibers**- smaller in size, but better capillary network and an increased number of mitochondria than fast twitch fibers. These fibers contract more slowly, but have great endurance. Slow twitch fibers often look darker in color than fast twitch fibers, due to the red pigment myoglobin. Myoglobin helps the slow twitch muscle store oxygen. Slow twitch fibers can also be called *red muscle fibers* or *Type I fibers.*
    *   **Intermediate Fibers**- (aka *Type II-B fibers*) are in-between fast and slow fibers. They are lighter colored and look like fast fibers, but have a better blood supply, much like slow fibers.
2. Physical Conditioning
    *   **Anaerobic endurance**- is the increase in time that muscle contractions can be sustained by CP and glycolysis. Usually muscle fatigue will begin within 2 minutes of activity. This is used for fast powerful activities (sprints, powerlifting, pole vault)
    *   **Aerobic endurance**- is the increase in time activities can be supported by mitochondria. Oxygen and nutrients (glucose, proteins or fats) are needed. Usually seen in lower intensity activities (jogging, distance swimming), but these activities can be performed for a longer time.

Hormones can also affect muscle performance and development. *Growth hormone* and *testosterone* will stimulate growth of the muscle fibers. *Thyroid hormone* and *epinephrine* will increase the metabolic activity in muscle cells

Trigger and Motor Points

A **motor point** is the area in a muscle where the motor nerve enters. If this region becomes irritated, it can become a **trigger point**. These trigger points can be palpated as tight bands of fibers. Some trigger points will create referred pain (pain sensations located in another area of the body away from the trigger point), while other trigger points will be locally sensitive. Causes of trigger points vary. It can be caused by trauma, psychological stress, muscle fatigue and overload, disease processes, inflammatory conditions or other homeostatic imbalances. *Active trigger points* create pain at all times. *Latent trigger points* only create pain when pressure is applied. This pressure can come from palpation of the point, or from strain on the muscle while the muscle is in use during activity. Treatment of trigger points can involve direct manual pressure (ischemic compression), ultrasound, needling, vibration, stretching the muscle, cryotherapy or low level laser therapy. Many trigger point locations also correspond to acupuncture points. Dr. Janet Travell was one of the first medical doctors to research and study trigger point theory.

Physical and Orthopedic Examination of the Musculoskeletal System

✓ Range of Motion tests should be performed using a goniometer or inclinometer
✓ During Range of Motion tests, measure the amount of range of motion and note any reported pain or tenderness when performing the test
✓ If an orthopedic test is warranted in an area (other than the spine), the test should be performed bilaterally. Test the non-painful side first, then the painful side (for example: in a patient with reported right elbow pain, perform the orthopedic tests first on the uninjured left elbow, then proceed with testing the painful right elbow.)
✓ Please note: the orthopedic tests listed here are just a small sampling of orthopedic tests that can be performed on a patient. Please consult an orthopedic examination text for more tests, if needed.

Head and Cervical Spine (Neck)

1. Inspect the head and neck for deformities (torticollis, immobility)
2. Palpate the temporomandibular joint (TMJ)
3. Palpate the cervical spine and musculature and feel for tenderness, swelling, atrophy of muscles
4. Test for **Active Range of Motion of the Cervical Spine**
   ➢ **flexion (45-50°)**
   ➢ **extension (55- 70°)**
   ➢ **left and right rotation (70-90°)**
   ➢ **left and right lateral flexion (20-45°)**
5. If there is any pain or discomfort in the neck (or radiating into the arm), orthopedic examinations of the cervical spine may be performed to try to determine the underlying cause of the pain or could indicate the need for additional diagnostic tests.

Orthopedic Tests for the Cervical Spine	Test indicates
Distraction test	If pain is relieved or decreased during distraction of the cervical spine, this indicates foraminal occlusion of spinal nerve root or facet irritation
Foraminal Compression test (aka Spurling's test)	Radiating pain during compression indicates foraminal occlusion or facet irritation
Soto-Hall	Pain during this test can indicate fracture or sprain. If knees bend while performing test, this could indicate meningitis
Valsalva test	Pain during this test may indicate disc herniation or mass (in all areas of the spine) at the area of discomfort
Shoulder Abduction (Relief) Test (aka Bakody's sign)	A decrease or relief of symptoms when this test is performed indicates herniated disc or nerve root compression (often of C4/C5 or C5/C6 area)
Adson's test	Upon inhalation, if pulse disappears, this indicates thoracic outlet syndrome- usually due to a cervical rib

Thoracic and Lumbar Spine

1. Inspect the thoracic and lumbar spine. Look for any abnormal curvatures (lordosis, hypolordosis, kyphosis, scoliosis)
2. Test for **Active Range of Motion in the Thoracolumbar Spine.** (Use goniometer, inclinometer or measuring tape)
   - ➤ **flexion (80°)**
   - ➤ **extension (35°)**
   - ➤ **left and right rotation (35°)**
   - ➤ **left and right lateral flexion (35°)**
3. Palpate spinous processes for tenderness.
4. Palpate paraspinal muscles for tenderness, hypertonicity or atrophy.
5. If there is any pain or discomfort in the thoracolumbar spine, orthopedic examinations may be performed to try to determine the underlying cause of the pain or could indicate the need for additional diagnostic tests.

Orthopedic Tests for the Thoracolumbar Spine	Test indicates
Straight leg raiser (SLR)	Pain in lumbar spine or pain radiating into leg indicates disc herniation or L4, L5, S1 nerve root injury
Bragard's sign	Pain on dorsiflexion of the foot tests for sciatica and disc herniation
Sicard's sign	Pain in the low back or radiating down the leg during toe movement tests for sciatica
Becterew's Sitting (Sitting Knee Extension)	Pain in the low back or extending into the legs indicate sciatica and/or disc herniation
Fajersztajn's test (Well leg raiser tests)	If pain is triggered on the symptomatic side (while moving the uninvolved leg), this test indicates disc herniation and nerve root irritation

Shoulder (Glenohumeral Joint)

1. Inspect shoulder area (look for bruising, swelling, deformation, atrophy)
2. Test for **Active Range of Motion of the Shoulder**
   - ➤ **flexion (160-180°)**
   - ➤ **extension (50-60°)**
   - ➤ **adduction (50-75°)**
   - ➤ **abduction (170-180°)**
   - ➤ **internal (medial) rotation (60-100°)**
   - ➤ **external (lateral) rotation (80-90°)**
3. Palpate for tenderness in the bicipital groove, subacromial area, acromioclavicular joint and sternoclavicular joint
4. Palpate shoulder muscles for tenderness, hypertonicity or atrophy.
5. If there is any pain or discomfort in the shoulder, orthopedic examinations may be be performed to try to determine the underlying cause of the pain or could indicate the need for additional diagnostic tests.

Orthopedic Tests for the Shoulder	Test indicates
Codman's (Drop Arm) test	If painful, or if the patient is unable to do the movement, this indicates a rotator cuff tear (often supraspinatus muscle)
Empty Can test (aka Jobe's Test)	Pain or weakness indicates possible supraspinatus tendonopathy or tear
Apprehension test	Apprehension on the face of the patient during this test indicates anterior shoulder instability
Sulcus sign	A positive sulcus sign (a gap greater than 1 cm appearing between the humeral head and the undersurface of the acromion) indicates inferior instability of the shoulder.
Apley's scratch test	Decreased movement on Apley's scratch test can indicate mobility restrictions of the shoulder. Muscles that perform internal rotation or external rotational movements should be addressed for spasms or hypertonicities.
Speed's test ("Straight-arm" test)	Increased pain in the bicipital groove indicates bicipital tendinitis
Yergason's test	Increased pain in the bicipital groove indicates bicipital tendinitis
Dugas Test	Inability to perform the test indicates unreduced anterior dislocation of the shoulder

Elbow (Radioulnar Joint)

1. Inspect elbow joint- looking for swelling, inflammation, nodules
2. Test for **Active Range of Motion of the Elbow**
   - ➤ **flexion (140-150°)**
   - ➤ **extension (back to anatomical position)**
   - ➤ **supination (90°)**
   - ➤ **pronation (80-90°)**
3. Palpate for tenderness or nodules on the olecranon process, medial and lateral epicondyles, and extensor surface of the ulna
4. Palpate muscles around the elbow for tenderness, hypertonicity or atrophy.
5. If there is any pain or discomfort in the elbow, orthopedic examinations may be be performed to try to determine the underlying cause of the pain or could indicate the need for additional diagnostic tests.

Orthopedic Tests for the Elbow	Test indicates
Cozen's test	Pain over the lateral epicondyle of the humerus during this test indicates lateral epicondylitis (tennis elbow)
Mills test	Pain over the lateral epicondyle of the humerus during this test indicates lateral epicondylitis (tennis elbow)
Golfer's elbow test	Pain over the medial epicondyle of the humerus during this test indicates medial epicondylitis (golfer's elbow)
Tinel's sign (at elbow)	Recreation of pain, numbness, or paresthesia indicates neuropathy
Ligamentous Instability Tests	Laxity compared to the contralateral (uninjured) elbow indicates a partial or complete tear of medial or lateral collateral ligament.

Wrist (Radiocarpal Joint) and Hand

1. Inspect wrist joint, hand and fingers- looking for swelling, inflammation, deformation, nodules
2. Test for **Active Range of Motion of the Wrist**
    - ➢ **flexion (80-90°)**
    - ➢ **extension (70-90°)**
    - ➢ **adduction (30-45°)**
    - ➢ **abduction (15°)**
3. Measure movement of the hand and fingers by having the patient make a fist and straighten fingers.
4. Test grip strength of each hand using a *grip dynamometer*. If dynamometer is not available, patient can grip the index and middle finger of the examiner and squeeze. Compare grip strength bilaterally.
5. Palpate wrist, metacarpophalangeal joints, proximal interphalangeal joints and distal interphalangeal joints and examine for swelling, tenderness, nodular masses (example Heberden's nodes)
6. Palpate muscles around the wrist and fingers for tenderness, hypertonicity or atrophy.
7. If there is any pain or discomfort in the wrist or hand, orthopedic examinations may be be performed to try to determine the underlying cause of the pain or could indicate the need for additional diagnostic tests.

Orthopedic Tests for the Wrist	Test indicates
Tinel's sign (at wrist)	Tingling or paresthesia into the thumb, index and middle finger during this test indicates ulnar neuropathy or carpal tunnel syndrome (median nerve)
Phalen's sign	A positive sign (burning, tingling or numb sensation over the thumb, index, middle and ring fingers) produces paresthesia in the distribution of the median nerve indicates carpal tunnel syndrome
Finkelstein's sign	Pain during this test indicates de Quervain's disease/syndrome (tenosynovitis of the thumb)
Allen's test	An increase in the time to achieve a flushing effect indicates arterial stenosis of the radial and/or ulnar arteries

Pelvis and Hip (Coxal Joint)

1. Inspect hip joint- looking for swelling, inflammation, deformation,
2. Test for **Active Range of Motion of the Hip**
    - ➢ **flexion (110-120°)**
    - ➢ **extension (10-15°)**
    - ➢ **abduction (30-50°)**
    - ➢ **adduction (20-30°)**
    - ➢ **internal (medial) rotation (30-40°)**
    - ➢ **external (lateral) rotation (40-60°)**
3. Palpate the hip joint and examine for swelling, tenderness
4. Palpate muscles around the hip for tenderness, hypertonicity or atrophy.
5. If there is any pain or discomfort in the hip, orthopedic examinations may be be performed to try to determine the underlying cause of the pain or could indicate the need for additional diagnostic tests.

Orthopedic Tests for the Pelvis and Hip	Test indicates
Thomas test	A positive test indicates flexion contractures
Trendelenburg test	A positive test indicates instability of the hip (usually as a result of a prior dislocation) or gluteal and abductor weakness
Patrick's test (aka FABER or Figure Four test)	A positive test indicates iliopsoas spasm, sacroiliac pathology or hip pathology (often osteoarthritis)
Yeoman's test	Pain in sacroiliac region indicates sacroiliac joint involvement. Pain in lumbar spine indicates lumbar involvement.

Knee (Tibiofemoral Joint)

1. Inspect the knee, looking for any swelling, inflammation, deformation
2. Test for **Active Range of Motion of the Knee**
   - ➢ **flexion (130°)**
   - ➢ **extension (knee fully straight)**
3. Palpate the knee (with patient lying supine) and the patella
4. Palpate the tibiofemoral joint (with patient seated with legs over the side of the table)
5. Palpate muscles around the knee for tenderness, hypertonicity or atrophy.
6. If there is any pain or discomfort in the knee, orthopedic examinations may be be performed to try to determine the underlying cause of the pain or could indicate the need for additional diagnostic tests.

Orthopedic Tests for the Knee	Test indicates
Abduction (valgus) stress test	Excessive movement during this test indicates medial collateral ligament (MCL) injury
Adduction (varus) stress test	Excessive movement during this test indicates lateral collateral ligament (LCL) injury
Lachman's test (aka Ritchie or Trillat test)	A "soft" or "mushy" end feel, or increased movement of the tibia indicates anterior cruciate ligament (ACL) injury
Anterior Drawer test	A "soft" or "mushy" end feel, or increased movement of the tibia indicates anterior cruciate ligament (ACL) injury
Posterior Drawer test	A "soft" or "mushy" end feel, or increased movement of the tibia indicates posterior cruciate ligament (PCL) injury
Apley's compression and distraction	Pain on distraction may indicate ligament injury. Pain on compression may indicate meniscus injury.
McMurray's sign (aka McMurray's Click)	A palpable, audible, or painful click over the medial or lateral joint line indicates a meniscal tear.
Bulge Sign	If a wave of fluid returns after 2 seconds, this test can indicate patellar effusion.
Peripatellar Swelling Test (aka Balloon Sign)	Feeling fluid moving to the infrapatellar area indicates patellar effusion.

Ankle (talocrural) Joint and Foot

1. Inspect the ankle and feet for swelling, deformities, redness and nodules.
2. Test for **Active Range of Motion of the Ankle**
   - **dorsiflexion (20°)**
   - **plantar flexion (50°)**
   - **inversion (45-60°)**
   - **eversion (15-30°)**
3. Test for toe movement by having patient flex and extend toes. Note any restricted motion or pain on movement.
4. Palpate ankle joints for tenderness, swelling, inflammation. Palpate foot and feel for tenderness, swelling, corns and calluses
5. Palpate along Achilles tendon for rheumatoid nodules. Palpate muscles around the ankle, calf and foot for tenderness, hypertonicity or atrophy.
6. If there is any pain or discomfort in the ankle/foot, orthopedic examinations may be be performed to try to determine the underlying cause of the pain or could indicate the need for additional diagnostic tests.

Orthopedic Tests for the Ankle	Test indicates
Drawer test	If a dimple or suction sign is present, this indicates an anterior talofibular ligament tear and possibly a calcaneofibular ligament tear
Thompson's test	If the foot does not move, this indicates an Achilles tendon tear
Tinel's percussion sign	Tingling and/or paresthesia in the foot can indicate neuritis of the deep peroneal nerve or posterior tibial nerve.
Morton's test	Pain when the forefoot is squeezed can indicate foot neuroma, stress fracture or metatarsalgia

Muscle Strength Grading:

1. Assess muscle strength (have patient contract muscle while the examiner applies resistance):

Muscle Strength Grading Scale	
5/5	Normal Strength or Resistance
4/5	Good Strength or Resistance
3/5	Fair Strength or Resistance
2/5	Poor Strength or Resistance
1/5	Trace Strength or Resistance
0/5	Zero Strength or Resistance

SUMMARY CHART

Range of Motion:

Cervical Spine	Thoracolumbar Spine	Shoulder (Glenohumeral Joint)	Elbow (Radioulnar Joint)
• Flexion= **45-50°** • Extension= **55- 70°** • Left and Right rotation= **70-90°** • Left and Right lateral flexion= **20-45°**	• Flexion= **80°** • Extension= **35°** • Left and Right rotation= **35°** • Left and Right lateral flexion= **35°**	• Flexion= **160-180°** • Extension= **50-60°** • Adduction= **50-75°** • Abduction= **170-180°** • Internal (medial) rotation= **60-100°** • External (lateral) rotation= **80-90°**	• Flexion= **140-150°** • Extension= back to anatomical position • Supination= **90°** • Pronation= **80-90°**

Wrist (Radiocarpal Joint)	Pelvis and Hip (Coxal Joint)	Knee (Tibiofemoral Joint)	Ankle (Talocrural Joint)
• Flexion= **80-90°** • Extension= **70-90°** • Adduction= **30-45°** • Abduction= **15°**	• Flexion= **110-120°** • Extension= **10-15°** • Abduction= **30-50°** • Adduction= **20-30°** • Internal (medial) rotation= **30-40°** • External (lateral) rotation= **40-60°**	• Flexion= **130°** • Extension= **knee fully straight**	• Dorsiflexion= **20°** • Plantar flexion= **50°** • Inversion= **45-60°** • Eversion= **15-30°**

General Abnormal Findings of Musculoskeletal System

Abnormal findings, if necessary, should be referred to patients PCP or an orthopedic surgeon, osteopath, chiropractor, rheumatologist, physiatrist.

Crepitus- abnormal crunching or grating sensation with movement of a joint. Often seen in rheumatoid arthritis, osteoarthritis, or when two fractured ends of a bone rub together

Footdrop- unable to lift foot up during gait. Due to weakness or paralysis of dorsiflexor muscles- either due to muscle damage, peripheral nerve damage, or spinal nerve root damage.

Muscle flaccidity- no muscle tone, usually due to a lower motor neuron lesion.

Muscle weakness- can be detected in any of the active range of motion testing. This could be due to a muscle injury, stroke, multiple sclerosis, or due to damage of the nerve which would serve the muscle.

Muscle Atrophy- muscle loses visible size and strength (muscle wasting). Can be due to neuronal pathology, prolonged immobility, metabolic disorders, and aging

Arm pain- usually due to musculoskeletal injuries (sprains and strains), BUT also could be referred pain from another area. For example:
- left arm pain which can be severe and crushing, with dyspnea, pallor and weakness- could be *myocardial infarction (heart attack)*
- radiating pain with crepitus and swelling over a specific bone in the arm- these symptoms could indicate a *fracture*

Leg pain- usually due to musculoskeletal injury (sprains and strains), but also could be:
- shooting, aching, tingling which radiates often down the back side of the leg- this could indicate *sciatica*
- discomfort in calf (tenderness or pain), edema, and a feeling of heaviness in the leg- possibly indicates *thrombophlebitis* or *deep vein thrombosis (DVT)*

Muscle Spasms- strong painful contractions which can occur in virtually any muscle. Most common in the calf and foot. Spasms typically occur after exercise, during pregnancy, and during muscle fatigue. Can also be a result of electrolyte imbalance (hypocalcemia, hyponatremia) or as a result of certain drugs

Muscle rigidity- Increased muscle tone- possibly caused by upper motor neuron lesions, such as during a stroke.

Heberden's Nodes- appear on the distal interphalangeal joints, usually hard and painless- seen in patients with osteoarthritis

Bouchard's Nodes- appear on proximal interphalangeal joints, also seen in osteoarthritis

Scoliosis- abnormal lateral curvature of the spine

Lordosis- increased lumbar curve of the spine ("swayback")

Kyphosis- increased thoracic curve of the spine ("hunchback")

Hallux Valgus- (a *bunion*) lateral deviation of the big toe

Rheumatoid arthritis- Can cause ulnar deviation of the fingers with swelling at metacarpophalangeal joints, soft tissue nodules, boutonnière and swan-neck deformities of the fingers.

Dupuytren's contracture- finger stuck in flexion, with a node palpable near the distal palmar crease

Step defect- seen at acromioclavicular joint- indicates shoulder separation or acromioclavicular joint sprain.

Trigger point- inflammation of a motor point (the area of the muscle where a motor nerve enters). Creates a taut, hyperirritable band in the muscle. Can be caused by injury, overuse, and build-up of metabolic wastes. Pain can be localized to the area of the trigger point, or can radiate (spread) or refer (show up in another area of the body). Ice and compression may help alleviate.

Swan Neck Deformity- seen in fingers. Uncontrollable flexion of metacarpophalangeal joint, hyperextension of the proximal interphalangeal joint, and flexion of the distal interphalangeal joint.

Boutonnière Deformity- seen in fingers. Proximal interphalangeal joint is flexed, and distal interphalangeal joint is extended.

DeQuervain's syndrome/disease- pain at base of the thumb (often due to overuse)

Torticollis "wryneck"- unilateral spasm of the sternocleidomastoid muscle.

Advanced Imaging and Diagnostic Tests of the Musculoskeletal System

Arthroscopy- inserting a tube fitted with a camera to view the inside of a joint surface. Surgical tools can also be fitted to assist in repair or removal of damaged structures (commonly done on the knee).

Bone Scan (Radionuclide scan) - This is a nuclear scan, also called a *radionuclide scan*. In a bone scan, a radioactive tracer is injected into the body, and accumulates in places in the patient's bones that are undergoing a lot of repair activity. This test identifies areas that might be injured due to a fracture, bone infection, arthritis, or invading cancer. In the bone scan images, bright spots appear in the areas where the tracer has collected. Bone scans are most frequently done for people with cancer to see if the cancer has spread to bones.

Computed Tomography (CT scan) - CT scans are a specialized x-ray machine. Can be used to visualize soft tissue (muscles, ligaments) and solid structures like bone.

Dual X-ray Absorptiometry (DEXA) - This is the most accurate way to measure bone density. It is a low dose x-ray used to measure bone density for possible osteoporosis. Often this is used to examine a specific portion of the skeleton (commonly hip, spine, wrist).

Electromyography- Electromyography (EMG) tests analyze nerve and muscle electrical activity. For the EMG, thin needles are inserted one by one into the muscles being tested. Each needle is attached to a wire that detects electrical patterns inside the muscle and the nerves that are attached to that muscle. Most patients find this test mildly uncomfortable. Testing times vary, depending on how many muscles are being tested. EMG testing takes 20 to 30 minutes

Goniometry- use of a goniometer to measure range of motion in a joint.

Grip Dynamometer- a handheld device that the patient squeezes. Measures grip strength.

Inclinometry- use of an inclinometer to measure range of motion in a joint

Joint Aspiration- A needle is inserted into the joint capsule and fluid is removed. The synovial fluid is assessed for blood cells, crystals formed from minerals or toxins (example: uric acid), and microorganisms.

Lumbar puncture- A lumbar puncture, also known as a spinal tap, uses a needle to remove a sample of cerebrospinal fluid from the space surrounding the spinal cord. The test is used to diagnose meningitis infections and some neurological conditions.

Magnetic Resonance Imaging (MRI) - MRI is a noninvasive technique for visualizing many different body tissues. Can be used to view intervertebral discs, spinal stenosis, tumors, muscular trauma, tendon and ligament damage.

Myelogram- A myelogram is an x-ray test in which radiopaque dye is injected directly into the spinal canal via a spinal tap to help show places where the vertebrae in the spine may be pinching the spinal cord. May be used to help diagnose back or leg pain problems, especially if surgery is being planned.

Nerve conduction studies are tests that are often used in combination with the EMG evaluation. For nerve conduction studies, the muscles and nerves are stimulated with small bursts of electricity to see whether the nerves and muscles respond in a normal way. Small pads are taped to the skin of the hands or feet. These pads can both deliver mild electric shocks and detect electric signals coming through the skin (similar in sensation to a "shock" that might be felt from static electricity). Muscles might twitch when the electricity is delivered.

X-ray- commonly used to assess fractures, dislocations.

Pathologies of the Muscular System

For additional infectious diseases that may affect this system, please refer to the Communicable/Infectious Disease Chart in Chapter 10.

Chronic Fatigue Syndrome (CFS): This condition usually has sudden onset (often after a viral infection), disabling fatigue, muscle weakness and pain, sleep disturbance, fever, and enlargement of cervical lymph nodes. Almost twice as many women are diagnosed with CFS than men.

Delayed Onset Muscle Soreness (DOMS)- muscle pain and stiffness that occurs the day after physical exertion. Any pain or soreness immediately after exercise is not DOMS, it is probably discomfort due to biochemical events from muscle fatigue. DOMS will begin several hours after exercise and can last for 3-4 days. DOMS is not fully understood, but there are three proposed mechanism which cause it. The first theory is that there are microtears in the muscle as a result of the exertion. The second theory is that it is due to muscle spasms after exercise. The third is that there are tears in the connective tissue around the muscle (tendons and ligaments). Evidence supports each of these theories, and DOMS may very well be a combination of them.

Duchenne's Muscular Dystrophy: an inherited disease (70% of the time), or may be the result of a spontaneous genetic mutation (30% of the time). Symptoms begin in childhood, usually between the ages of 3-7, and usually in males. *Gower's sign* is an early signal of muscular dystrophies (Gower's sign is when the child must use their arms to push themselves up from sitting to standing- usually by placing hands on their knees and pushing up). Incidence is roughly 30 per 100,000 male births. In these children, the muscles only contain 0-5% of the dystrophin fibers needed. Dystrophin is a protein which attaches the internal cytoskeleton of the muscle cell to the sarcolemma (cell membrane). This lack of dystrophin causes progressive muscular weakness, and the children are usually wheelchair bound by the ages of 8-12. Most children die before age 20 from cardiovascular or respiratory complications. Prenatal genetic testing is available for fetal diagnosis at week 8 of gestation.

Fibromyalgia – a connective tissue disorder that causes pain, tenderness, "tender spots," and stiffness in the muscles, tendons, and surrounding soft tissues. It may be caused or aggravated by stress, trauma, dampness/cold, or a lack of sleep, and it affects far more women than men. Diagnosis requires tenderness in 11 of 18 pre-determined spots, and widespread musculoskeletal pain for more than three months. Often times irritable bowel syndrome, depression and sleep disorders occur alongside fibromyalgia.

Flaccid paralysis – if the nerve supply to a muscle is destroyed (such as in an accident), the muscle becomes unable to contract, loses tone, becomes soft, and begins to decrease in size (*atrophy*).

Golfer's Elbow (Medial Epicondylitis)- Pain and inflammation (usually due to overuse) of the muscles that attach on the medial epicondyle of the humerus. These muscles are used in flexion and abduction of the wrist. Testing with resisted wrist flexion and/or abduction will cause pain at the medial epicondyle of the humerus.

Myasthenia gravis – an autoimmune disease in which there is a progressive destruction of ACh receptors at the neuromuscular junction. This will cause droopy eyelids (*ptosis*), difficulty swallowing and talking, and generalized muscle weakness. After affecting the face and head muscles, the disease spreads to the upper extremity and chest. In 5-10% of victims, respiratory muscles will become paralyzed and death occurs. Roughly 70% of people with myasthenia gravis have a problem with their thymus gland, which programs the immune system incorrectly- thus the autoimmune disease. More common in women than men- average age of onset for women is 20-30 years old, whereas for men it is usually over the age of 60.

Myositis Ossificans: abnormal deposition of bone in and around muscles. A muscle trauma can lead to calcification within the muscle tissue. In other very severe cases, the cause is unknown. In these severe cases, the muscles of the neck, back, and upper limb are gradually replaced by bone.

Myotonic Dystrophy: Another inherited muscular dystrophy disease. This type of muscular dystrophy occurs more commonly after puberty. Incidence of 13.5 per 100,000. Gradual loss of muscle strength occurs. Cardiovascular, digestive, and respiratory complications will develop.

Polio (Poliomyelitis): caused by the *polio virus*. In 95% of infected people, the virus causes no effects. In 5% of the people, symptoms will occur. In some people the infection presents as a mild flu, from which they recover. In others, it may cause meningitis. In some individuals, the effects can be more severe. In the severe cases (paralytic polio), the virus attacks somatic motor neurons (the nerves that carry messages from your brain to your muscles), causing paralysis. In this severe form, usually a person will develop a very high fever 10-14 days after infection, muscle pain and paralysis will then occur. If the respiratory muscles are affected, this can be fatal. In individuals who survive paralytic polio, they may suffer from *postpolio syndrome* later in life- where muscles not paralyzed by polio earlier, start to lose their strength. A vaccine is available for prevention of polio.

Rhabdomyolysis- When muscle tissue is injured, the muscle fibers break down. The fibers release their contents (proteins, enzymes, etc.) into the bloodstream. These materials must be removed from the bloodstream by the kidney. If the kidney is overwhelmed with the muscle breakdown by-products, renal failure can occur.

Spasm – a sudden, involuntary muscle contraction that can cause pain, and is often brought about by chemical imbalances in the muscle. A prolonged spasm is called a ***cramp***.

Strain – occurs when a muscle or its tendon is stretched or torn, causing inflammation. A chronic inflammation of a tendon is called ***tendonitis***.

Tennis Elbow (Lateral Epicondylitis)- Pain and inflammation (usually due to overuse) of the muscles that attach on the lateral epicondyle of the humerus. These muscles are used in extension and adduction of the wrist. Pain can be seen with shaking hands, using a screwdriver, hitting a backhand in tennis, carrying suitcases and/or heavy grocery bags. Testing with resisted wrist extension and/or adduction will cause pain at the lateral epicondyle of the humerus. Tennis elbow is more common than golfers elbow.

Tetanus: caused by the bacteria *Clostridium tetani.* The bacteria thrives in areas with low oxygen levels, so deep puncture wounds are more likely the type of injury where tetanus could occur. The bacteria will release a neurotoxin which affects the motor neurons, and this causes the skeletal muscles served by those motor neurons to go onto a sustained powerful muscular contraction. Incubation period from time of injury is usually less than 2 weeks. Most common early complaints are headache, muscle stiffness, difficulty in swallowing. Soon it may become difficult to open the jaw ("lockjaw"). Widespread muscle spasms occur 2-3 days after initial symptoms- and can last for 2-4 weeks. 40-60 people out of 100 with severe tetanus will die. Immunization is recommended, with booster shots every 10 years.

Torticollis (wryneck) – a chronic rotation and lateral flexion of the neck, usually due to an injury to the sternocleidomastoid (SCM) muscle.

Trigger point- inflammation of a motor point (the area of the muscle where a motor nerve enters the muscle). This inflammation creates a taut, hyperirritable band in the muscle. Can be caused by injury, overuse, and/or a build-up of metabolic wastes. Pain can be localized to the area of the trigger point, or can radiate (spread) or refer (show up in another area of the body). Ice and compression may help alleviate. Many trigger points also are located in the same location as acupuncture points. Please see discussion earlier in this chapter on trigger points.

Whiplash- most commonly a result of a motor vehicle accident (usually being rear-ended)- but can also occur in falls or during sporting activities. This injury can damage the muscles and ligaments which support the cervical spine. Neck pain, stiffness, headaches, and vision troubles are most common symptoms. Common treatments can vary from rest, ice, NSAIDs, prescription painkillers and muscle relaxants, acupuncture, chiropractic, massage therapy, and/or physical therapy.

Practice Study and Test Questions:

1) The Krebs (Citric Acid) Cycle and oxidative phosphorylation will produce
  A) ATP
  B) muscle spasm
  C) glycogen
  D) myosin

2) A viral infection which attacks somatic motor neurons is called
  A) Myasthenia gravis
  B) Polio
  C) Duchenne's muscular dystrophy
  D) Tetanus

3) A positive Adson's Test could indicate
  A) herniated disc
  B) bursitis of the shoulder
  C) medial meniscus tear
  D) thoracic outlet syndrome

4) A tennis player comes in complaining of elbow pain. Where on the elbow would the practitioner expect to find tenderness upon palpation?
  A) medial epicondyle
  B) olecranon process
  C) lateral epicondyle
  D) mastoid process

5) For the patient listed above in question #4, what orthopedic test might be useful in confirming a diagnosis?
  A) Cozen's test
  B) Finkelstein's sign
  C) Mill's test
  D) both A and C

6) What device can be used to measure range of motion?
  A) goniometer
  B) DEXA
  C) EMG
  D) Arthroscope

7) Normal active range of motion for glenohumeral abduction is
  A) 90-100 degrees
  B) 40-50 degrees
  C) 170-180 degrees
  D) 120-130 degrees

8) Having tenderness upon palpation in 11 of 18 per-determined places on the body is one dignostic key for
  A) fibromyalgia
  B) bursits
  C) torticollis
  D) rhabdomyolysis

9) When performing muscle strength testing, how would you document normal strength or resistance?
    A) 1/5
    B) 10/10
    C) 5/5
    D) 5/10

10) The neurotransmitter used to stimulate skeletal muscle contraction is
    A) norepinephrine
    B) serotonin
    C) dopamine
    D) acetylcholine

11) A step defect visible on observation during an examination could indicate
    A) anterior cruciate ligament tear
    B) thrombophlebitis
    C) shoulder separation or acromioclavicular joint sprain
    D) sternocleidomastoid muscle spasm

12) Gower's sign is a common sign of
    A) Myasthenia gravis
    B) Duchenne's Muscular dystrophy
    C) Chronic fatigue syndrome
    D) Fibromyalgia

13) Inflammation of the region of a muscle where a motor nerve enters the muscle is called a
    A) trigger point
    B) tetanus
    C) flaccid paralysis
    D) myositis ossificans

14) The diagnostic test which involves injecting radioactive dye into the spinal canal is called
    A) electromyography
    B) inclinometry
    C) MRI
    D) myelogram

15) Heberden's nodes usually are visualized on the physical examination in the
    A) proximal interphalangeal nodes
    B) distal interphalangeal nodes
    C) acromioclavicular joint
    D) distal palmar crease

Answers: 1) A 2) B 3) D 4) C 5) D 6) A 7) C 8) A 9) C 10) D 11) C 12) B 13) A 14) D 15) B

CHAPTER 6: THE NERVOUS SYSTEM

Our nervous system is a very large and complex system. It is the primary control system of the body and is able to offer very speedy analysis and instruction for body activities.

The nervous system is divided into two anatomical divisions. One, the *central nervous system (CNS)*, is composed of your brain and spinal cord. It is responsible for integrating, processing, and coordinating sensory information and motor commands. The other division is called the *peripheral nervous system (PNS)*. It is composed of spinal nerves and cranial nerves. The PNS takes care of bringing sensory information from the body to the CNS, and carrying motor instructions from the CNS out to body parts. The autonomic nervous system (sympathetic and parasympathetic) is also considered a part of the PNS.

Structure and Functions of the Neuron:

The main functional cell in the nervous system is called the **neuron**. The most common shape of a neuron is called a *multipolar neuron*. There are three main parts to a basic multipolar neuron. 1.) The **cell body** contains the nucleus and most organelles (mitochondria, ribosomes, rough endoplasmic reticulum, etc.). The cytoplasm in the cell body of neuron is called the perikaryon. 2.) **Dendrites** of a neuron are highly branched sensitive processes that extend off of the cell body. Dendrites detect and then carry messages toward the cell body. 3.) An **axon** is a long process which extends off of the cell body and is able to carry an action potential (electrical nerve message). The cytoplasm which fills an axon is called the axoplasm. Axoplasm contains neurofibrils, neurotubules, lysosomes, mitochondria, and enzymes. The axon is attached to the cell body at a widened area called the axon hillock. At the tip of the axon there are enlargements called synaptic terminals. The axon will conduct messages away from the cell body of a neuron.

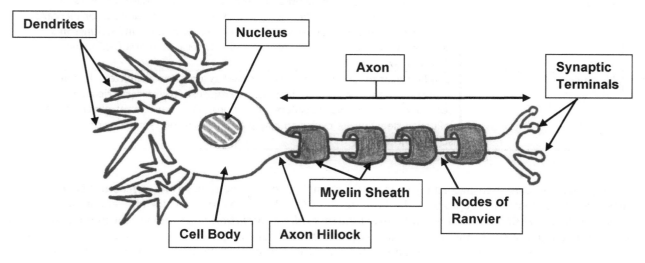

Usually information is detected and received at the dendrites. The dendrites send the information to the cell body. The cell body integrates the information and passes it into the axon. The axon generates an action potential, which can then be sent to another cell.

A **synapse** (also called a synaptic cleft) is the area where a neuron communicates with another body cell or another neuron. The synapse is a fluid filled gap between the pre-synaptic neuron (the neuron sending the message) and the post-synaptic cell (the next cell receiving the message). In order for the message being sent by the neuron (the pre-synaptic cell) to reach the post synaptic cell, a messenger must be created that can cross the synapse. This messenger is a chemical called a **neurotransmitter**. The neurotransmitter is made in the synaptic terminal of the neuron and packaged in the form of synaptic vesicles. Our neurons make many different types of neurotransmitters. Many pharmaceutical medications have been developed and create their effects by altering the levels or potency of neurotransmitters (SSRI's, benzodiazepines). Some illegal and recreational drugs also create an effect in our bodies by altering neurotransmitter levels and actions (amphetamines, marijuana).

SOME COMMON NEUROTRANSMITTERS

Neurotransmitter	Uses in the Body
Norepinephrine	Used in the brain and autonomic nervous system (especially in triggering sympathetic nervous system "fight or flight" bodily responses). Is usually excitatory.
Dopamine	A neurotransmitter in the brain. Dopamine can be used to prevent overstimulation of muscles (therefore, lack of dopamine can lead to Parkinson's Disease symptoms). In the limbic system of the brain, high levels of dopamine can increase mood, and even give a "high" sensation (for example, in cocaine use). Low levels of dopamine may trigger depression.
Serotonin	In the brain, low serotonin levels may decrease mood (cause depression) and decrease attention span. Along with norepinephrine and histamine, it may influence sleep and awake cycles.
Gamma-aminobutyric Acid (GABA)	Usually has an inhibitory effect in the brain and can decrease anxiety
Acetylcholine	Stimulates skeletal muscle contractions and is used in parasympathetic nervous system ("resting and digesting") bodily responses
Glutamate	Is the main excitatory neurotransmitter in the brain. Excessive levels of glutamate in the brain can be damaging. High levels of glutamate (or increased glutamate sensitivity) mat possibly be a contributing factor in Huntington's Disease, Alzheimer's Disease, Amyotrophic Lateral Sclerosis (ALS), and fibromyalgia.
Histamine	Can be released locally or can be released as a neurotransmitter. It is an important mediator in the inflammatory response, triggers gastric acid secretion, and is present in allergic reactions. As a neurotransmitter, it can influence sleep/awake cycles an may play a role in the symptoms of schitzophrenia.

Neurons can be classified according to their functions. **Sensory Neurons (aka *afferent neurons*)** carry messages from sensory receptors in the body to the CNS. **Motor Neurons (aka *efferent neurons*)** carry messages from the CNS out to the body. **Interneurons (aka *association neurons*)** are located mostly within the brain and spinal cord- and are the most common functional category type of neuron. Interneurons are used to allow sensory neurons to communicate with the motor neurons and are involved with all higher learning functions in the brain.

There are many different types of sensory neurons. Each kind can detect a different type of stimuli. Some examples of the different sensory receptors are as follows:

- **Nociceptors:** "pain receptors". These receptors detect pain caused by temperature extremes, mechanical damage, chemicals. *Type A fibers*: carry pain messages quickly to the CNS and can often trigger reflexes. Pain is often able to be localized more easily. *Type C fibers*: *slow pain* (burning and aching pain). Messages travel slower to the CNS and are felt over a more general region. Neurotransmitters released by nociceptors in the CNS are: *glutamate* and *Substance P.*

- **Thermoreceptors**- detect temperature and are located in the dermis of the skin, skeletal muscles, liver, and hypothalamus. *Cold Receptors*- detect cold stimuli. *Warm Receptors*- detect warm/hot stimuli
- **Mechanoreceptors**: detect stretching, tearing, compression, touch vibration, pressure. *Tactile receptors*- detect touch, pressure, and vibration (some examples: root hair plexus, tactile disc, tactile corpuscles, and lamellated corpuscles). *Baroreceptors*- monitor change in pressure, often found inside of organs (for example, the bladder). *Proprioceptors*- monitor the position of joints, muscle tension, tension in tendons and ligaments and muscle contraction force. Three main types: muscle spindles, Golgi Tendon Organs, and receptors in joint capsules
- **Chemoreceptors**- detect changes in the concentration of specific chemicals. For example, these receptors can monitor pH, carbon dioxide levels, and oxygen levels.

Structure and Function of Neuroglia

Neuroglia are the "helper" cells of the neuron. They do not transmit electrical impulses; instead they help take care of the neuron. In the Central Nervous System (CNS), there are 4 main types of neuroglia (glial cells).
- *Ependymal Cells*- line the central canal of the spinal cord and the ventricles of the brain. These cells circulate cerebrospinal fluid, a clear liquid which cushions the brain and spinal cord.
- *Astrocytes*- the largest and most numerous of the neuroglia in the CNS. These cells create the *blood-brain barrier*. They provide a physical framework in the CNS, feed the neuron, and regulate nutrients and chemicals in the fluids around the neuron.
- *Oligodendrocytes*- are cells with long processes which extend off of it and wrap themselves around the axons of neurons. This creates a white-colored membranous wrap called *myelin*. Myelin is composed mostly of lipids (fats). Myelin insulates the neuron and increases the speed in which action potentials are sent. Many oligodendrocytes will wrap their processes along the length of an axon. These oligodendrocytes will not touch one another; there will be a small gap between them called the *Nodes of Ranvier*. Not every neuron in the CNS has myelin wrapped around it. Neurons that have myelin are called *myelinated neurons* (or *white matter*); neurons that do not have myelin are called *unmyelinated neurons* (or *gray matter).*
- *Microglia*- least numerous and smallest neuroglial cell in the CNS. They clean and protect the neuron

In the Peripheral Nervous System (PNS), there are two main types of neuroglia.
- *Satellite Cells*- surround neuron cell bodies in the PNS and act much like the astrocytes did in the CNS.
- *Schwann Cells*- act much like the oligodendrocytes did in the CNS. They wrap around small sections of an axon in the PNS and form myelin. Whenever a Schwann cell wraps around part of an axon, the outer surface of the Schwann cell is called the *neurilemma*. Many Schwann Cells cover the surface of one axon, with Nodes of Ranvier between them.

Generating an Action Potential:

The inside of a resting neuron (the intracellular fluid) is composed of many negatively charged proteins and some potassium (K+). The extracellular fluid outside of the neuron is composed of mostly sodium (Na+). The cell membrane surrounds the neuron and keeps these two fluids separate. The intracellular and extracellular fluids both contain positive and negatively charged ions. These extracellular and intracellular ions exhibit a "pull" against one another, but are kept separated by the cell membrane. This "pull" of the charged ions is called the *transmembrane potential* and is measured at -70mV (millivolts) in a resting neuron. (The dominance of the negatively charged proteins in the intracellular fluid causes the transmembrane potential to be negatively charged.)

If a neuron is going to send a message (called the *action potential*) it must be in the resting potential state. When a stimulus occurs, the message usually enters the cell body through the dendrite. This stimulus causes the resting potential of the neuron cell body to change. During a stimulus, the channels of the membrane allow some of the Na+ to flow inside. This causes the resting potential to shift from its normal reading of -70mV moving towards a more positive reading. As the positive ions move across the membrane, the membrane potential shifts and moves from -70 mV to -60 mV to -30 mV, and so on. For a neuron to actually send a message (the action potential), it must be stimulated to the point it reaches its *threshold level* (usually around -55mV).

If the stimulus is small, only a slight temporary shift in the resting potential may occur- this is called a *graded potential*. Any shift in the resting potential from -70 to -60 will trigger a graded potential. This single graded potential will not be strong enough to cause the neuron to fire (send an action potential). The stimulus must be strong enough to make the resting potential shift past the range of -60mV to -55mV (the threshold level) for an action potential to be triggered and sent out of the neuron cell body and through the length of the axon. It often takes multiple graded potentials in a row to generate a stimulus strong enough to bring the neuron to its threshold level. Once this threshold of -55mV has been passed, the neuron will automatically fire. Any stimulus that does not reach -55mV will not trigger an action potential. This is called the **All or None Principle**. For example, a stimulus that causes the resting potential to shift to -65mV will not be strong enough to send an action potential. The neuron will not fire. However, if the stimulus causes the membrane potential to shift past -55mV (let's say it shifts to -35 mV) the neuron will automatically fire, always.

Let's look at the basic steps involved in generating an action potential

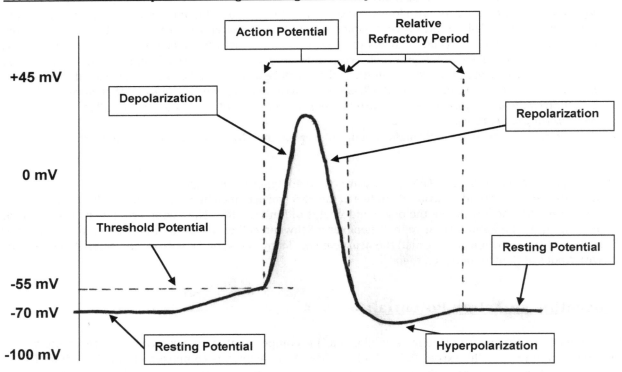

1. The neuron is at its resting potential of -70mV. Remember, when the neuron is in this resting state, the outside of the neuron is surrounded by Na+, while the inside of the neuron contains K+ and negatively charged proteins.

2. A stimulus occurs, and Na+ begins to flow into the neuron cell body. This causes the threshold level (-55mV) to be reached and/or passed

3. Once we pass the threshold, a flood of voltage regulated Na+ channels open and large amounts of Na+ rushes inside the axon of the neuron, beginning at the axon hillock (the end of the axon near the cell body). As sodium rushes inside the cell, **depolarization** occurs. During depolarization, the inside of the neuron becomes more positively charged as Na+ ions rush in. The *action potential* (nerve message) is being generated when the neuron enters depolarization. During depolarization, the membrane potential rapidly goes from -55mV to -45mV to -20mV and can even swing into the positive readings +10mV, +20mV (see graph). When the peak has been reached, Na+ channels will close and Na+ stops entering the neuron

4. After the inside of the neuron is swamped with Na+, the neuron now tries to get back to its original resting state. It needs to start to remove some of the + charged ions in the intracellular fluid. To remove the + charges, K+ channels in the neuron cell membrane begin to open in the neuron membrane and allow K+ to flow out of the neuron. This phase is called **repolarization.** The voltage reading starts to move back towards the resting state of -70mV. During depolarization and repolarization, the neuron is unable to be stimulated to send another message- this is called **absolute refractory period**

5. When we get to about -90mV the K+ channels close and K+ stops leaving the neuron. This is called **hyperpolarization.** At this point, there are more K+ ions on the outside of the neuron and there are many Na+ ions on the inside of the neuron. Now, remember, in a resting neuron we want the *opposite* ratio of Na+ and K+ to be present (more Na+ on the outside and more K+ on the inside). Hmmm, what should we do here? Well, the neuron will go into the next step.....

6. The neuron goes into the **relative refractory period**. This is where it works to switch the position of the + charged ions across the membrane. The Sodium/Potassium pump kicks in and it pumps Na+ and K+ back to their original sides of the membrane. Na+ gets pumped back to the outside of the cell and K+ gets pumped back to the inside of the cell. The pump is pretty efficient- in one pump cycle it can pump 3 Na+ outside the cell while pumping 2 K+ inside the cell. During this relative refractory period, the neuron is highly unlikely to send another message. After the relative refractory period has re-set all of the + charges back to their original positions, the neuron will finally return to its resting state. At this point the neuron could be re-stimulated.

These steps will continue to occur down the entire length of the axon. Once the action potential reaches the end of the axon, it will trigger the release of a neurotransmitter- which can be passed on to the next cell- thus passing the message on.

There are two methods in which an action potential can be carried down the length of an axon. **Continuous propagation** occurs in *unmyelinated* neurons. The wave of depolarization begins at the cell body and moves from the cell body out to the end of the axon involving all sodium channels along the length of the neuron. **Saltatory propagation** occurs in *myelinated* neurons. In a myelinated neuron, sections of the neuron will be covered with myelin (a fatty insulation); with small gaps of uncovered neuron membrane between the insulated sections (the Nodes of Ranvier). In saltatory propagation, the action potential gets to rapidly hop over (or skip) the sections of myelin- therefore the action potential travels down the length of the neuron at a very fast speed. This method is much faster than continuous propagation.

Axons are classified into three groups according to their diameter, myelination, and propagation speed. **Type A Fibers** are the largest diameter of axons, myelinated, and the fastest of the three types of fibers. These neurons carry information about proprioception, touch, and pressure to the CNS and can carry motor messages from the CNS to the muscles. In **Type B Fibers**, they are smaller in diameter, but still myelinated. **Type C Fibers** are the smallest in diameter and are unmyelinated. Both Type B and Type C fibers carry information about pain, temperature, general touch. They also carry messages to our smooth muscle, cardiac muscle, organs, and glands. Type B and Type C fibers carry messages at a slower speed than Type A fibers.

The Spinal Cord, Spinal Nerves, and Spinal Reflexes

The spinal cord acts a bridge or communicating pathway between the brain and the nerves in the body. Sensory messages travel from the peripheral spinal nerves (the ones that go to all of your muscles and organs) through the spinal cord and up to the brain. Motor messages leave the brain, travel down the spinal cord, and exit out of the spinal cord through the peripheral spinal nerves to return back to our muscles and organs.

The spinal cord begins at the vertebral level of C1 and between the L1 and L2 vertebra. There are 31 pairs of spinal nerves that exit off of the spinal cord. These spinal nerves are **mixed nerves**- meaning that they can carry both sensory information and motor information.

Spinal and Cranial Meninges:

The spinal cord and brain is surrounded by three protective layers of membranes called **meninges (spinal meninges** and **cranial meninges).** Both the spinal and cranial meninges are composed of the same three layers:
1. **Dura Mater**- This is the outer layer of meninges, sitting just underneath the skull. It is the thickest layer, and literally means "hard mother". This layer contains dense collagen fibers. Between the dura mater and the inside walls of the vertebra or skull bones is the *epidural space* (which contains blood vessels and a layer of adipose for cushioning).
2. **Arachnoid Mater**- This middle layer of meninges has a network of fibers (called the *arachnoid trabeculae*) which extend off of it. There is a space between the arachnoid mater and the innermost layer, the pia mater. This space is called the *subarachnoid space*. The subarachnoid space is filled with *cerebrospinal fluid (CSF)*, which acts as a cushion/shock-absorber to protect the brain and spinal cord from bumping against the inside of the vertebra and the skull. A spinal tap may be performed in the subarachnoid space to extract some CSF for analysis.
3. **Pia Mater**- This is the innermost layer of the meninges and will be firmly connected to the surface of the brain or spinal cord. The pia mater is the thinnest and most delicate of the three meninges.

Sectional Anatomy of the Spinal Cord:

If the spinal cord is cut in cross section, we can see that there are two different colored regions of the spinal cord. The inner area is gray in color and is somewhat shaped like a butterfly. This area is called the *gray matter* and is composed of *unmyelinated* neurons. The outer area is white in color- so is conveniently called the **white matter**. White matter is composed of mostly *myelinated neurons*. In the gray matter, the "tips" of the butterfly wings are called "horns"- posterior gray horns, lateral gray horns, and anterior gray horns. The central canal is a small canal in the center of the spinal cord where cerebrospinal fluid circulates.

Spinal nerves will attach into the spinal cord. As the spinal nerve approaches the spinal cord, it divides into two sections. One section, the *dorsal spinal root*, reaches around towards the posterior side of the spinal cord. It carries incoming afferent sensory messages from the spinal nerve into the spinal cord. The other section, the *ventral spinal root*, will reach toward the anterior surface of the spinal cord. The ventral root carries the efferent motor messages that will travel out from the spinal cord to the body.

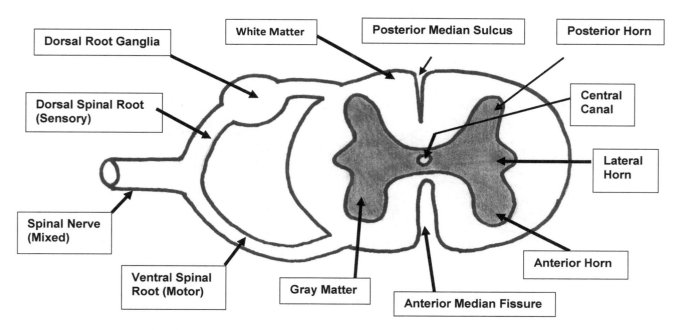

In the white matter, the spinal cord tissue can be divided into pathways which transmit messages to and from the brain. The **ascending pathways** carry sensory messages. The **descending pathways** carry motor messages. Most of these pathways will *dessutate* (cross over), meaning messages from the right side of the body will be processed in the left side of the brain. Please see your anatomy text for an illustration of the location of these pathways in the spinal cord.

The common ascending (sensory) pathways in the spinal cord are the ***posterior column***, ***anterolateral***, and ***spinocerebellar pathways***. These pathways can be divided into smaller tracts. The posterior column pathway is divided into *fasciculus gracilis* and *fasciculus cuneatus* (which carry fine touch, pressure, vibration, and proprioception from the upper and lower halves of the body to the thalamus). The anterolateral pathway is composed of the *anterior spinothalamic tract* (carries crude touch and pressure sensation from the spinal cord to the brain) and the *lateral spinothalamic tract* (carries pain and temperature sensations from spinal cord to the thalamus). The spinocerebellar pathway is divided into the *posterior spinocerebellar tract* and *anterior spinocerebellar tract*. Both tracts carry proprioceptive information about muscles, tendons and ligaments from spinal cord to the cerebellum.

Motor messages are movement messages being sent from the CNS out to the skeletal muscles in the body. These motor messages will travel through specific descending motor pathways in the spinal cord- much like the sensory messages traveled through ascending pathways. There are usually two neurons through which motor messages will travel in the CNS. The ***upper motor neuron*** starts in the brain and passes the outgoing message to a lower motor neuron which is located in the brain stem or spinal cord. The ***lower motor neuron*** then leaves the CNS and heads out to a specific motor unit in a muscle and stimulates it to contract.

Here are the common pathways in the spinal cord responsible for carrying motor (descending) messages. The **corticospinal pathway** (also called the *pyramidal system)*, the **medial pathway** and **lateral pathway**. The corticospinal pathway is composed of the following tracts: the *corticobulbar tracts, lateral corticospinal tracts*, and *anterior corticospinal tracts*. These tracts control conscious muscle movements and carry motor messages to cranial nerves III, IV, V, VI, IX, XI, and XII. The medial pathway is made up of the *vestibulospinal tract, tectospinal tract*, and *reticulospinal tracts*. These tracts control movements of head, neck, and upper limbs. The lateral pathway is composed of one tract- the rubrospinal tract, which controls muscle tone and precise movements in the distal joints of the limbs (precise finger and toe movements).

DERMATOMES OF THE BODY

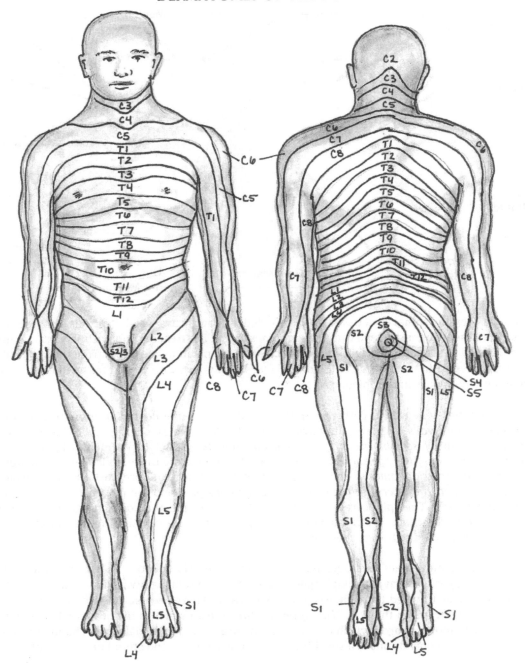

A **dermatome** is a specific bilateral area of the skin surface monitored by a single pair of spinal nerves. Dermatomes are relatively consistent from person to person, so they are used in a medical setting for help in isolating damage to specific nerve levels. Nerves exiting off of the cervical spinal region are abbreviated as C1, C2, C3, and so on. Thoracic, Lumbar and Sacral nerve roots are abbreviated the same way. In a clinical setting, if a patient presents with numbness around the nipples, the T4 spinal nerve would likely be involved. If numbness was present in the pinky finger, the nerve roots involved would most likely be C8. Numbness along the outside of the foot would indicate the S1 nerve root. All areas of skin on the body have dermatomes mapped out, and these dermatomes can be tested during a physical examination. (Please note: the skin of the face is innervated by cranial nerves- this diagram above illustrates only spinal nerve dermatome distribution)

Dermatomes and Nerve Plexuses:

The 31 pairs of spinal nerves exit the spinal cord at specific levels of the spine. One spinal nerve exits between each vertebra, and nerves will also exit out through openings of the sacrum and coccygeal area. There are 8 pairs of cervical nerves (C1-C8), 12 pairs of thoracic nerves (T1-T12), 5 pairs of lumbar nerves (L1-L5), 5 pairs of sacral nerves (S1-S5) and one coccygeal nerve.

Each spinal nerve is composed of many neurons bundled together. Every nerve is wrapped in protective layers of connective tissue- much like the muscles and muscle fibers were. The three layers of connective tissue are:
- **Epineurium**- the outermost layer, covers the outside of the nerve
- **Perineurium-** wraps groups of neuron axons into bundles (fascicles)
- **Endoneurium-** wraps around each individual neuron axon.

Spinal nerves are what we call "mixed" nerves. Each nerve contains some sensory neurons which carry sensory information from various muscles organs and skin segments. And, every spinal nerve also contains additional motor neurons which carry motor messages to specific muscles and organs in the body. All of us are "wired" very similarly- therefore the 2nd thoracic spinal nerve carries sensory and motor messages to and from the same area of the body in everyone. Because of this consistency, we have been able to track and chart nerve distribution patterns.

For sensory distribution of nerve roots, please see the dermatome diagram.

Ventral roots of the spinal nerves can be bundled together into a **plexus**. There are four major spinal plexuses:
1. The **Cervical Plexus** (roots of C1-C5) controls the diaphragm (controlled by the **phrenic nerve**) and muscles of shoulder, larynx, and neck. If damaged, respiratory paralysis (death if not treated), and/or limited movement of neck and shoulder can occur.
2. The **Brachial Plexus** (roots of C5-T1) exits the neck, runs under clavicle, and into the arm. There are 5 major nerves which come off of the brachial plexus. The **Axillary Nerve** controls the deltoid and teres minor muscles; therefore damage to the axillary nerve would result in paralysis and atrophy of those muscles. The **Radial Nerve** controls the triceps muscle and extensor muscles of forearm. Damage here could cause *wristdrop* (inability to extend wrist). The **Median Nerve** controls flexor muscles of forearm and some muscles of the hand. Injury to the median nerve can cause decreased ability to flex and abduct hand, flex and abduct thumb and index finger (inability to pick up small objects). The **Musculocutaneous Nerve** controls flexor muscles of arm, and damage would decrease the ability to flex forearm. The **Ulnar Nerve** controls the wrist and many hand muscles. *Clawhand,* the inability to spread fingers apart, would result with damage to the ulnar nerve.
3. **Lumbar Plexus** (Roots of L1-L4) controls the lower abdomen, anterior thigh, and hip adductors. Damage to this plexus could cause the inability to extend leg, flex hip, and/or the inability to adduct hip.
4. The **Sacral Plexus** (roots of L4-S4) will form the **Sciatic Nerve** (L4-S3). This nerve will control the posterior thigh and glutes, lateral aspect of leg and foot, posterior aspect of leg and foot. Damage to the sacral plexus would result in the inability to flex knee and extend hip. In addition, foot motion such as plantar/dorsiflexion can be limited. Pain can also result in the posterior gluteal region and thigh, called sciatica.

The following chart shows some of the main nerves associated with the four plexuses. Please refer to your antomy text for a full list of nerves and their distributions if you would like more details.

SPINAL NERVES AND PLEXUSES

Nerve	Spinal Nerve Roots	Structures in the body served by the nerve
Cervical Plexus		
Lesser occipital	C2/C3	Skin sensation on posterior/lateral neck
Greater auricular	C2/C3	Skin sensation of ear and anterior to TMJ
Transverse cervical	C2/C3	Skin sensation on anterior and lateral neck
Supraclavicular	C3/C4	Skin sensation of shoulder and clavicular region
Ansa Cervicalis	C1-C3	Omohyoid, sternohyoid, and sternothyroid muscles
Phrenic	C3-C5	Diaphragm
Brachial Plexus		
Musculocutaneous	C5-T1	Flexor muscles on anterior arm, skin sensation on lateral forearm
Median	C6-T1	Most flexor muscles on anterior forearm; skin sensation of anterior and lateral 2/3 of the hand
Ulnar	C8-T1	Flexor carpi ulnaris, most muscles in the hand; skin sensation on medial 1/3 (anterior and posterior) hand
Radial	C5-T1	Posterior muscles of arm and forearm; skin sensation on posterior and lateral arm, forearm and hand
Axillary	C5-C6	Deltoid and teres minor muscles; skin sensation on shoulder
Dorsal scapular	C5	Rhomboid major, rhomboid minor, and levator scapulae muscles
Subscapular	C5-C6	Teres major and subscapularis muscles
Suprascapular	C5-C6	Supraspinatus and infraspinatus muscles; sensation from shoulder joint
Long Thoracic	C5-C7	Serratus anterior muscle
Pectoral	C5-T1	Pectoralis major and minor muscles
Lumbar Plexus		
Iliohypogastric	L1	External oblique, internal oblique and transversus abdominus muscles; skin sensation on lower abdomen and gluteal region
Ilioinguinal	L1	Assists iliohyogastric innervating abdominal muscles; skin sensation of upper inner thigh and genital region (along with genitofemoral nerve).
Genitofemoral	L1-L2	Skin sensation on upper to mid anteriomedial thigh and genetalia
Femoral	L2-L4	Anterior thigh muscles (quadriceps, sartorius) pectineus and iliacus muscles; skin of mid-lower anteriomedial thigh and medial knee, leg and foot.
Lateral femoral cutaneous	L2-L3	Skin sensation of lateral thigh
Obturator	L2-L4	Adductor muscle group, gracilis, and obturator externus muscles; sensation of hip and knee joints
Sacral Plexus		
Sciatic	L4-S3	Two of the hamstring muscles (semimembranosus and semitendinosus muscles). Just above the knee, the sciatic nerve splits into the tibial nerve and common fibular (peroneal) nerve
Tibial	L4-S3	Part of biceps femoris muscle, plantar flexor muscles (muscles in the calf), flexor muscles of the toes; skin sensation over posterior surface of leg and plantar surface of foot.
Common fibular (peroneal) nerve	L4-S2	Part of biceps femoris muscles, muscles on anterior and lateral leg; skin sensation on anterior leg, lateral foot and dorsal surface of foot
Superior gluteal	L4-S1	Tensor fascia latae, gluteus medius and minimus muscles
Inferior gluteal	L5-S2	Gluteus maximus muscle

Spinal Reflexes:

A **reflex** is a rapid, automatic (involuntary) response to specific stimuli. A **reflex arc** involves all of the body segments a reflexive message must travel through. Here is a pathway of a reflex arc:

Step 1: Sensory receptor in a body part detects stimulation *(touch a hot stove)*
Step 2: The sensory receptor sends a message to the CNS
Step 3: The information is processed in the CNS. *("Ouch! Danger, hot!")*
Step 4: A motor neuron is activated, and sends a response message back out to the body
Step 5: The effector (body part) responds *(muscles in the arm contract to pull the hand off of the hot stove)*

There are many types of reflexes and they can be classified in many different ways:

- **Innate reflexes-** form during development of the CNS (withdrawal from pain, suckling, tracking objects with the eyes). Will be tested at different ages in newborn development to assess nervous system development.
- **Acquired Reflexes-** learned reflexes that occur later in life. Sporting reflexes, reflexive responses when driving, etc.
- **Somatic Reflexes-** allow for involuntary control of the muscular system (patellar reflex or deep tendon reflexes)
- **Visceral Reflexes-** reflexes which regulate autonomic (involuntary) control of internal organs.
- **Monosynaptic Reflexes-** only one synapse is present in the circuit. This is a very simple and fast responding reflex. The sensory message enters the CNS via a sensory nerve, and is passed through a synapse directly to a motor nerve and heads right back out to the body.
- **Polysynaptic reflexes-** involve more than one synapse in the reflex arc. These reflexes are a little more complex and the response time may be slightly slower. A sensory neuron passes the information to an interneuron in the CNS, which will then pass the message onto the motor neuron.
- **Spinal reflexes** are processed in the spinal cord. For example: *stretch reflexes, postural reflexes, tendon reflexes, withdrawal/flexor reflexes, crossed extensor reflexes*
- **Cranial Reflexes** are processed in the brain. For example: *corneal reflex, tympanic reflex.*

Many of these reflexes can occur simultaneously to protect the body. For example, if a person steps on a thorn with the right foot, the withdrawal reflex will automatically kick in and cause the flexor muscles in the right leg to contract and create the movement of flexion (to pull the foot off of the thorn). At the same time, the crossed-extensor reflex will occur to cause the extensor muscles in the left leg to contract and create the movement of leg extension (to take all of the body weight)- so the person can remain standing.

The Brain and Cranial Nerves

The brain contains about 98% of the neural tissue. It weighs about 3 pounds and is similar to the texture of cold oatmeal. The brain contains white matter (myelinated neurons) and gray matter (unmyelinated neurons), just like the spinal cord. The brain is composed of many different regions, and each of these regions will be responsible for carrying out important bodily functions.

The four main regions of the brain are the *cerebrum, cerebellum, diencephalon, and brain stem.* **Ventricles** are hollow chambers deep inside the brain tissue, and produce *Cerebrospinal Fluid (CSF).* There are two lateral ventricles, one third ventricle and the fourth ventricle.

The brain is protected and supported in three main ways. The most obvious of the protective structures are the *bones* of the skull. Under the bones are the *cranial meninges* (dura mater, arachnoid mater, and pia mater). The dura mater will fold in between gaps and spaces in the brain tissue to provide additional stabilization and support. These folds of tissue are called the *dural folds* (the falx cerebri, tentorium cerebelli, and falx cerebelli.) Lastly, the *Cerebrospinal Fluid (CSF)* is used to cushion and support the brain, as well as transporting nutrients and waste products. The cerebrospinal fluid is made in the ventricles by a tissue called the choroid plexus. CSF will circulate through the ventricles of the brain and then into the central canal of the spinal cord. CSF also will leave the fourth ventricle through the lateral and median apertures and flow into the subarachnoid space in the meninges of the brain and spinal cord.

Now, let's take some time and look at the main areas of the brain. We will look at the composition, location, and functions of the brain stem (medulla oblongata, pons, mesencephalon/midbrain), cerebellum, diencephalon (thalamus, hypothalamus, limbic system), and cerebrum (cerebral cortex, cerebral white matter, basal nuclei, frontal lobe, temporal lobe, occipital lobe, and parietal lobe).

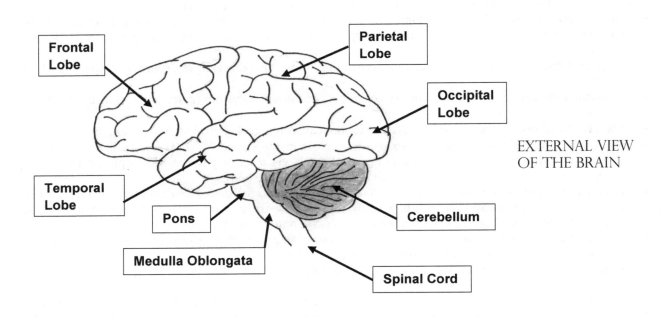

EXTERNAL VIEW
OF THE BRAIN

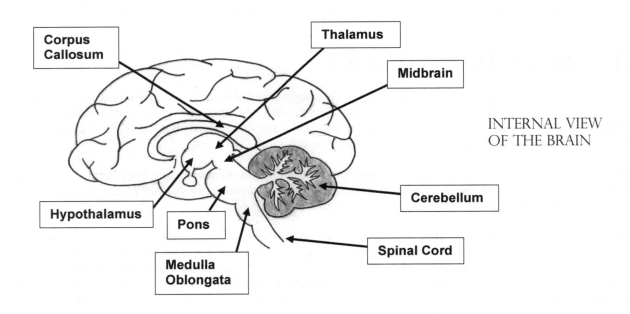

INTERNAL VIEW
OF THE BRAIN

Brain Stem:

The brain stem is composed of three main regions- the medulla oblongata, the pons, and the mesencephalon (also known as the midbrain).

The **medulla oblongata** is located in the lowest area of the brain stem and will actually transition into the spinal cord. Because the medulla oblongata becomes the spinal cord, all messages traveling up or down the spinal cord must pass through the medulla oblongata on their way to and from other regions of the brain. 5 of the 12 pairs of cranial nerves will attach here. Important functions of the medulla oblongata are: regulation of heart rate, force of heart contraction, regulating distribution of blood flow, and pace (rate) of breathing

The **pons** is located directly on top of the medulla oblongata. It acts as a bridge and helps to connect your cerebellum to other areas of the brain and the spinal cord. The pons serves as an attachment site for 4 of the 12 pairs of cranial nerves. The pons also acts as the respiratory *rhythm center*- it assists the medulla oblongata in respiration and manages the depth of breath and the transition from inspiration to expiration.

The **mesencephalon** (also known as the **midbrain**) is located on top of the pons. It is composed of a few regions. The *tectum* helps to coordinate visual stimuli and generate visual and auditory reflexes. The *red nucleus* works with the cerebellum and helps to coordinate the position of the upper limbs. The *substantia nigra* regulates the basal nuclei. The *Reticular Activating System (RAS)* maintains consciousness (damage here can result in a coma).

Cerebellum:

The cerebellum sits on the underside of the larger cerebrum region of the brain. It has a left and right hemisphere. The *superior, middle*, and *inferior cerebellar peduncles* connect the cerebellum with other areas of the brain. The cerebellum will receive proprioceptive input from the spinal cord. The cerebellum will also monitor all proprioceptive, visual, tactile, balance, and auditory sensations received by the brain. In addition, it also assists in coordinating motor movements, adjusting the postural muscles, and maintains balance and equilibrium. Internally, the cerebellum is composed of an outer region of gray matter with an internal layer of white matter (called the *arbor vitae*). The arbor vitae is so named due to its tree branch shaped appearance.

Diencephalon:

The diencephalon sits atop the brainstem and is composed of three main areas.

The **Epithalamus**- contains the pineal gland (which produces the hormone melatonin) and part of the choroid plexus.

The **Thalamus**- contains many nuclei which function to: generate emotions and relay them to the higher brain for processing; relay sensory information (touch, pressure, pain, temperature, and proprioception) to the higher areas of the brain for processing; relays visual stimuli to the occipital lobe for processing; relays auditory information to the temporal lobe of the brain. Basically, the thalamus is a relay center for sensory information (stimuli) and generates an emotional response to those stimuli.

The **Hypothalamus** is important in regulating many vital activities in the body to keep us alive. The hypothalamus controls our ability to swallow, regulates our hunger and thirst mechanisms, regulates body temperature, regulates heart rate and blood pressure, coordinates our circadian rhythms, assists in motor responses during heightened emotional states, and regulates the release of some hormones in our body from other endocrine glands.

In addition to the main three areas of the diencephalon, a not as easily delineated region called the **limbic system** is located between the cerebrum and diencephalon. It uses neurons from both regions to accomplish its functions. Generally speaking, the limbic system assists in establishing emotions, links our conscious functions with our autonomic (involuvtary) responses, and facilitates memory storage and retrieval. There are some main regions of the limbic system: the Amygdaloid body, Hippocampus, and Hypothalamic nuclei. These areas are used in giving us emotions and urges such as rage, fear, pain, sexual arousal, pleasure, and alertness.

Cerebrum:

The cerebrum is the largest area of the brain. It is covered with ridges and grooves (gyri and sulci). The cerebrum is composed of gray matter (the cerebral cortex and the deep basal nuclei), and white matter (which lies underneath the cerebral cortex). The cerebrum is divided into two hemispheres (left and right) by a deep *longitudinal fissure*.

Each cerebral hemisphere can be divided into four separate lobes. These lobes are named according to the skull bone they sit underneath. Deep grooves (sulci/sulcus) separate the different lobes. The *central sulcus* separates the frontal lobe from the parietal lobe. The *lateral sulcus* separates the frontal lobe from the temporal lobe. The *parieto-occipital sulcus* separates the parietal and occipital lobe. Here are the four lobes and a brief discussion on the functions they carry out.

Frontal Lobe- is located under the frontal bone. It is the *primary motor cortex* (meaning it controls all voluntary movements of skeletal muscles) and it also contains the *somatic motor association area* (which helps us with the coordination of learned movement). The left frontal lobe also contains *Broca's area* (or the *motor speech area*) which controls the muscle movements in our lips, tongue, cheeks, and jaws when speaking. The *prefrontal cortex* is located in both the left and right frontal lobe and is used for intellectual reasoning. The prefrontal cortex allows us to process our emotions, interpret current events, is used in predicting future situations or consequences, problem solving, and placing a time relationship on events.

Parietal Lobe- is located under the parietal bone. It contains the *primary sensory cortex* and the *somatic sensory association area* which receives sensory messages pertaining to touch, pressure, pain, vibration, taste, and temperature.

Temporal Lobe- located under the temporal bone. The *auditory* and *olfactory cortex*- receives hearing and smell stimuli. And, the *Auditory* and *Olfactory association area* allows us to process what we smell and hear.

Occipital Lobe- located under the occiput. The occipital lobe contains the *visual cortex* and *visual association area*, which receives and processes visual stimuli

There are two other areas of the cerebrum worth mentioning that do not fit exactly into one of the above lobes. The **Insula** is located between the frontal lobe and temporal lobe and contains the *gustatory cortex* (taste). **Wernicke's area** overlaps the parietal, temporal and occipital lobes in the left hemisphere. It is also known as the **general interpretive area**. It integrates all of the sensations handled by the parietal, temporal, and occipital lobes.

In the cerebrum, the left hemisphere usually handles movements and sensations that are occurring on the right side of the body, and the right hemisphere handles movements and sensations on the left side of the body. Each hemisphere also specializes in a few other activities. This specialization is called **hemispheric**

lateralization. The left hemisphere specializes in general interpretation and speech, language based skills, reading, writing, analytical tasks (math), and logical decision making. The right hemisphere plays a dominant role in recognizing faces, analyzing emotional contexts in conversations, identifying objects by our senses (touch, smell, taste, sight), and spatial visualization.

If you were to cut one of the cerebral hemispheres open, you would see that it contains both white matter and gray matter. The outer layer of the cerebrum is gray matter (called the *cerebral cortex*) - much like the rind on the outside of an orange. The gray matter is where the majority of the lobes are located. This is where all of our information processing occurs. Deep to the gray matter is white matter. The white matter is like a superhighway. The white matter connects all of the lobes and the gray matter so that all of the areas of the cerebrum can talk to one another. *Association fibers* allow lobes on the same side of the brain to talk to one another (for example: left occipital lobe talking to the left frontal lobe). *Commissural fibers* (the corpus callosum and anterior commissure) allow the left and right hemisphere to talk to one another. *Projection fibers* allow the cerebrum to talk to the diencephalon, cerebellum, and brainstem.

Located deep inside the white matter are tiny islands of gray matter called the *basal nuclei*. The basal nuclei are involved with the subconscious control of muscle tone and the coordination of learned muscle patterns. The basal nuclei work with the muscles in the arms and legs to control proper muscle tone during movements. The basal nuclei are inhibited by the neurotransmitter dopamine. Dopamine is released by the substantia nigra in the diencephalon. If dopamine levels drop, the basal nuclei become over-stimulated. This causes muscle tone to increase, and makes voluntary muscle movements very difficult. This is what occurs in Parkinson's disease.

Cranial Nerves:

There are 12 pairs of cranial nerves. These nerves connect directly onto the brain and do not use the spinal cord. Most of the cranial nerves will attach onto the brainstem region of the brain. Cranial nerves are named in two ways. One way is using Roman numerals. The numerals are given according to the order in which the nerves attach onto the brain. The other name is a word name. Often, the word name tries to give you a hint as to the function of that nerve. For example: *Oculomotor nerve-* "Oculo" means "eye" and "Motor" means "movement", therefore a good guess as to the function of this nerve is eye movement. Here is a chart summarizing the 12 pairs of cranial nerves.

THE CRANIAL NERVES

Nerve # and Name	Function	Physical Exam
I. Olfactory	Sense of Smell	Patient asked to smell and identify aromatic substances (such as coffee, vanilla, essential oils)
II. Optic	Sense of Vision	*Snellen* and *Rosenbaum* eye charts Test Visual Fields
III. Oculomotor	Controls 4 out of 6 eye muscles (Superior Rectus, Inferior Rectus, Inferior Oblique, Medial Rectus) involved in eye movement. Pupil constriction and dilation.	Planes of Gaze Test Pupillary Reflex Exam
IV. Trochlear	Controls the Superior Oblique eye muscle used in eye movement	Planes of Gaze Test
V. Trigeminal (contains three branches: ***Opthalmic, Maxillary*** and ***Mandibular***)	Facial skin sensation (chin, cheek, forehead). Controls muscles of mastication.	Facial Sensation (touch patient's face with cotton swab and pin/toothpick). Have them identify type of sensation and location Open mouth against resistance
VI. Abducens	Controls the Lateral Rectus eye muscle used in eye movement	Planes of Gaze Test
VII. Facial	Controls muscles of facial expression. Controls taste on anterior 2/3 of tongue.	Ask patient to smile, frown, blink. Taste and detect sweet, sour, salty and bitter solutions placed on the tongue
VIII. Vestibulocochlear (Also known as the ***Acoustic Nerve.***)	Balance (Vestibular Branch) Hearing (Cochlear Branch)	Tuning fork tests: *Weber Test* (tests lateralization) *Rinne Test* (tests bone and air conduction)
IX. Glossopharyngeal	Taste on posterior 1/3 of tongue Swallowing, saliva production, and throat sensations.	Taste and detect sweet, sour, salty and bitter solutions placed on the tongue Gag and swallowing reflexes
X. Vagus	Pharynx, larynx, digestive organs and heart activity	Gag and swallowing reflexes
XI. Accessory (also known as ***Spinal Accessory Nerve***)	Motor control of sternocleidomastoid muscle and trapezius muscle	Rotate head and shrug shoulders against resistance.
XII. Hypoglossal	Tongue movements and tongue sensations (pain and temperature)	Stick out tongue, press tongue into cheek bilaterally

The Autonomic Nervous System

Overview of the Autonomic Nervous System-

The **Autonomic Nervous System (ANS)** controls our involuntary body activities. This involves controlling most of our internal organs (digestive system, respiratory system, cardiovascular system, urinary system, digestive system). The ANS has control over cardiac muscle, smooth muscle, organs, and glands. Control and activities of our skeletal muscles (walking, talking, waving, etc.) are conscious activities and were controlled by our **Somatic Nervous System.**

The main control center of our ANS is an area of the brain called the *hypothalamus.* Messages originate here, travel from the hypothalamus, down the brain stem and usually out through the spinal cord. After traveling down the spinal cord, the messages will leave the spinal cord through the spinal nerves.

After the spinal nerves leave the spinal cord, they will enter the ***autonomic ganglia***. Ganglia are big clusters of neuron cell bodies- they act as junction boxes. Many messages leaving the spinal cord will enter the ganglia, and then the ganglia will route them out the correct nerve that is heading to the appropriate body part or organ. Neurons which run from the spinal cord out to a ganglion are called **preganglionic neurons** (or **preganglionic fibers**). Neurons which leave the ganglion and run out to specific organs in the body are called **postganglionic neurons** (or **postganglionic fibers**).

There are two main divisions of the ANS: the **Sympathetic Division** and the **Parasympathetic Division**. Both of these divisions often control the same organs in the body, but usually they will have opposite effects on the body parts. For example, one part of the ANS may be responsible for speeding up the heart rate, while the other division may be responsible for slowing down the heart rate. The effector organ (responding body part) knows whether it is receiving instructions from the sympathetic or parasympathetic division by the type of neurotransmitter it receives from the sympathetic neuron or the parasympathetic neuron.

The Sympathetic Division

The sympathetic division has the nickname as the "fight or flight" division. Nerve fibers which carry sympathetic division messages leave the spinal cord at the spinal levels of T1-L2. Because of this, the sympathetic division is also called the *thoracolumbar division.* The ganglia on the sympathetic division are usually located very near the spine. The three main ganglia are the Sympathetic Chain Ganglia, Collateral Ganglia and Adrenal Medullae. Sympathetic preganglionic fibers are *short* in length, due to most of the ganglia being located near the spinal cord. This will then require a longer length for the postganglionic neuron as it travels from the ganglion all the way out to the target organ.

Most of the neurotransmitters released by the sympathetic postganglionic fibers are **norepinephrine (NE).** Neurons which use norepinephrine as their neurotransmitter are called *adrenergic.* The neurotransmitter will be received at the target organ by receptors. There are two main types of sympathetic adrenergic receptors:

- **Alpha (α) Receptors-** Alpha-1 receptors are more common than Alpha-2 and usually excite the target cell. Alpha-2 receptors inhibit activity. Alpha-2 receptors are usually used by the sympathetic nervous system to inhibit the parasympathetic nervous system.
- **Beta (β) Receptors-** located on the membranes of cells in many organs including the skeletal muscles, heart, lungs, and liver. Beta-1 receptors will usually increase the metabolic activity of those organs. Beta-2 receptors will usually inhibit, or relax, the muscles along the respiratory tract, thus widening the air passageways so you can breathe easier. These receptors are sometimes targeted by pharmaceuticals prescribed by medical physicians (ex: Beta blockers).

Side note: Sympathetic nervous system stimulation will also cause Norepinephrine (NE) and Epinephrine (E) to be released by the adrenal medulla into the bloodstream and act as <u>hormones,</u> not as neurotransmitters. (A <u>hormone</u> is a chemical which can create a bodily response that is carried in the bloodstream. A <u>neurotransmitter</u> is a chemical which is released by a neuron to trigger a bodily response.) When functioning as hormones, NE and E will then travel through the bloodstream to the target organ. This hormonal method causes NE and E to have a much longer lasting effect on the target organs.

Physiological changes caused by the Sympathetic Division are: Increased state of arousal and awareness, heightened mental alertness, increased metabolic rate, reduced digestive and urinary function, activation of energy reserves, increased respiratory rate and dilation of respiratory passageways, increased heart rate and blood pressure and activation of sweat glands

The Parasympathetic Division

The parasympathetic division is a time for rest and rejuvenation of the body. It is here when we get to replenish any energy stores and reserves that may have been depleted by the sympathetic division activities. The parasympathetic division is sometimes called the "resting and digesting" or the "rest and repose" division. Nerve fibers which carry parasympathetic division messages leave the brainstem and spinal cord through the cranial nerves and spinal nerves exiting the sacrum. Because of this, the parasympathetic division is also called the *craniosacral division.* Cranial Nerve X (the Vagus nerve) carries **75%** of parasympathetic outflow.

The ganglia on the parasympathetic division are usually located very near the organs they are serving. The main ganglia are ciliary ganglion, pterygopalatine and submandibular ganglia, otic ganglion, and intramural ganglia, The parasympathetic preganglionic fibers are *longer* in length, due to most of the ganglia being located near the organs. Preganglionic fibers will leave the brainstem and spinal cord from the cranial nerves (III, XII, IX, and X) and the sacral spinal nerves (S2, S3, and S4). Postganglionic fibers are *shorter* in length.

The neurotransmitter which is released by all parasympathetic postganglionic fiber is **Acetylcholine (ACh).** ACh is quickly broken down by acetylcholinesterase, so it has short lived effects- only a few seconds or so. The receptors on the target organ which will receive the acetylcholine are *Cholinergic Receptors.* There are two main types of cholinergic receptors: the **Nicotinic Receptors** (will excite or increase organ activity when exposed to ACh) and the **Muscarinic Receptors** (can either have an excitatory or inhibitory effect on the organs). Usually muscarinic receptors will cause a slightly longer lasting response than a nicotinic receptor when exposed to ACh.

The physiological changes caused by the Parasympathetic Division are: A state of energy conservation, decreased metabolic rate, increased digestive and urinary function, increased secretion of digestive enzymes and saliva, increased motility and blood flow to the digestive tract, decreased heart rate and blood pressure, stimulation of urination and defecation, pupil constriction, increased sexual arousal and stimulation of sexual glands.

COMPARISON CHART FOR SYMPATHETIC AND PARASYMPATHETIC NERVOUS SYSTEMS

	Sympathetic	Parasympathetic
Common Nickname	Fight or Flight	Resting and Digesting
Nerve Source	Thoracolumbar (Thoracic and Lumbar Nerves)	Craniosacral (Cranial and Sacral Nerves)
Ganglia Location	Near the spine	Near the target organs
Preganglionic Neuron	Short in length	Long in length
Postganglionic Neuron	Long in length	Short in length
Neurotransmitter (used to stimulate the target organ)	Norepinephrine (NE)	Acetylcholine (ACh)
Receptor type	Adrenergic (Alpha and Beta receptors)	Cholinergic (Nicotinic and Muscarinic receptors)
Physiologic Changes	• Increased state of arousal and awareness • Heightened mental alertness • Increased metabolic rate • Reduced digestive and urinary function • Activation of energy reserves • Increased respiratory rate and dilation of respiratory passageways • Increased heart rate and blood pressure • Activation of sweat glands	• A state of energy conservation • Decreased metabolic rate • Increased digestive and urinary function • Increased secretion of digestive enzymes and saliva • Decreased heart rate and blood pressure • Stimulation of urination and defecation • Pupil constriction • Increased sexual arousal and stimulation of sexual glands

Physical Examination of the Nervous System

Assess Speech

1. During health history and intake, the examiner will also be making notes of the patient's speaking ability. Are they able to speak clearly? Watch for Broca's aphasia, Wernicke's aphasia, global aphasia, dysphonia, dysarthria

Assess Mental Status

1. During health history and intake, the examiner will also be making notes of the patient's mental status.
2. How is the appearance of the patient? (behavior, dress, grooming)
3. How are their behaviors? Nervous, depressed, anxiety, paranoia, delusions, hallucinations?
4. What is the patient's level of consciousness? (Alert, lethargic, comatose, falling asleep). Use the **Glasgow Coma Scale** to rate level of consciousness if concerned. Maximum score is a 15, minimum score is a 3. Total score of 7 or less indicates severe neurological damage.
5. Assess cognitive function- Are they able to comprehend questions asked of them that test higher brain functions? Assess orientation to person, orientation to time, orientation to place, memory (remote and recent), general knowledge, abstract thought, attention span and calculation skills
   o What is your name?
   o What year is it?
   o How old are you?
   o Where are you right now?
   o What is your mother's name?
   o What year were you born?
   o What did you have for breakfast?
   o Who is the current President of the United States?
   o Can you count backward from 20 to 1?
   o The examiner will tell the patient a sentence or name 5 objects. Can they repeat it back correctly immediately? Can they repeat it back correctly after 5 minutes?
   o The examiner may ask a hypothetical question to how the patient responds- "What would you do if the fire alarm went off while you were in a public place?"
   o The examiner may ask the patient to interpret a well-known proverb like "People who live in glass houses shouldn't throw stones."

Assess Cranial Nerves

1. Please refer to the Cranial Nerve chart earlier in the chapter.

Assess the Motor System

1. Inspect for any involuntary movements: muscle tremors, fasciculation, tics
2. Inspect muscles for any signs of atrophy (compare muscles bilaterally)
3. Assess muscle strength using the following grading scale:
    - 0 = no muscular contraction detected
    - 1 = barely detectable contraction
    - 2 = able to move, but not strong enough to move against gravity
    - 3 = active movement against gravity, but no resistance
    - 4 = active movement against gravity with some resistance from the examiner
    - 5 = Normal muscle strength- active movement against gravity with full resistance from the examiner

Muscle movements	Nerves involved
Shoulder abduction	C5
Elbow flexion	C5, C6
Elbow extension	C6, C7
Wrist extension	C6, C7, C8, radial nerve
Grip	C7, C8, T1
Finger abduction	C8, T1, ulnar nerve
Thumb opposition	C8, T1, median nerve
Hip flexion	L2, L3, L4
Hip adduction	L2, L3, L4
Hip abduction	L4, L5, S1
Hip extension	S1
Knee extension	L2, L3, L4
Knee flexion	L4, L5, S1, S2
Ankle dorsiflexion	L4, L5
Ankle plantar flexion	S1

Assess Cerebellar Functioning

1. Have the patient walk and observe their gait. Look for unsteadiness, deviation to one side or another
2. Have patient walk heel to toe and observe for unsteadiness
3. Perform **Romberg's test**- instruct patient to stand with feet together and eyes open. Observe patient's balance. Then have them remain standing and close their eyes for 20-30 seconds. Watch for swaying or unsteadiness
4. Perform **Pronator Drift test**.
5. Test for patient's coordination
6. Test for the patient's ability to perform rapid alternating movements in arms and legs

Assess the Sensory System

1. Dermatomal testing- Assess pain sensation bilaterally in the major dermatome areas (fingers, shoulders, trunk, thighs and toes).
2. Dermatomal testing- Assess light touch sensation using a wisp of cotton to assess sensation bilaterally in the major dermatome areas (fingers, shoulders, trunk, thighs and toes).
3. Assess vibration sensation bilaterally using a vibrating tuning fork.
4. Assess joint position sensation
5. Assess discriminative sensations
    a. Test **Stereognosis**- have patient close eyes and identify a commonly used object placed in the palm of their hand (a key, comb, closed safety pin, paperclip)
    b. Test **Graphesthesia**- have patient close eyes while the examiner draws a number on the palm of their hand (with the blunt end of a pen)
    c. Test **Point Localization**- have patient close eyes. The examiner will touch the patient briefly on their body. Have patient open eyes and point to the area that the examiner touched.
    d. Test **Two Point Discrimination**- have patient close eyes. Simultaneously touch the patient's fingertip of their index finger with a caliper or two pins. Begin with pins together and gradually move them apart. Alternate touching the patient's skin with one point of the caliper or touching the skin simultaneously with both points. Note when patient can feel both pins. Test bilaterally. Assesses parietal lobe.

Assess Reflexes

1. Test reflexes bilaterally. Begin superiorly and proceed inferiorly.
2. Use the following rating scale for the reflexes
    - ➢ 0 = No response
    - ➢ 1+ = Diminished or low normal response
    - ➢ 2+ = Normal response
    - ➢ 3+ = Slightly increased response, but not necessarily abnormal
    - ➢ 4+ = Hyper-reflexive, with clonus

Reflex	Nerves involved
Biceps	C5, C6
Triceps	C6, C7
Brachioradialis (Supinator)	C5, C6
Knee (Patellar)	L2, L3, L4
Ankle	S1
Plantar	L5, S1
Upper Abdominal	T8, T9
Lower Abdominal	T10, T11

SUMMARY CHARTS

Comparison of Rating Scales for Muscle Testing and Reflex Testing:

Reflex Grading		Muscle Strength Grading	
0	No Response	0	No response
1+	Diminished or Low Normal Response	1	"Trace strength"- Barely detectable contraction
2+	**Normal Response**	2	"Poor strength"- Able to move, but not strong enough to move against gravity
3+	Slightly increased response	3	"Fair strength"- active movement against gravity, but no resistance
4+	Hyper-reflexive, with clonus	4	"Good Strength"- active movement against gravity with some resistance from examiner
		5	**Normal Response**

Nerve Levels Involved in Muscle Movements and Reflexes

Nerves involved	Muscle movements	Reflexes
C5	Shoulder abduction	
C5, C6	Elbow flexion	Biceps reflex
C6, C7	Elbow extension	Triceps reflex
C5. C6	Supination	Brachioradialis reflex
C6, C7, C8, radial nerve	Wrist extension	
C7, C8, T1	Grip	
C8, T1, ulnar nerve	Finger abduction	
C8, T1, median nerve	Thumb opposition	
L2, L3, L4	Hip flexion	
L2, L3, L4	Hip adduction	
L4, L5, S1	Hip abduction	
S1	Hip extension	
L2, L3, L4	Knee extension	Knee/Patellar reflex
L4, L5, S1, S2	Knee flexion	
L4, L5	Ankle dorsiflexion	
S1	Ankle plantar flexion	Ankle/Achilles reflex
L5, S1		Plantar reflex
T8, T9		Lower abdominal reflex
T10, T11		Upper abdominal reflex

General Abnormal Findings of the Nervous System

Abnormal findings, if necessary, should be referred to patients PCP or a neurologist

Altered level of consciousness- may result from several factors, including toxic encephalopathy, hemorrhage, extensive cortical atrophy, compression of brainstem from tumor/swelling/hemorrhage, drugs (opioids, sedatives)

Broca's Aphasia (expressive) - comprehension is fine, but speech sounds are not formed properly (non-fluent speech) or difficulty in finding words. Due to damage to frontal lobe in brain

Wernicke's Aphasia (receptive) - poor comprehension (inability to understand written words or speech), words are formed (fluent speech) but are often meaningless. Due to damage at the junction of the parietal and temporal lobes of the brain

Global Aphasia- lack of comprehension and lack of fluent speech. Involves both expressive and receptive aphasia.

Dysphonia- unable to produce sounds due to larynx/vocal cord problem

Dysarthria- words are not formed properly due to difficulty with mouth, tongue movements. Could be neurologically based or muscular based.

Agnosia- inability to identify objects (can be visual, auditory, or body image)

Anosmia- loss of sense of smell. Can be in one nostril or bilaterally. Often involving Cranial Nerve I.

Pupillary changes- unusual dilation, non-response to light stimulation, unusual constrictions, and unilateral differences can all indicate different neurological problems

Hemianopia/Hemianopsia- loss of vision in either the left field of vision or right field of vision in both eyes. Can be caused by stroke or brain injury.

Aniscoria- pupil size does not change with changes in light levels.

Nystagmus- rapid uncontrollable movements of the eye. Can be up and down ("vertical nystagmus") or from side to side ("horizontal nystagmus")

Trigeminal neuralgia- (also called **tic douloureux**) sharp stabbing facial pain over one or more of the facial dermatomes innervated by Cranial Nerve V

Bell's palsy- paralysis of the facial muscles (unilaterally), due to irritation to Cranial Nerve VII. Usually temporary- last a few weeks and then resolves.

Froment's Sign: tests for palsy of the ulnar nerve, specifically, the action of adductor pollicis. To perform the test, a patient is asked to hold an object, usually a piece of paper, between the thumb and a flat palm or side of finger. The object is then is pulled away. A normal individual will be able to maintain a hold on the object without difficulty. However, with ulnar nerve palsy, the patient will experience difficulty maintaining a grasp. and will compensate by flexing the FPL (flexor pollicis longus) of the thumb. Clinically, this will appear as flexion of the DIP joint of the thumb (rather than extension, as would occur with correct use of the adductor pollicus)

Vertigo- inappropriate sense of motion- often felt as a spinning sensation or "dizziness". Abnormal conditions in the inner ear, CNS infections, high fever, endolymph movement, alcohol and drugs, viral infection of the vestibular nerve, and motion sickness can all be causes. In some cases, the cause is unknown.

- If vertigo is present with nystagmus, hearing loss, and/or nausea; increases with movement and then decreases after change in body position indicates a *peripheral lesion (lesion in the labyrinth or cranial nerve IX)*
- If vertigo does not change with movement or when the patient is still- can indicate a *central lesion (lesion in the vestibular nucleus or brainstem)*

Apraxia- inability to perform purposeful movements and make proper use of objects

Tics- sudden uncontrollable movements of the face, shoulders and extremities

Tremors- involuntary repetitive movements. Examples: "pill rolling" (Parkinson's), intention tremor (hand shaking which worsens on movement), essential tremor (disappears with relaxation)

Fasciculation- slight twitching of muscle fibers that can be seen under the skin- usually due to a lower motor neuron dysfunction

Upper Motor Neuron Lesion- Results from brain or spinal cord damage to an Upper Motor Neuron. This will result in muscular dysfunction. Muscles will be spastic and reflexes will be hyper-reflexive. *(Messages from the brain heading out to the muscles in the body travel on two nerve cells. The first nerve cell is called the Upper Motor Neuron, and usually carries the messages from the brain down into the spinal cord. The Upper Motor Neuron will then synapse with a Lower Motor Neuron, who picks up the message in the spinal cord and then carries the message out into the body to the appropriate muscle)*

Lower Motor Neuron Lesion- Results from damage to a Lower Motor Neuron. Muscles will be flaccid, unresponsive, and reflexes will be hyporeflexive or absent.

Babinski's sign/response- Abnormal response in an adult when performing the plantar reflex. In this sign, the big toe extends and other toes flare. This sign is abnormal in an adult (but normal in infants). Can indicate upper motor neuron damage.

Increased reflex (hyperreflexive) or clonus- Clonus is involuntary muscular contraction and relaxation in a rhythmic pattern. This can indicate an upper motor neuron lesion or hyperthyroidism

Hypotonia- poor muscle tone and strength

Foot drop- patient is unable to maintain dorsiflexion (for example, if attempting to walk on their heels). Often causes a ***Steppage Gait***- where the patient lifts knees higher than normal and then "slaps" foot down on the ground. Can be caused by a lesion to L5 or peripheral neuropathy.

Parkinsonian (or propulsive) Gait- patient has a stooped over posture and takes small shuffling steps. May have difficulty starting and stopping walking. Caused by Parkinson's disease.

Scissoring Gait- patient has normally spaced paces, but the feet cross over each other when stepping. Could indicate multiple sclerosis, cerebral palsy, spinal cord compression

Waddling gait- patient walks or "waddles" similar to a duck, due to pelvis rotating excessively. This indicates weakened proximal muscles (muscles close to the trunk). Classic sign of muscular dystrophy or could indicate hip dysplasia.

Hemiplegic gait- an asymmetrical gait in which the strong leg is used as a pivot and the weaker (often spastic) leg is swung around as a step is taken. Often caused by corticospinal tract damage.

Cerebellar Ataxia- a staggering gait with a wide stance and uncoordinated leg movements. Indicates cerebellar damage or excessive alcohol use

Dysdiadochokinesia- inability to perform rapid alternating movements. Often due to a cerebellar lesion.

Dysmetria- Loss of ability to precisely control muscle movements while reaching or grasping. They have lost the ability to anticipate and stop a movement precisely. Hands may oscillate back and forth as a person tries to reach or grasp objects. This oscillating movement is called an intention tremor.

Neuropathy- often creates sensory loss or weakness in extremities (toes and fingers) and can increase to involve the entire hands or feet. This is usually occurring bilaterally. Often described as a "glove-like" pattern of loss of function or sensation.

Anaesthesia- loss of all sensation

Hypoesthesia- decreased sensation (can be localized or diffuse)

Dysesthesia- an uncomfortable burning sensation

Paresthesia- the patient feels a sensation that is not actually being stimulated. Usually a "pins and needles" or "prickly" sensation.

Flaccid paralysis – if the nerve supply to a muscle is destroyed (such as in an accident), it is unable to contract, loses tone, becomes soft, and begins to decrease in size (atrophy). This is caused by damage to the lower motor neuron.

Battle's sign- also called mastoid ecchymosis, is an indication of fracture of the base of the posterior portion of the skull and may suggest underlying brain trauma. It consists of bruising immediately behind the ears

Brudzinski Sign- is the appearance of involuntary lifting of the legs when the physician lifts a patient's head while the patient is lying supine. Can be indicative of meningitis

Kernig's Sign is positive when patient is lying supine and the leg is fully bent in the hip and knee, and subsequent extension in the knee is painful (leading to resistance). Patients may also show *opisthotonus*-spasm of the whole body that leads to legs and head being bent back and body bowed forward. A sign of meningitis

Lhermitte's Sign- sometimes called the **Barber Chair phenomenon**, is an electrical sensation that runs down the back and into the limbs, and is produced by bending the neck forward. Although often considered a classic finding in multiple sclerosis, it can be caused by a number of conditions which compress the spinal cord in the neck, such as cervical spondylosis, disc herniation, tumor, and Arnold-Chiari malformation

Raccoon Eyes- the purplish discoloration around the eyes following fracture of the frontal portion of the skull base

Romberg's test- A sign indicating loss of proprioceptive control. Increased unsteadiness occurs when standing with the eyes closed compared with standing with the eyes open. Could indicate possible cerebellar damage among other things

Weber test- see discussion on performing this test in the Special Senses Chapter

Rinne test- see discussion on performing this test in the Special Senses Chapter

Abnormal pupillary responses and other eye responses- see discussion in the Special Senses Chapter

Advanced Imaging and Diagnostic Tests of the Nervous System

Cerebral Angiography- A contrast liquid is injected into the bloodstream and then monitored by X-ray. Allows the physician to look for stenosis of blood vessels in the neck and brain or to look for aneurysms.

Computed Tomography (CT scan) - CT scans are a specialized x-ray machine. It generates a collection of black-and-white pictures, each showing a slightly different "slice" or cross-section of your internal organs (about ¼ inches apart). Used most often when diagnosing a stroke patient.

CT angiography- A technician or other health care professional inserts an IV and injects contrast dye through it. This dye outlines blood vessels in the brain which is then detected on a CT scan. Often used in suspected stroke patients, to detect aneurysms, and TIA's.

Electroencephalogram (EEG)- Used to diagnose brain lesions (in epilepsy, tumors, and abscesses). Normal brain function involves the continuous transmission of electrical impulses by neurons. EEG's are accomplished by placing electrodes on various points on the scalp and recording electrical impulses. The electrical impulses recorded are "brain waves". Sleep and coma result in brain waves slower than normal. Fright, epileptic seizures, and some kinds of drug overdose can result in abnormally fast brain waves.

Electromyography- Electromyography (EMG) tests analyze nerve and muscle electrical activity. For the EMG, thin needles are inserted one by one into the muscles being tested. Each needle is attached to a wire that detects electrical patterns inside the muscle and the nerves that are attached to that muscle.

Lumbar puncture- A lumbar puncture, also known as a spinal tap, uses a needle to remove a sample of cerebrospinal fluid from the space surrounding the spinal cord. The test is used to diagnose meningitis infections and some neurological conditions (spinal cord tumor, multiple sclerosis, Guillain- Barre).

Magnetic Resonance Imaging (MRI) - uses radio waves, a large magnet, and a computer to create images. Each MRI picture shows a different "slice," or cross-section, of the area being viewed. Often used to look for tumors in the brain or myelination changes in multiple sclerosis.

Myelogram- A myelogram is an x-ray test in which radioopaque dye is injected directly into the spinal canal via a spinal tap to help show places where the vertebrae in the spine may be pinching the spinal cord. It is sometimes used to help diagnose back or leg pain problems, especially if surgery is being planned

Nerve conduction studies are tests that are often used in combination with the EMG evaluation. For nerve conduction studies, the muscles and nerves are stimulated with small bursts of electricity to see whether the nerves and muscles respond in a normal way. If nerve conduction studies are done, small pads are taped to the skin of the hands or feet. These pads can both deliver mild electric shocks and detect electric signals coming through the skin (similar in sensation to a "shock" you might feel from static electricity).

PET scan- Used to localize lesions that generate epileptic seizures and is also used in some cases to diagnose Alzheimer's disease. PET scans can also be utilized to monitor heart conditions. PET scans take a substance necessary for proper health (oxygen, glucose) and label it with a radioactive molecule and inject the substance into a vein. It is then watched to see how the substance is transported through the body and used by body tissues.

Reflex tests (Deep Tendon Reflexes) - often done using a small hammer, tapping on muscle tendons. Tests proper functioning of spinal nerves

X-Ray- may be performed if the physician is concerned with a skull fracture.

Pathologies of the Nervous System

For additional infectious diseases that may affect this system, please refer to the Communicable/Infectious Disease Chart in Chapter 10.

Alzheimer's Disease- chronic progressive illness with memory loss, impairment in thinking, judgment and personality changes. 5.2 million people in the US have Alzheimer's. By 2025, the projected number of people with Alzheimer's disease is expected to grow to 7.1 million. Neurofibrillary tangles and plaques occur in the nucleus basalis, hippocampus, and parahippocampal gyrus. The plaques are caused by the build-up of amyloidβ protein. Why this occurs is not fully understood. No cure for Alzheimer's disease.

Amnesia- memory loss. Can be partial or complete, permanent or temporary. Often caused by trauma. *Retrograde amnesia-* loss of memories of past events, usually events preceding the trauma *Anterograde amnesia-* old memories are intact, but they may be unable to store new memories. Magazines can be re-read over and over. New people must constantly re-introduce themselves. *Post-traumatic amnesia-* has characteristics of both retrograde and anterograde amnesia.

Amyotrophic Lateral Sclerosis- ALS (also known as **Lou Gehrig's disease**)- progressive disease which affects motor neurons. Sensory neurons are normal and intellectual processing is normal. Motor neurons throughout the CNS are destroyed. Symptoms usually begin over the age of 40. More common in males than females. 3-5 cases out of 100,000 worldwide. Loss of muscle tone occurs and the muscles will atrophy. Average survival is 3-5 years after diagnosis. The person remains alert and fully aware during the disease. Cause is uncertain. 5-10% is genetic. Treatment to slow respiratory paralysis is the drug riluzole.

Anorexia Nervosa- an eating disorder where the person loses an unhealthy amount of weight. <u>*Red Flag symptoms:*</u> *having a very strong fear of gaining weight (even if they are already underweight), refuse to stay at a healthy weight, have a distorted body image, missed 3 or more menstrual cycle (women).* They may refuse to eat, eat only very small amounts, exercise all the time, take diuretics or laxatives, or make themselves vomit after eating. It is more common in females than males.

Anxiety Disorder- The causes of anxiety disorders are not fully understood. Anxiety disorders come in many forms:
- *Generalized Anxiety Disorder-* may show constant worrying, restlessness, irritability, sleep changes, shortness of breath, rapid heartbeat. More often in women than men.
- *Post-Traumatic Stress Disorder (PTSD)-* as a result of a traumatic event. Nightmares, flashbacks and uncontrollable thoughts about the event may occur in addition to anxiety symptoms. Most common events triggering PTSD are combat, abuse, rape, physical attack.
- *Obsessive Compulsive Disorder (OCD)-* recurrent upsetting thoughts cause the person to perform a ritual, which temporarily alleviates the anxiety
- *Panic Disorder-* sudden, repeated intense fear reaction. Can cause strong physical symptoms- racing heartbeat, shortness of breath, chest pain.

Treatment may involve medication and/or psychotherapy.

Aphasia: disorder that affects language. *Global aphasia-* loss of comprehension and expression of both verbal and written language. Often due to damage to left frontal and temporal brain areas. *Major motor aphasia* (non-fluent aphasia, Broca's aphasia, expressive aphasia) can comprehend language and knows how to respond, but lacks the ability to find the right words to say. Due to damage to frontal lobe of the brain. *Fluent aphasia-* does not understand what is heard, does not make sense while speaking. They can easily form words and sounds, but have no meaning. Damage to temporal lobe of the brain

Ataxia- loss of coordination and maintenance of balance due to cerebellar damage. The person may stagger and sway as if they were drunk.

Attention Deficit Disorder (ADD)/Attention Deficit Hyperactivity Disorder (ADHD)- This can be diagnosed as an adult or child. Symptoms can involve inability to pay attention, difficulty concentrating, hyperactivity, and impulsive behavior. The hyperactivity is more pronounced as a child and may fade as the person matures- but the inability to pay attention and concentration difficulties may persist for the person's entire life. The cause of ADHD is not fully understood. Risk factors for developing ADHD- family history, environmental toxin exposure, and stresses on the fetus during development (maternal drug use or alcohol use, maternal exposure to environmental toxins- such as PCB's). There is no cure. Treatment can involve medications, counseling and behavior therapy.

Autism Spectrum Disorder (ASD)- a very complicated range of symptoms. Usually people diagnosed on the Autism Spectrum may exhibit problems with communication, social interaction, and/or repetitive behaviors. The severity of the condition can range from person to person. Autistic Disorder or Classical ASD is the most severe form, whereas Asperger's is a milder form. Males are four times as likely to develop ASD as females.

Bell's Palsy- irritation of the facial nerve (Cranial Nerve VII). Usually unilateral. Causes facial drooping on the side affected. Often resolves after a few weeks.

Bi-polar Disorder (also known as **manic-depressive illness**)- an illness in which the patient oscillates between extreme mood states (a manic state and a depressive state). *Red flag symptoms: The patient will have episodes of mania and depression. For the manic state, symptoms include: an overly happy feeling, sleeping little, agitation, impulsive behaviors, being easily distracted, engaging in risky behaviors. For the depressive state: sleep changes, feeling low, sadness, worthlessness, irritability, loss of interest in activities, and possible suicidal thoughts.* The degree of severity of symptoms of the manic and depressive states can vary from individual to individual as well as the length of time of each episode. In between manic and depressive episodes, the patient may have relatively normal periods of time. Treatment may include medications (antidepressants, antipsychotics or mood stabilizing drugs) and/or psychotherapy.

Bulimia Nervosa- an eating disorder in which the person commonly binges on food and then purges the food (either through vomiting or laxative use). It can share some symptoms with anorexia nervosa. *Red Flag symptoms: being preoccupied with weight, eating large amounts of food in private, visiting the bathroom during meals, excessive exercise, weight fluctuation, bad breath, tooth decay, sores in the mouth or throat, feeling shame about eating, and depression.* Women are more likely to develop bulimia than men.

Carpal Tunnel Syndrome- entrapment of the median nerve in the wrist region. May be unilateral or bilateral. Pain and paresthesia in the first 3 fingers of the hand most common symptom- but pain can occasionally radiate back up the arm towards the neck. Patient may exhibit weakness in hand and wrist movements. Phalen's sign and Tinel's test may increase symptomatology.

Cerebrovascular accident- CVA (also known as a **"stroke"**) – one of the leading causes of death in the United States. A stroke will occur when blood flow to a section of the brain is disrupted, either by a blood clot (ischemic stroke) or a ruptured blood vessel (hemorrhagic stroke). The brain tissue supplied by that blood vessel will die due to lack of nutrients. 85 percent of strokes are ischemic. Symptoms of stroke victims will vary, depending on the region of the brain that has been damaged. *Red Flag symptoms can include: speech difficulties, muscle weakness in face, arm or leg (often one-sided), blurred vision, loss of balance, sudden severe headache or confusion. A TIA (transient ischemic attack) is a red flag of an impending stroke* You can remember F.A.S.T.- *F*ace drooping on one side, *A*rm weakness, *S*peech difficulty (slurred or incoherent speech, *T*ime- note the time the symptoms started and then it is time to call 911 . Risk factors include: being over age 55, high blood pressure, high blood cholesterol, smoking, diabetes, sleep apnea, being overweight and family history of stroke or cardiovascular disease. Treatment varies on whether the stroke is hemorrhagic or ischemic. Ischemic strokes may be immediately treated with thrombolytic medications. Call 911 right away if a stroke is suspected.

Delirium- variations in degrees of wakefulness. Hard to grasp reality and may have hallucinations. Can be caused by high fever, infections, drugs, withdrawal from drugs, or brain tumors.

Dementia- chronic state of memory loss, decreased spatial orientation, loss of language, changes in personality.

Depression- The exact cause of depression is not fully known. It may be a neurotransmitter imbalance issue. It can run in families (although not always) and is more common in females than males. And, it can be seen more commonly with other illnesses (for example PTSD). _Red flag symptoms: feelings of sadness, hopelessness, worthlessness, anxiety, guilt, or suicide. Irritability, loss of interest in usual activities, insomnia or excessive sleeping, fatigue, body aches, changes in appetite or difficulty in making decisions can also be seen._ Symptoms can vary from person to person. There are different forms of depression:
- _**Major Depressive Disorder (Major Depression)**_ - disabling- prevents person from functioning normally and carrying out normal daily activities.
- _**Dysthymic Disorder-**_ symptoms present for over 2 years, but the person is still somewhat functional in daily activities and not completely disabled.
- _**Minor Depression-**_ symptoms for 2 weeks or longer, but not severe enough to be diagnosed as Major Depression. Includes _postpartum depression_ (depression after delivering a baby) or _seasonal affective disorder_ (onset of depression in the winter months, when there is less natural sunlight). Minor Depression can progress into Major Depression without treatment.

Treatments may include medications (antidepressants) and/ or psychotherapy. Electroconvulsive Therapy (ECT) may be done for patients who do not respond to medications and psychotherapy.

Disconnection Syndrome- occurs when the corpus callosum has been cut. This means the left and right hemispheres of the brain cannot communicate with one another. Motor movements on both sides of the body cannot be coordinated. Other sensory interpretation and responses may be affected.

Dysmetria- Loss of ability to precisely control muscle movements while reaching or grasping. They have lost the ability to anticipate and stop a movement precisely. Hands may oscillate back and forth as a person tries to reach or grasp objects. This oscillating movement is called an intention tremor.

Epilepsy- a neurological disorder which causes seizures. There are three main types of seizures:
- _**Absence (petit mal) seizure-**_ occur most often in children. The seizure may look like the person is staring off into space or not paying attention. There is usually no muscular movement during this type of seizure and the person remains conscious during the seizure. A person may have many of these per day and they only last a few seconds.
- _**Grand Mal (tonic-clonic) seizure-**_ these seizures have strong, uncontrollable muscular contractions and the person will lose consciousness. (This is the type of seizure most people are thinking of when they hear the term epilepsy). These seizures can affect large areas of the brain.
- _**Partial (focal) seizure-**_ occur in limited parts of the brain. Symptoms can vary, depending on which part of the brain is affected. There may be muscular contractions, repetitive movements, vision changes, abnormal sensations, or hallucinations. The person remains conscious during the seizure.

Diagnosis of seizure activity is done with an EEG. A CT scan or MRI may also be used. Treatment may involve anti-seizure medications or surgery (if there is a tumor or abnormal blood vessel causing the seizures)

Flaccid paralysis – if the nerve supply to a muscle is destroyed (such as in an accident), the muscle is unable to contract, loses tone, becomes soft, and begins to decrease in size (atrophy).

Guillain Barre Syndrome- a peripheral nervous system autoimmune disease. This is a type of _acute idiopathic demyelinating polyneuropathy_ (the immune system attacks and destroys myelin in multiple nerves in the body). Main symptom: _ascending paralysis_ (paralysis beginning in feet and hands and then progressing toward the trunk). This condition can be fatal. This condition can appear days or weeks after symptoms of a gastrointestinal or respiratory infection- most commonly an infection with _Campylobacter jejuni_ or _Cytomegalovirus._ Diagnostic tests can include nerve conduction studies or a spinal tap. Treatment can include physical therapy, plasmapheresis ("plasma exchange") and intravenous immunoglobulin (receiving antibodies from a donor).

Hansen's disease (leprosy)- caused by a bacterium. The bacterium destroys cutaneous nerve endings which are sensitive to pain, touch, heat, and cold. Damage to the distal tissues occurs, due to the fact the individual no longer feels pain in the area.

Headache- There are many types of headaches. Some common ones are:
- **Tension Headache-** The most common types of headache. Pain is a constant ache and is commonly located at the back of head, neck, or around the temples.
- **Cluster Headache-** Affects more men than women. Pain usually comes on very suddenly and is severe and one sided. The eye may water and nasal congestion can occur also. These headaches can appear in groups or "clusters"
- **Migraine Headache-** The moderate to severe pain of this headache can be one sided, throbbing, trigger nausea, can last 4-72 hours, and can interfere with activities or functions. A migraine attack that lasts for more than 72 hours is called "*status migrainosus*".
- **Sinus Headache-** due to a sinus becoming infected. There may be pain and tenderness over the sinus
- **Post-Traumatic Headache-** occurs after a trauma and can last for weeks or months. Dizziness, difficulty concentrating or irritability can accompany a post-traumatic headache.

Herniated disc – the shock-absorbing intervertebral discs are located between the vertebrae, and are composed of an outer ring of fibrocartilage (called the annulus fibrosis) with water-filled, jelly-like centers (called the nucleus pulposus). If the discs lose water and the spinal ligaments stiffen and weaken (both of which tend to happen as we get older), the nucleus pulposus may bulge out through the annulus fibrosus and possibly press on the spinal cord or spinal nerve roots, causing pain and numbness.

Horner's syndrome- sympathetic innervation to one side of the face is interrupted. The affected side of the face may be flushed, is unable to sweat, and has pupil constriction with drooping eyelid.

Huntington's Disease- inherited fatal disease. Progressive decreased motor function and dementia. 30,000 Americans have this condition, 75,000 have the gene for this condition and will develop it in their adult years. Basal nuclei and frontal lobe have degenerative changes. No effective treatment is available.

Hydrocephalus ("Water on the Brain")- Fresh cerebrospinal fluid (CSF) is constantly being made, while old CSF is constantly being removed. If CSF production increases while the rate of removal remains the same, excess CSF will build up and increase the pressure in the skull (intracranial pressure). This can compress the brain, and if occurring in a child can cause the developing skull bones to deform. Can cause permanent mental retardation. Treatment can involve inserting a shunt to drain the excess CSF.

Insomnia- difficulty falling asleep or staying asleep. Can be caused by many different conditions and may be a symptom of other diseases.

Lower Motor Neuron Lesion- Results from damage to a Lower Motor Neuron (LMN). LMN are neurons which carry messages from the brain and spinal cord out to the skeletal muscles. As a result of damage to a lower motor neuron, muscles will be flaccid/unresponsive and reflexes will be hyporeflexive or absent.

Meningitis: infection of the meninges of the spinal cord or the brain. *Red Flag symptoms can be a fever, fatigue, and a very stiff neck. The neck will be very painful when asked to perform cervical flexion and movement will be very limited.* Diagnosis is often completed by performing a spinal tap and analyzing the CSF extracted for the presence of viruses or bacteria. Meningitis comes in two forms: viral meningitis or bacterial meningitis. The severity of the infections will vary, depending on the strength of the pathogen, age of the victim, overall health of the victim, and other factors. Mortality rate for meningitis will range from 1-50 %. Bacterial meningitis may be treated with antibiotics, while viral meningitis will not.

Motion Sickness- headache, sweating, nausea, vertigo, flushing of the face, vomiting, and changes in mental perspectives can be symptoms. Researchers think that the processing centers in the mesencephalon receive conflicting sensory information from sensory receptors in the body. Often times, using your eyes to focus on a steady point (like the horizon) can give the mesencephalon strong signals to focus on and decrease motion sickness symptoms. Medications such as Dramamine, scopolamine, promethazine appear to depress the vestibular nuclei.

Multiple Sclerosis (MS): demyelination of the neurons in the CNS. Symptoms are muscular paralysis and sensory losses. A person may start with temporary symptoms, damage occurs to the myelin, but the body can recover and symptoms improve. But during subsequent attacks, the symptoms increase and may remain and not resolve. Gradual paralysis and sensory loss may occur. It is considered an autoimmune disease, with a number of environmental and genetic factors causing the immune system to attack and destroy myelin. The exact causes are unknown. Some leading theories are that cold and temperate climates increase the risk, lack of vitamin D, and heredity. On average in the US 1 in 2000 people develop it. The Pacific Northwest has one of the highest incidences of MS in the US with over 1 in 700 people developing the condition.

Myasthenia gravis – an autoimmune disease in which there is a progressive destruction of ACh receptors at the neuromuscular junction, causing droopy eyelids (ptosis), difficulty swallowing and talking, and generalized muscle weakness. After affecting the face and head muscles, the disease spreads to the upper extremity and chest. In 5-10% of victims, respiratory muscles will become paralyzed and death occurs. Roughly 70% of people with myasthenia gravis have a problem with their thymus gland, which programs the immune system incorrectly- thus the autoimmune disease. More common in women than men- average age of onset for women is 20-30 years old, whereas for men it is usually over the age of 60.

Narcolepsy- extreme fatigue and uncontrollable sleeping at inappropriate times. Genetic predisposition, possibly an autoimmune disease are cited as causes. Cataplexy, sleep hallucinations, and sleep paralysis can be seen. REM sleep patterns begin immediately when a person with narcolepsy falls asleep and can be seen on an EEG.

Parasomnias- abnormal behaviors during sleep such as sleepwalking, talking in sleep, bruxism (night grinding of teeth).

Parkinson's Disease (also known as ***paralysis agitans***)- loss of activity of the basal nuclei. Basal nuclei help to inhibit excess unwanted muscle contractions. When the basal nuclei are not functioning, these excess muscle contractions are able to be exhibited. This disease is chronic and progressive. The increased muscle tone causes spasticity (rigidity, stiffness, and jerky movements). They may also have a continual tremor. These people will have difficulty starting voluntary movements, and movements will usually be slower and labored. Posture will be rigid, and the gait will be a slow, shuffling gait. Gradually muscle movements become so taxing and exhausting, that the person's mobility is lost. They will lose the ability to control facial muscles, which will cause difficulty in speaking clearly and masked facies (a blank stare). Treatment often involves administering dopamine to the basal nuclei via the drug levodopa (LDOPA). Surgeries may also be done as the effectiveness of the drug therapies decrease over time.

Peripheral Neuropathy- damage to the peripheral nervous system (cranial and spinal nerves). Most commonly involves the spinal nerves. Spinal nerves can carry both motor and sensory information, so peripheral neuropathy can cause both motor and/or sensory symptoms. Symptoms will vary widely from patient to patient, but some common symptoms include: pain, numbness, tingling, burning, paresthesia (pricking sensations) or muscle weakness. *Mononeuropathy-* involves only one nerve. *Polyneuropathy-* involves more than one nerve. Causes of peripheral neuropathy: physical injury to the nerve, diabetes mellitus, Guillain Barre, nutritional deficiencies (for example: Thiamine B1), repetitive stress, HIV infection, viral and bacterial infections, and Lyme Disease.

Polio (Poliomyelitis): caused by the polio virus. In 95% of infected people, the virus causes no effects. In 5% of the people, symptoms will occur. In some people the infection presents as a mild flu, from which they recover. In others, it may cause meningitis. In some individuals, the effects can be more severe. In the severe cases (paralytic polio), the virus attacks somatic motor neurons (the nerves that carry messages from your brain to your muscles), causing paralysis. In this severe form, usually a person will develop a very high fever 10-14 days after infection, muscle pain and paralysis will then occur. If the respiratory muscles are affected, this can be fatal. In individuals who survive paralytic polio, they may suffer from postpolio syndrome later in life- where muscles not paralyzed by polio earlier, start to lose their strength. A vaccine is available for prevention of polio.

Radiculopathy- irritation of the nerve roots. Can occur at any level of the spinal cord. Can be caused by pressure being placed on the nerve roots by disc herniation, foraminal stenosis, osteophytes, or swelling. _Red Flag symptoms: Pain, tingling or numbness that follows the distribution of the dermatomal level of that spinal nerve root. Muscle weakness may also occur in the muscles served by that nerve root._ Treatment can involve decompression therapy, physical therapy, medications (oral or injection near affected nerve root), acupuncture, chiropractic care, or surgery (laminectomy, discectomy). An example of a radiculopathy is sciatica.

Raynaud's phenomenon (Raynaud's disease)- Affects women more often than men. Sympathetic nervous system causes excessive constriction of small arteries in the hands, feet, ears, and nose. This phenomenon is often triggered by exposure to the cold. Skin in the area changes color as blood flow is disrupted. First it becomes pale, and then turns blue. Eventually the skin will turn red once blood flow returns.

Sciatica- irritation and inflammation of the sciatic nerve (spinal nerve roots L4-S3). _Red Flag symptoms include: low back pain, pain in the gluteal region, pain down the back of the leg- possibly into the foot, muscle weakness or numbness in leg or foot._ Sciatica can be caused by disc herniation, piriformis spasm, and can be seen during pregnancy.

Seizure- temporary disorder of the cerebrum, causing abnormal involuntary movements, unusual sensations, and/or inappropriate behavior. They may lose consciousness. In 50% of people, no known cause. In others the cause could be due to infection, brain trauma, brain damage, stroke, genetic factors, poisoning. Drugs like barbiturates, Dilantin, and other anticonvulsants can be used for treatment. Two main types of generalized seizures: **Grand mal seizure-** powerful uncontrollable contractions of the eye, face, limbs. Loss of consciousness. Seizure begins in one area of the brain but then spreads to the rest of the brain. There may be no warning. After the attack the individual may be disoriented or exhausted. **Petit mal seizure-** very brief, less than 10 seconds. Involve few motor abnormalities. May have loss of consciousness, with no warning. Can occur up to hundreds of times per day.

Shingles – an infection by the *Varicella-Zoster virus*—the same virus that causes chicken pox. After having chicken pox, some of the virus may remain alive but become dormant and live in the dorsal root ganglia. Later (years) during times of stress or if an individual becomes immunocompromised the virus may become active. It will cause painful red blisters along the entire dermatome of the infected nerve.

Sleep Apnea- Obstructive Sleep Apnea- occlusion of the throat or upper airway. **Central Sleep Apnea** is caused by dysfunction in the respiratory area of the brain (brain stem). Symptoms may be snoring, dry mouth at night, gasping, choking, and pauses in breathing. Oxygen levels in the blood can plummet while carbon dioxide levels can climb. Drugs, obesity, alcohol use can increase symptoms. This can cause cardiac problems. Is often treated with a machine called the CPAP (continuous positive airway pressure). On a physical examination of the throat, enlarged pharyngeal tonsils may be seen in some individuals.

Spina Bifida: This is the most common neural tube defect and will begin in the third week of embryonic development. This condition occurs as the vertebrae are forming around the neural tube. In this condition, the spinal cord grows in an abnormal shape, and the vertebral arches are unable to form around the spinal cord. The vertebra now does not offer protection to the spinal cord, and the meninges (the outer membranes which cover the spinal cord) bulge outwards. Most common in the thoracic, lumbar or sacral regions. Heredity and maternal diet play a role. It is now recommended that a pregnant woman take 400-800 micrograms of folic acid a day. In mild cases, the open gap in the vertebra can be corrected surgically. In severe cases, the brain or spinal cord may not develop properly and death may occur.

Spinal Trauma: Trauma to the spine can cause different pathologies. **Spinal Shock**- trauma to the spinal cord, may cause a period of sensory loss and motor paralysis. Recovery depends on the severity of trauma and location of injury. **Spinal Concussion**- trauma near the spine may cause temporary spinal shock. There is no actual damage to the spinal cord, so recovery usually occurs. **Spinal Contusion**- damage to the spinal cord from hemorrhages in the meninges. The pressure may damage some of the white matter of the spinal cord. Partial recovery may occur. **Spinal laceration**- part of the spinal cord is cut, and the area damaged will lose its function. Recovery is more difficult. **Spinal Transection**- the entire spinal cord is severed. There are no surgical methods to repair this. Damage is permanent. **Paraplegia**- loss of the use of both legs, usually due to spinal cord damage in the thoracic region. **Quadriplegia**- loss of the use of arms and legs, usually due to cervical spinal cord damage.

Suicidal Depression- _Red Flag symptoms_ *that a person may be suicidal: they appear sad, depressed, anxious, hopeless about life, talking about death, sleep difficulties (insomnia or sleeping all the time), feeling failure, mood swings, withdrawing from family/friends, and abusing drugs/alcohol. They may give away important possessions, get affairs in order, start purchasing things that may harm themselves (weapons, pills), engage in reckless behavior and call/post messages that may insinuate saying goodbye.* Suicide hotlines (local and national) are available for immediate help for someone who is feeling that they may harm themselves (1-800 SUICIDE, for example). Calling 911 is appropriate if you are concerned that another person may harm themselves.

Tic Douloureux (Trigeminal Neuralgia)- severe, often debilitating facial pain. Occurs very suddenly and then disappears. This condition is caused by irritation of the trigeminal cranial nerve (usually unilateral). Usually evaluated by a MRI or CT scan to look for a tumor as a potential cause.

Transient ischemic attack (TIA) – a temporary restriction of blood flow to a part of the brain. _Red Flag symptoms_ *are: temporary numbness, paralysis, and impaired speech.* TIAs could indicate an impending CVA (cerebrovascular accident- "stroke").

Traumatic Brain Injuries (TBI) - 1.5 million cases of TBI every year in the US. Of those, approximately 50,000 people die, and 80,000 have long term disability. There can be varying degrees and types of brain injuries.
- **Concussion**- is a transient condition. _Red Flag symptoms_: *may have temporary loss of consciousness, headache, difficulty with mental processes (thinking clearly, memory, and concentration), nausea/vomiting, blurred vision, vertigo, fatigue and sleep changes.* Often times no permanent damage. Usually the mildest form of injury to the brain. X-ray or CT may be used in assessment.
- **Contusion**- more severe concussion or brain injury. Brain tissue is actually bruised. Internal bleeding may occur. Possibility of recovery will vary according to the amount of damage sustained.
- **Laceration**- a cut or tear of the brain tissue. Possibility of recovery will vary according to the amount of damage sustained

Upper Motor Neuron Lesion- Results from brain or spinal cord damage to an Upper Motor Neuron. This will result in muscular dysfunction. Muscles will be spastic and reflexes will be hyper-reflexive.

Vertigo- is an inappropriate sense of motion. _Red Flag symptoms_- *often felt as a spinning sensation or "dizziness".* Some causes of vertigo are: abnormal conditions in the inner ear, CNS infections, high fever, endolymph movement, Meniere's disease, alcohol and drugs, viral infection of the vestibular nerve, and motion sickness. Some cases of vertigo have an unknown cause.

Practice Study and Test Questions:

1) What symptoms might a patient have if they suffered a stroke in the left frontal lobe?
   A) blindness in the left eye
   B) left side weakness and/or paralysis in the body
   C) the loss of the sense of smell
   D) right side weakness and/or paralysis in the body

2) Which physical examination test is performed to assess cerebellar functioning?
   A) dermatomal testing
   B) sterognosis
   C) Glascow scale
   D) Romberg's test

3) What imaging test might be used in diagnosis of a stroke patient?
   A) myelogram
   B) electroencephalogram
   C) CT angiography
   D) PET scan

4) There are ___ pairs of cranial nerves and ___ pairs of spinal nerves.
   A) 31; 12
   B) 12; 31
   C) 10; 24
   D) 15; 9

5) Brudzinski's sign can be indicative of
   A) a stroke
   B) meningitis
   C) multiple sclerosis
   D) Bell's palsy

6) The Planes of Gaze test will evaluate which cranial nerves?
   A) trochlear
   B) cranial nerve VI
   C) occulomotor
   D) all of the above

7) Spastic muscles and hyperreflexia may be signs of a/an
   A) cerebellar tumor
   B) lower motor neuron lesion
   C) stroke in the occipital lobe
   D) upper motor neuron lesion

8) Bell's palsy is a pathology involving cranial nerve
   A) V
   B) VII
   C) III
   D) IX

9) Pain, tingling or numbness following the path of a single dermatomal level can indicate
   A) stroke
   B) concussion
   C) multiple sclerosis
   D) radiculopathy

10) Sensation of the thumb is controlled by which spinal nerve
   A) C6
   B) C3
   C) T4
   D) L1

11) What condition causes the patient to fluctuate between feelings of deep sadness, lethargy, guilt; and then periods of time where they feel overly happy, energized, and have impulsive behaviors?
   A) bipolar disorder
   B) depression
   C) ADHD
   D) generalized anxiety disorder

12) What can cause vertigo?
   A) Meniere's disease
   B) ear infection
   C) high fever
   D) all of the above

13) A patient has a diminished patellar reflex on physical examination. How should this finding be documented?
   A) 4+
   B) 2+
   C) 1+
   D) 0

14) Levodopa or Sinemet (levodopa/carbidopa) may be used to treat
   A) Myasthenia gravis
   B) Raynaud's disease
   C) Multiple sclerosis
   D) Parkinson's disease

15) The insulating substance which covers the axon region in some neurons is called
   A) troponin
   B) myelin
   C) ganglion
   D) axoplasm

16) The diaphragm is controlled by the
   A) sciatic nerve
   B) phrenic nerve
   C) femoral nerve
   D) radial nerve

Answers: 1) D 2) D 3) C 4) B 5) B 6) D 7) D 8) B 9) D 10) A 11) A 12) D 13) C 14) D 15) B 16) B

CHAPTER 7: THE SPECIAL SENSES: OLFACTION, GUSTATION, VISION, EQUILIBRIUM AND HEARING

The five special senses discussed in this chapter are: olfaction (smell), gustation (taste), vision, equilibrium, and hearing.

Olfaction:

The sense of smell (olfaction) begins with the olfactory organs in the nasal cavity. The olfactory organs contain two layers. The more superficial layer is the **olfactory epithelium**. This layer contains the *olfactory receptors* (neuron receptors from Cranial Nerve I) and *basal cells* (regenerative stem cells). Deep to the olfactory epithelium lies the lamina propria. Here you will find blood vessels, nerves, and olfactory glands (mucus producing glands).

Olfactory Pathway:

The olfactory receptors detect odorant molecules. Axons leaving the olfactory epithelium will bundle together, penetrate through the ethmoid bone of the skull and end in the olfactory bulb in the brain. The message is then passed from the olfactory bulb to the olfactory cortex in the temporal lobe of the brain. Olfactory messages will also pass through the hypothalamus and limbic system on their way to the temporal lobe for final processing. The olfactory system can discern between 2000-4000 chemical stimuli. Olfactory receptor cells can regenerate and be replaced by basal cells in the olfactory epithelium. However, this process slows with age, and as we get older, we are less able to produce new receptor cells to maintain olfaction. Therefore, the sense of acute olfaction in an elderly person is less than someone in their younger years.

Gustation (Taste)

The surface of the tongue is covered with epithelial projections called **lingual papillae**. There are three types of lingual papillae. **Filiform papillae** are thread-like papillae which do not contain taste buds, but assist in moving food in the mouth. **Fungiform papillae** are mushroom shaped papillae and each papillae contains about 5 taste buds. **Circumvallate papillae** are large rounded papillae that contain as many as 100 taste buds. They form a V near the posterior aspect of the tongue.

Taste Receptors

Taste receptors (specialized nerve endings) and specialized epithelial cells form the *taste buds*. An adult has an average of 3000 taste buds. These cells begin as *basal cells* (stem cells) and gradually mature into *gustatory cells*. Each gustatory cell only survives for about 10 days before it is replaced. Three cranial nerves monitor the activity of the taste buds. Cranial Nerve VII (Facial Nerve) carries messages from taste buds on the anterior 2/3 of the tongue. Cranial Nerve IX (Glossopharyngeal Nerve) carries messages from the posterior 1/3 of the tongue. The Vagus Nerve (Cranial Nerve X) detects messages from a small number of taste receptors on the epiglottis in the larynx. These cranial nerves carry their messages into the medulla oblongata, then the thalamus, and on to final processing in the insula region of the cerebral cortex.

There are five taste sensations that the tongue can detect: sweet, salty, sour, bitter and umami. Out of the taste sensations, we are almost a thousand times more sensitive to acids (sour) tasting substances than sweet or salty, and 100 times more sensitive to bitter than sweet or salty. This is because acidic substances potentially could burn our digestive lining and bitter substances often are toxic. We begin life with more than 1000 taste buds, but the number begins to dramatically decline by age 50.

Vision

The Eye:

The wall of the eye consists of three distinct layers, or tunics: The outer layer is called the **fibrous tunic**. It is composed of the *sclera*, or the white area of the eye. The six muscles of the eyeball attach onto the sclera. There are blood vessels and nerves that penetrate the sclera and go deeper into the eye. The *cornea* is also a part of the fibrous tunic and is a transparent covering over the iris and pupil. It is continuous with the sclera. It has no blood vessels, but a lot of nerve endings and is the most sensitive structure of the eye. Damage here can cause blindness.

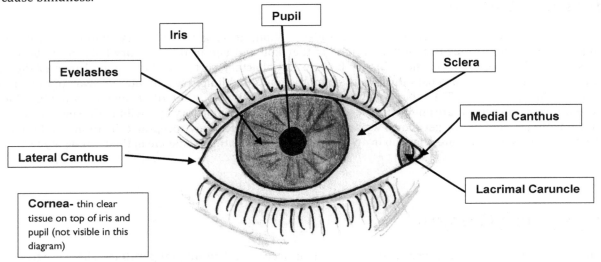

The intermediate (middle) layer is called the **vascular tunic** (or **uvea**). It contains the *iris* (pigmented/colored area of eye), *ciliary body* (muscles and ligaments which hold the lens, and also produces aqueous humor), and *choroid* (blood rich vascular layer which delivers oxygen to the retina).

The innermost layer of the eye is the **neural tunic** or **retina**. This layer contains the visual receptors (photoreceptors). *Rods* detect levels of light (to help us see in a dimly lit room) and are located more around the periphery of the retina. *Cones* help us detect color- and are located more towards the center of the retina. The cones need a significant amount of light in order to work properly. Cones give us sharper images than rods. The *Macula Lutea* (yellow spot) is an area in the retina where there are no rods, only cones. The center of the macula lutea is called the *fovea* (or *fovea centralis*), and this is the area of sharpest vision. The optic disc is the origin of the optic nerve (Cranial Nerve II) and contains no photoreceptors. Therefore it is called the *blind spot*.

INTERIOR VIEW OF THE EYE

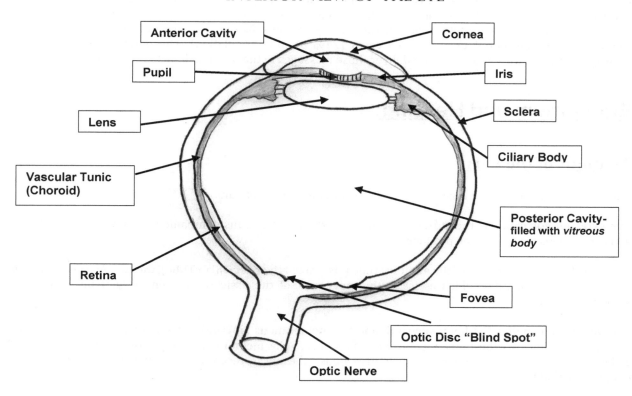

The inside of the eyeball is hollow and can be divided into two cavities. These spaces are separated by the ciliary body/muscle and lens. The **posterior cavity** is a large cavity, which sits behind the lens of the eye-and is also called the *vitreous chamber*. It contains a gelatinous substance called the *vitreous body/humor*. The vitreous body helps to stabilize the shape of the eye. The **anterior cavity** is anterior to the lens, is smaller in size and is subdivided into the anterior and posterior chamber. Both chambers are filled with a fluid called *aqueous humor*. Pressure from the aqueous humor helps to hold the retina in place.

The transparent **lens** of the eye is posterior to the cornea and iris, and is held in place by the suspensory ligaments of the ciliary body. The function of the lens is to focus an image on the focal point of the photoreceptors in the retina (the fovea of the macula lutea). Focusing the image onto the focal point is a changing process which depends on the distance of the object to the lens and the shape of the lens. Therefore, the lens must be able to adapt and change shape depending on the distance of the object we are looking at. The lens will be pulled by the ciliary body and suspensory ligaments to change its shape. For an object that is close to the eye, the lens becomes rounder in shape to focus the image on the focal point in the retina. For an object further away from the eye, the lens will flatten to focus the object appropriately. This process is called *accommodation*. When the image is transmitted to the retina it is reversed. The image will look upside down and backwards. The brain then re-orients the image properly when it processes the visual image.

Visual Physiology:

The **photoreceptors** (**rods** and **cones**) each contain two main anatomical segments: the outer and inner segment. The *outer segment* of the rods and cones is what gives them their names. The outer segment of the rod is more oblong shaped, while the cone tapers at the top. Visual pigments such as *rhodopsin* (opsin and retinal) are stored here. Rhodopsin is sometimes called "visual purple" and is composed of Vitamin A. The *inner segment* of the photoreceptors contain all of the cellular organelles (ribosomes, mitochondria, Golgi apparatus, etc.).

Rods provide images that are less clear and detailed- more "fuzzy" images, and only deliver images in black and white. They are used for seeing in low light levels. Cones provide images that are more crisp, detailed, and in color. Color vision is determined by three types of cones: *blue cones* (16% of cone population), *green cones* (10% of cone population) and *red cones* (74% of cone population). The optic nerve will pick up messages from the rods and cones and deliver those messages to the occipital lobe of the cerebral cortex.

Equilibrium and Hearing:

Anatomy of the Ear:

The ear is divided into three regions: the external, middle, and inner ear.

The **external ear** contains the auricle, external acoustic canal, meatus, tympanic membrane "the eardrum", and ceruminous glands (which produce earwax).

The **middle ear** is composed of the auditory tube (also called the Eustachian Tube), the *ossicles* (*malleus, incus* and *stapes*), and muscles which assist in the movement of the ossicles- the tensor tympani muscle and stapedius muscle.

The **inner ear** contains the bony labyrinth and the membranous labyrinth. The bony labyrinth is the outer covering, and encases the inner membranous labyrinth. The membranous labyrinth is filled with a fluid called endolymph. These inner ear structures house the nerve receptors that will detect our senses of equilibrium and hearing.

Equilibrium

To measure our sense of equilibrium, we will utilize a few structures located in the inner ear. The **semicircular canals and ducts** measure rotational movement of the head. There are three ducts, each angled in a different directional plane: **anterior, posterior** and **lateral semicircular ducts**. These ducts are filled with a fluid called *endolymph. Hair cells* line the inside of the ducts and will detect movement of the endolymph. With the three semicircular ducts angled to detect three planes of motion, each one will have endolymph movement when the head rotates in a specific direction. Shaking your head "no", will create movement in the endolymph of the lateral semicircular duct, and stimulate the hair cells in that duct. Nodding "yes" will stimulate the hair cells in the anterior duct, and tilting your head from side to side will activate the posterior duct.

Two other structures are located in the **vestibule** of the inner ear- the **utricle** and **saccule**- are also used in equilibrium. They determine if the body is moving or stationary. The Utricle and Saccule also contain hair cells which are embedded in a gelatinous mass with calcium crystals. These calcium crystals are called *statoconia* (also can be called *otoliths* or *otoconia*). When the head is upright, the statoconia press directly down through the matrix on the hair cells. When your head is tilted, the statoconia press on the hair cells at an angle. Those messages tell the brain that your head is not level. Your brain will also use information from your eyes and musculoskeletal proprioceptors to fully process the position of the body. Hair cells from the semicircular ducts, utricle and saccule feed messages into the vestibular branch of the vestibulocochlear nerve (Cranial Nerve VIII). The vestibulocochlear nerve will carry messages to the vestibular nuclei in the brainstem, and finally to the cerebellum.

Hearing:

The main organ of hearing is the **cochlea.** The cochlea is a coiled, elongated tube-like structure and is filled with a fluid called *perilymph*. The cochlea contains hair cells, similar to the semicircular ducts. These hair cells are located in the **organ of Corti**. The organ of Corti and hair cells sit on top of the basilar membrane, and then the tectorial membrane sits like a roof on top of the hair cells. (The hair cells are basically sandwiched between the basilar membrane and tectorial membrane). When sound vibrations enter, they cause the basilar membrane to bounce, which pushes the hair cell up into the underside of the tectorial membrane. The stimulation of the hair cells will create an action potential. This action potential will be carried to the temporal lobe of the brain.

The hearing process occurs in six steps:
1. Sound waves arrive at the Tympanic Membrane, causing it to vibrate.
2. Movement of the tympanic membrane causes displacement of the Auditory Ossicles (malleus, incus and stapes). Tympanic membrane moves the malleus. The malleus then strikes the incus and causes it to move. The incus then moves the stapes.
3. Movement of the stapes at the oval window causes pressure waves in the perilymph of the vestibular duct.
4. The pressure waves distort and vibrate the basilar membrane in the cochlea
5. Vibration of the basilar membrane causes vibration of the hair cells against the tectorial membrane
6. This stimulation of the hair cells is relayed to the CNS via the Cochlear Branch of the Vestibulocochlear Nerve (Cranial Nerve VIII). The temporal lobe of the cerebral cortex does final processing of the auditory messages.

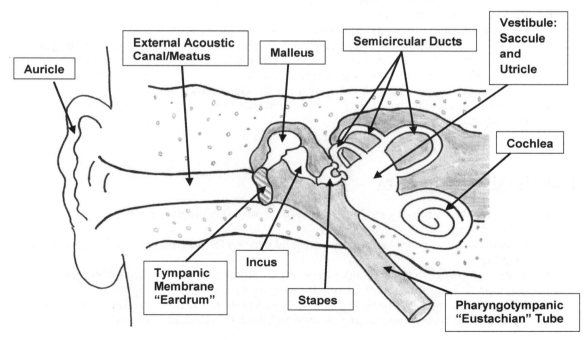

INTERIOR VIEW OF THE EAR

Physical Examination of the Head, Neck and EENT (Eyes, Ears, Nose, and Throat)

Examination of the Head

1. Inspect/observe the skull and face for contour, symmetry, facial expressions
2. Palpate the skull for any tenderness, lumps, nodules, edema

Examination of the Eyes

1. Inspect/observe the eyes for position and alignment of the eyes.
2. Inspect eyebrow position and skin around eyebrow
3. Inspect eyelids of each eye for swelling or redness, position of the upper eyelid on the eye and drooping of the lower eyelid
4. Inspect the conjunctiva, sclera, cornea and iris of each eye
5. Inspect the pupil of each eye for size, for direct and consensual response to light, and accommodation
6. Palpate the nasolacrimal duct
7. Test the extraocular muscles (the "planes of gaze"). This test evaluates the extraocular muscles and the cranial nerves that control them
   - Cranial Nerve IV- Superior Oblique muscle
   - Cranial Nerve VI- Lateral Rectus muscle
   - Cranial Nerve III- Medial Rectus, Superior Rectus, Inferior Oblique, Inferior Rectus
8. Perform corneal light reflex
9. Perform Visual Acuity Tests: Snellen Eye Chart and Rosenbaum Near Vision Chart
   - Visual acuity is recorded as a fraction. The top number is the distance the patient is from the object (20). The bottom number is the distance from which a normal person could read the letters in that line. The larger the bottom number, the poorer the patient's vision. This bottom number is obtained by using the charts listed above.
10. Examine intraocular structures (red reflex, cornea, lens, retina, retinal blood vessels, optic disc, macula) using an opthalmoscope

Examination of the Ears

1. Inspect/observe the outer ear structures for position, symmetry, masses, lumps, drainage, bleeding, inflammation
2. Palpate the outer ear structures and mastoid process for masses, pain on movement, warmth and swelling.
3. Examine internal structures of the ear using an otoscope. Note presence of cerumen, shape and color of tympanic membrane, malleus, and the tympanic light reflex.
4. Perform Hearing tests (using 512 Hz tuning fork): **Weber test** (tests lateralization) and **Rinne test** (tests air and bone conduction). These tests help assess Cranial Nerve VIII

Examination of the Nose and Sinuses

1. Inspect the external nose and observe position, symmetry, color, growths, lesions, swelling, discharge or nasal flaring
2. Palpate external nose for tenderness, swelling or deformity
3. Inspect internal nose structures using an otoscope with speculum or a penlight. Observe the color of the nostril and the patency of the airway, look for any masses or polyps and observe any secretions (mucus, blood)
4. Inspect and palpate the sinuses

Examination of the Mouth and Throat

1. Inspect the mouth: lips, oral mucosa, gums (gingiva), teeth, and tongue
2. Inspect the throat (oropharynx)
3. Palpate lips and tongue for any lumps or edema
4. Elicit gag reflex

Examination of the Neck

1. Inspect the patient's neck
2. Palpate patient's neck- the lymph nodes, trachea and thyroid
3. Auscultate the neck over the carotid arteries

General Abnormal Findings of EENT and Neck

Abnormal findings, if necessary, should be referred to patient's PCP, an ophthalmologist, or otolaryngologist (ENT specialist)

Eye

Ptosis- drooping of upper eyelid- could be a result of myasthenia gravis, Horner's syndrome, eye muscle weakness, damage to oculomotor nerve (Cranial Nerve III)

Direct Response (of the pupil): In a slightly darkened room, shine a penlight in the right eye. Watch the pupil on the right eye react (it should constrict). This is a direct response. Repeat and test the left eye. Abnormal response would be no pupil constriction. This could indicate a problem with Cranial Nerve III.

Consensual Response (of the pupil): In a slightly darkened room, shine a penlight in the right eye. Watch the pupil on the opposite side react (it should constrict). This is a consensual response. Repeat and test the left eye. Abnormal response would be no pupil constriction. This could indicate a problem with Cranial Nerve III.

Accommodation (of the pupil)- Place one finger 4" in front of the bridge of the patient's nose. Have the patient look at an object far away. Then have them look at your finger. The pupils should constrict in both eyes and the eyes should converge. Abnormal response would be no constriction and/or no convergence.

Miosis- constriction of the pupil

Mydriasis- dilation of the pupil

Enlarged Palpebral Fissure- increased space between upper eyelid and iris of the eye. Due to retraction of eyelids or exophthalmoses, both are a result of hyperthyroidism

Amblyopia- "lazy eye". Decreased vision in one eye because the brain is favoring the other. Most common vision impairment in childhood

Strabismus- "cross eye"

Nystagmus- rapid uncontrollable movements of the eye. Can be up and down ("vertical nystagmus") or from side to side ("horizontal nystagmus")

Arteriolar narrowing- narrowing of internal eye blood vessels, seen with ophthalmoscope- indicates hypertension

Myopia- (nearsightedness)- eye focuses visual image in front of the retina inside of the eye. Images close up are seen clearly, distant images are fuzzy

Hyperopia- (farsightedness)- eye focuses visual image behind the retina. Images farther away are seen clearly, closer images are fuzzy.

Diplopia- double vision

Presbyopia- similar to hyperopia, often seen as a result of aging. As we age, the lens loses the flexibility and ability to accommodate.

Decreased visual acuity- loss of vision, which can be caused by many factors.
- Gradual visual blurring, with halo vision, visual glare in bright light, and a gray colored pupil that eventually turns milky- is a result of *cataracts*
- Gradual vision loss, constant morning headache (which decreases throughout the day), restlessness, confusion, and/or seizures can all be a result of uncontrolled *hypertension*
- Decreased visual acuity with attacks of severe throbbing headache (either unilateral or bilateral), nausea and vomiting, sensitivity to light and noise, and/or visual auras can all be symptoms of *migraines*

Kayser Fleisher rings- a rusty brown ring around the edge of the iris of the eye. The most common sign of *Wilson's Disease* (a build-up of excessive copper levels in the blood).

Ear:

Earache- can be due to issues in external and middle ear usually.
- Earache with feeling of fullness or blockage, itching, partial hearing loss, possible dizziness- can be due to *cerumen impaction*
- Earache with tragus stimulation, low grade fever, sticky or purulent discharge from the ear, and swelling of the tragus and external meatus- can be due to *otitis externa*
- Earache with severe, deep pain, hearing loss, high fever, bulging eardrum (on otoscope exam) is usually- *acute otitis media*

Otorrhea- drainage from the ear. Can be bloody, purulent, or clear and may occur alone or with other symptoms (pain, hearing loss). Can be a result of trauma, allergies, infection, neoplasms

Weber test (tests lateralization)- Examiner will strike tuning fork (causing it to vibrate) and places it on top of the patients head in the midline position. In a sensorineural type of hearing loss, sound will travel and be heard more strongly in the good ear. In a conductive type of hearing loss, the sound will travel towards the poor ear.
- *Normal response=* patient hears sound equally in both ears
- *Right lateralization=* patient hears sound strongly in right ear
- *Left lateralization=* patient hears sound strongly in left ear

Rinne test (tests air and bone conduction). Examiner will strike tuning fork (causing it to vibrate) and places it on the mastoid process behind the ear. The examiner will ask the patient to report when they can no longer hear the sound- and note that time in seconds. This is the *bone conducted tone.* After the patient reports that they no longer hear the sound, the examiner will move the still vibrating tuning fork in front of the ear opening. The patient should be able to hear the sound again. The examiner will note the length of time the patient can hear the tuning fork in this position. This is the *air conducted tone.*
- *Normal response=* Air conducted tone should be twice as long as the bone conducted tone
- *Conductive Hearing Loss=* bone conducted tone is heard as long or longer than air conducted tone
- *Sensorineural hearing loss-* air conducted tone is longer than bone conducted tone, but not as long as in a normal scenario

Tympanic light reflex: using an otoscope, the examiner will view the tympanic membrane. Light will reflect off of the tympanic membrane.
- In the right ear, a band of light should reflect off of the tympanic membrane between the 4:00 and 6:00 position.
- In the left ear, a band of light should reflect off of the tympanic membrane between the 6:00 and 8:00 position.
- If the light reflex is positioned anywhere else, it can indicate that the eardrum could be bulged, retracted or inflamed

Mouth, Nose and Throat:

Cheilosis- fissuring and scales on the lips and the angles (corners) of the mouth.

Epistaxis- "nosebleed" Can occur spontaneously or be a direct result of: dry mucus membranes, trauma, septal deviation, coagulation or renal disorders, certain drugs and/or the as the result of medical treatments

Glossitis- swelling of the tongue. The tongue may also change color (pale or red) and the surface of the tongue may appear smooth.

Nasal obstruction- increased difficulty breathing through the nose. Many causes:
- Nasal obstruction with watery nasal discharge, sneezing, temporary loss of taste and smell, sore throat, malaise, and mild headache can all be a result of the *common cold*
- Nasal obstruction with loss of smell, watery discharge, presence of pear-shaped masses in nasal cavity, and history of allergies, trauma, or cystic fibrosis- can indicate *nasal polyps*
- Nasal obstruction with thick purulent discharge, pain over sinus area, fever, inflamed nasal mucosa- all can indicate *sinusitis*

Dysphagia- difficulty swallowing, could be a result of many things (example: cranial nerve IX or X damage, esophageal cancer)

Advanced Imaging and Diagnostic Tests of the Eyes, Ears, Nose and Throat

Audiometry- Patient wears headphones and listens to tones in different frequencies and volumes. This test assesses the ability to hear and distinguish sounds at specific pitches and volumes.

Auscultation- The examiner listens with a stethoscope for abnormal blood vessel sounds in the carotid artery

Non-contact tonometry- Used to help diagnose glaucoma. The tonometer produces a "puff of air" on the eye. The tonometer then measures eye pressure

Applanation tonometry- Used to help diagnose glaucoma. Is more specific than non-contact tonometry. Anesthetic drops are given to the eye and then the tip of the tonometer touches the eye, reading the pressure.

Corneal and Retinal Topography- These are computerized maps which show the surface of the cornea or retina. Used to show distortions of the eye (astigmatism, scarring, retinal detachment, macular degeneration). May be done before refractive surgery or for fitting of contact lenses.

Fluorescein Angiogram- evaluates blood circulation in the eye. Just like other angiograms, a dye (fluorescein) is injected into the bloodstream (usually through a vein in the arm). The dye travels through the bloodstream and can be viewed in the blood vessels in the back of the eye. Used in diagnosing or monitoring patients with diabetic retinopathy, retinal detachment and macular degeneration.

Sinus Endoscopy- A flexible viewing tube is inserted into the sinuses to view the inner lining and internal sinus chamber.

Rapid Strep Test- A throat infection with streptococcus bacteria ("strep throat") can be treated with an antibiotic. The traditional test for a strep throat has been a throat culture, which takes two to three days to produce results. Several different types of rapid strep tests, however, can produce results within minutes to hours. A rapid strep test can only detect the presence of Group A strep, the one most likely to cause serious throat infections; it does not detect other kinds of strep or other bacteria. A cotton swab is rubbed against the back of the throat to gather a sample of mucus. This takes only a second or two and makes some patients feel a brief gagging or choking sensation. The mucus sample is then tested for a protein that comes from the Group A strep bacteria.

Tympanometry- Measurement of the impedance of the middle ear, which helps in determining the cause of hearing loss.

Ophthalmoscopy- An ophthalmoscope is a hand held instrument with an angled mirror, lenses and a light source. The light is shone into the eye and the doctor can observe the internal structures in the eye by looking through the lenses.

Otoscope (also called **auriscope**)- a handheld device used to examine structures inside the ear. It can also be used to examine structures in the nose or mouth. It has a light source, a magnifying lens and a (usually disposable) speculum. The speculum portion is narrowed and is placed in the external canal of the ear.

Pathologies of the Special Senses, Throat and Neck

For additional infectious diseases that may affect this system, please refer to the Communicable/Infectious Disease Chart in Chapter 10.

Age Related Macular Degeneration- most commonly due to the thinning of the macula portion of the retina of the eye (called "dry" macular degeneration). As this thinning occurs, vision is gradually lost. Symptoms can include gradual loss of vision, vision becomes distorted, and/or a dark area appears in the center of the patient's visual field. This is the leading cause of vision loss in patients over the age of 50. No known treatment for "dry" macular degeneration. Nutritional supplementation of certain nutrients may lower the risk of developing some eye conditions (Vitamin C, E, zinc and lutein).

Allergies (*hypersensitivities*) – an abnormally vigorous immune response. This occurs when the immune system causes tissue damage as it fights off a perceived "threat" that would otherwise be harmless to the body. These "threats" or *allergens* can include pet dander, pollen, dust, etc. The immune system will release histamine as it fights and destroys the allergen. The histamine release can cause the symptoms of the allergic response. Symptoms in the head and neck typically include a runny nose, watery eyes, swollen eyes, and itching, reddened skin. If the allergen is inhaled, symptoms of asthma may appear. Scratch tests (see integumentary system) may be done for diagnosis. Treatment may include over the counter or prescription allergy medications (Benadryl, Claritin, Flonase, Nasonex). For an anaphylaxic reaction (a life threatening allergic reaction), epinephrine may be administered- usually in an injectable form ("EPI-pen").

Astigmatism- occurs when light passing through the cornea and lens is not refracted properly. This can be due to an abnormally shaped cornea or if the lens is curved abnormally and is not symmetrical. Corrective lenses or contacts are commonly prescribed for treatment

Cataracts- are when the lens of the eye loses its transparency, becoming cloudy. Can be due to injuries, radiation, drug reactions, and/or aging. A lens replacement may need to be done if significant loss of vision or blindness results.

Color Blindness- occurs when one or more classes of cones are non-functional. The most common type is red-green color blindness (where red cones are missing and a person cannot tell the difference between red and green colors). Inherited color blindness is a common cause. 10% of men show some color blindness, where only 0.67% of women do.

Conductive Deafness- is due to conditions in the outer or middle ear that block or dampen the transmission of sound waves. Wax build-up or trapped water in the external canal can be a cause of temporary conductive deafness. Scarring or perforation of the tympanic membrane may be a permanent cause. Fused ear ossicles could be another cause. Surgery to patch a tympanic membrane rupture or to repair fused ossicles may be done.

Conjunctivitis- (sometimes called "*pink eye*") - can be caused by an allergen (not contagious), bacteria (contagious) or viruses (contagious) and *discharge from the eye which can dry and form crusting on the eyelashes or eyelids.* Treatment depends on the cause. Viral conjunctivitis usually needs to just run its course. Bacterial conjunctivitis may be treated with antibiotics. Allergic conjunctivitis improves if the allergen is removed.

Glaucoma- Due to the aqueous humor being unable to drain from the anterior chamber of the eye. Usually is a result of a blockage of the canal of Schlemm. Eye pressure increases, which may damage the optic nerve. Drugs may be prescribed to help with the drainage of aqueous humor, or surgery can be done to perforate the wall of the anterior chamber to encourage drainage.

Goiter- an enlargement of the thyroid gland, often due to an iodine deficiency. If an enlargement is seen in the thyroid, it could be a goiter (non-cancerous enlargement) or possibly thyroid cancer. Further testing should be done to confirm cause of enlargement of the thyroid (usually done via a biopsy).

Hyperopia- occurs when the lens of the eye is too flat. The visual image entering the eye is projected behind the retina (making the image appear blurry or distorted). This person is "far-sighted"- can see far away, but not close up. Corrective lenses can be used for treatment. LASIK can be performed to reshape the lens.

Legal blindness- occurs when visual acuity falls below 20/200. Normal visual acuity is 20/20

Meniere's Disease- occurs when the membranous labyrinth of the inner ear is distorted by high fluid pressures. The wall of the membranous labyrinth may rupture and endolymph and perilymph may mix. Receptors in the vestibule and semicircular canals may become overly stimulated, leading to intense spinning or rolling sensations. It may also cause auditory disturbances such as "ringing" in the ears. Diuretics and low sodium diets may be prescribed to lower fluid levels in the inner ear.

Myopia- where the lens of the eye is too curved. This causes the visual image entering the eye to fall short of the retina (making the image appear blurry or distorted). This person is "near-sighted". Corrective lenses can be used for treatment. LASIK can be performed to reshape the lens.

Nerve Deafness- This type of hearing loss is due to a problem with the cochlea or somewhere along the auditory nerve pathway. Loud sounds can damage the hair cells in the cochlea causing them to be unable to respond to sound stimuli. Drugs such as the aminoglycoside antibiotics (neomycin and gentamicin) may kill hair cells in the cochlea. A cochlear implant may be done for treatment.

Otitis Media- infection of the middle ear, often caused by bacteria. Commonly seen in children and infants. Pain, dizziness can be a symptom. Bacterial otitis media can be treated with antibiotics. Viral otitis media (less common) cannot be treated with antibiotics. Rupture of the tympanic membrane can be a complication.

Presbyopia- "far-sightedness" in an elderly person. This is a result of the lens becoming inflexible as we age. This makes it difficult for the person to read items close up. (They might hold a book or menu far away from their body to try to read it). Corrective lenses might be prescribed, or the person might utilize "reading glasses" that can be purchased over the counter at a drug store.

Sinusitis- inflammation of a sinus. Most commonly caused by an infection (bacterial or viral) or allergies. Symptoms can include nasal discharge, post-nasal drip, feeling pressure in the head and/or headache. Sinusitis of the frontal sinuses gives pain in the forehead. Pain in the upper jaw or teeth may indicate sinusitis in the maxillary sinuses. Pain or pressure in the bridge of the nose (between the eyes), may indicate sinusitis of the ethmoid sinus. Sinusitis can last from days (acute) to weeks or months (chronic).

Sleep Apnea- occlusion of the throat or upper airway occurs in *obstructive sleep apnea. Central sleep apnea* is caused by dysfunction in the respiratory area of the brain. Symptoms may be snoring, dry mouth at night, gasping, choking, and pauses in breathing. Oxygen levels in the blood can plummet while carbon dioxide levels can climb. Drugs, obesity, and alcohol use can increase symptoms. This can cause cardiac problems. Is often treated with a machine called the *CPAP (continuous positive airway pressure)*. On a physical examination of the throat, enlarged pharyngeal tonsils may be seen in some individuals.

Strep Throat- an infection caused by *Group A Streptococcus.* Symptoms: a sore throat, redness and swelling in the throat, white patches (pus) may be visible in the throat or on the tonsils, fever, pain with swallowing, swollen lymph nodes in the neck, and sometimes a rash. Having a sore throat does not automatically mean a patient has "strep throat"- a rapid strep test must be done to confirm Group A streptococcal infection (other pathogens, including viruses, can cause a sore throat). Antibiotics can be prescribed for a bacterial infection, if needed.

Vertigo- is an inappropriate sense of motion. <u>*Red Flag symptoms*</u>- *often felt as a spinning sensation or "dizziness".* Many causes, and some cases have an unknown cause. Some causes of vertigo are: abnormal conditions in the inner ear, CNS infections, high fever, endolymph movement, Meniere's disease, alcohol and drugs, viral infection of the vestibular nerve, and motion sickness.

Wilson's Disease- a rare inherited disease where the body accumulates excessively high levels of copper in the body. Normally, the liver will clear out excessive levels (by putting it into the bile for excretion), but in Wilson's disease, the genetic mutation causes to liver to be unable to do so. The excess copper will start to accumulate in body tissues (such as the eyes, brain, and kidney) leading to: muscular weakness, clumsiness, speech difficulty, depression. *Kayser Fleisher rings* in the eyes is the most common abnormal sign for Wilson's Disease on a physical exam.

Xeropthalmia- is the inability to see in low light (for example, at night- aka *"night blindness"*). This is the most common symptom of Vitamin A deficiency in children and pregnant women. In order to recycle and re-use the visual pigment rhodopsin, stores of vitamin A must be available for conversion into retinal. In night blindness, the amount of rhodopsin in the photoreceptors begins to decline due to being unable to recycle and form new pigments. If light levels are low (like at night) there may not be enough light to stimulate the few rhodopsin pigments remaining. Treatment- ingesting vitamin A and carotene pigments (for example- found in carrots) in foods or supplementation.

Practice Study and Test Questions:

1) The drooping of the upper eyelid is called
    A) ptosis
    B) miosis
    C) diplopia

2) Which of the following is a normal response when performing the Rinne test?
    A) air conducted tone is equal to the bone conducted tone
    B) bone conducted tone is twice as long as the air conducted tone
    C) bone conducted tone is three times as long as the air conducted tone
    D) air conducted tone is twice as long as the bone conducted tone

3) Semicircular ducts are used in
    A) detecting movements of our head
    B) our sense of hearing
    C) our sense of smell
    D) our sense of taste

4) Which diagnostic test may be used to diagnose glaucoma?
    A) tympanometry
    B) non-contact tonometry
    C) tympanic light reflex
    D) endoscopy

5) A distorted tympanic light reflex could indicate
    A) hypertension
    B) conduction deafness
    C) nerve deafness
    D) ear infection

6) Hyperopia is
    A) when the lens is too curved, causing the patient to be unable to see objects farther away
    B) when the lens is too flat, causing the patient to be unable to see objects farther away
    C) when the lens is too curved, causing the patient to be unable to see objects close up
    D) when the lens is too flat, causing the patient to be unable to see objects close up

7) Which structure of the eye detects color and higher detailed vision?
   A) cones
   B) rods
   C) cornea
   D) lens

8) Redness on the sclera of the eye, eye itching, and eye discharge may be signs of
   A) conjunctivitis
   B) myopia
   C) presbyopia
   D) night blindness

9) CPAP machines may be used in the treatment of
   A) glaucoma
   B) strep throat
   C) night blindness
   D) sleep apnea

10) Conductive deafness may be caused by
   A) wax build-up in ear canal
   B) scarring of tympanic membrane
   C) fused ear ossicles
   D) all of the above

11) An abnormally shaped cornea can cause
   A) "dry" macular degeneration
   B) cataracts
   C) astigmatism
   D) glaucoma

12) Legal blindness is when visual acuity falls below
   A) 20/100
   B) 20/200
   C) 20/50
   D) 20/20

13) What is the most common cause of blindness in patients over the age of 50?
   A) hyperopia
   B) presbyopia
   C) "dry" macular degeneration
   D) myopia

14) Dysphagia is noted during the physical exam. This could indicate damage to
   A) cranial nerve IX or X
   B) the tympanic membrane
   C) the lens
   D) cranial nerve II

15) The malleus is located in
   A) the inner ear
   B) the olfactory epithelium
   C) the middle ear
   D) the internal eye

Answers: 1) A 2) D 3) A 4) B 5) D 6) D 7) A 8) A 9) D 10) D 11) C 12) B 13) C 14) A 15) C

CHAPTER 8: THE ENDOCRINE SYSTEM

The two main control systems of the body are the Nervous System and Endocrine System. The nervous system is the primary control system of the body. It is very rapid, and uses electrical impulses to control bodily activity. The endocrine system is the second most important control system. It is slower acting, but longer lasting. To exert its effects, it uses chemical messengers called *hormones*

Hormones are produced by endocrine glands. Endocrine glands are ductless glands- meaning they release their secretions into the bloodstream or lymph for delivery. There are two main categories of hormones: **Amino Acid based** hormones are composed of proteins, peptides, or amines. **Steroid Based** hormones are composed of cholesterol. Once hormones are created, they are released into the blood or lymph. They then circulate through the entire body, reaching all organs and tissues. But, not every organ/tissue in contact with hormone-filled blood will respond. Protein markers on the cell membrane surface of tissues determine which hormones will have an effect on that specific tissue. The *Target tissue/ Target Organ* is the specific body tissue which responds to a specific hormone.

After a hormone binds to a target tissue/organ, these changes can occur: changes in plasma membrane permeability, protein synthesis, activation or inactivation of enzymes, and stimulation of mitosis. Most hormones are not produced continuously. Their production and release are under regulation. Negative feedback is the main regulator of hormone production and release. But, other stimuli can also influence the hormone levels in the body. The methods of stimulation for hormone release are as follows: *Hormonal stimuli* occurs when other hormones can stimulate an endocrine gland. *Humoral stimuli* is where levels of substances in the blood (ex: glucose, Na+, calcium) can influence endocrine gland and stimulate it to produce a hormone. *Neural stimuli* occurs when the nervous system can control endocrine gland production.

There are nine major endocrine glands in the body. In the brain region we have the: **Hypothalamus, Pituitary Gland** (divided into the **Anterior Lobe** and **Posterior Lobe**), and **Pineal Gland.** In the neck and thorax region we have the: **Thyroid Gland, Parathyroid Glands,** and **Thymus.** And, finally in the abdominopelvic region are located the: **Adrenal Glands** (divided into the **Adrenal Cortex** and the **Adrenal Medulla**), **Pancreas,** and **Gonads (Ovaries** and **Testes).**

HYPOTHALAMUS HORMONES

Hormone	Produced by / in:	Target cell or tissue	Hormonal effects
Releasing and Inhibiting Hormones	Hypothalamus	Anterior Lobe of the Pituitary	Regulate secretions of hormones by the anterior pituitary

PITUITARY GLAND HORMONES

Hormone	Produced by / in:	Target cell or tissue	Hormonal effects
Thyroid Stimulating Hormone (TSH)	Anterior Pituitary	Thyroid	Stimulates production of thyroid hormones
Adrenocorticotropic Hormone (ACTH)	Anterior Pituitary	Adrenal cortex	Stimulates secretion of adrenal cortex hormones
Follicle Stimulating Hormone (FSH)	Anterior Pituitary	Ovaries/ Testes (Gonadotropic)	♀: Estrogen & Egg Dev. ♂: Sperm Development
Luteinizing Hormone (LH)	Anterior Pituitary	Ovaries/ Testes (Gonadotropic)	♀: Ovulation and Progesterone ♂: Testosterone
Prolactin (PRL)	Anterior Pituitary	Mammary Glands	Stimulates milk *production*
Growth Hormone (GH)	Anterior Pituitary	Skeletal Muscle, Bones	Stimulates growth
Antidiuretic Hormone (ADH)	Produced by the *Hypothalamus*, but stored and released by the *Posterior Pituitary*	Kidneys (collecting ducts)	Stimulate H_2O reabsorption (decreases urine production)
Oxytocin (OT)	Produced by the *Hypothalamus*, but stored and released by the *Posterior Pituitary*	Uterus Mammary glands	Stimulates contraction (labor) Stimulates milk *ejection*

PINEAL GLAND HORMONES

Hormone	Produced by / in:	Target cell or tissue	Hormonal effects
Melatonin	Pinealocytes in Pineal Gland	Hypothalamus	Sleep rhythm. Makes you "drowsy"

THYROID GLAND HORMONES

Hormone	Produced by / in:	Target cell or tissue	Hormonal effects
Thyroxine (T4) and Triiodothyronine (T3)	Follicle cells in the Thyroid Gland	All body cells	Metabolic rate, essential for normal growth and development
Calcitonin (CT)	Parafollicular cells in Thyroid Gland	Bones	Lowers blood calcium levels by depositing calcium in bones

PARATHYROID GLAND HORMONE

Hormone	Produced by / in:	Target cell or tissue	Hormonal effects
Parathyroid Hormone (PTH)	Chief cells of the Parathyroid Gland	Bone, Renal tubules (nephron) of kidney	Raises blood calcium levels (removes calcium from bones and urine and places it in the blood)

ADRENAL GLAND HORMONES

Hormone	Produced by / in:	Target cell or tissue	Hormonal effects
Aldosterone (mineralocorticoid)	Adrenal Cortex	Renal tubules (nephron) of kidney	Causes reabsorption of sodium out of urine, into bloodstream (↑ blood Na+ levels)
Cortisol (glucocorticoid)	Adrenal Cortex	All body cells	Cope with stress, ↑ blood glucose, ↓ inflammation
Sex Hormones	Adrenal Cortex	All body cells	Androgens and estrogens (small amounts) for opposite sex.
Epinephrine Norepinephrine	Adrenal Medulla	Skeletal Muscle, cardiac muscle, smooth muscle in blood vessels	Stimulates "fight or flight" mechanism. ↑ B.P., ↑H.R., reroutes blood

PANCREAS HORMONES

Hormone	Produced by / in:	Target cell or tissue	Hormonal effects
Glucagon	Alpha (α) cells of Pancreas	Liver, adipose stores	Raises blood glucose (sugar) levels
Insulin	Beta (β) cells of Pancreas	All body cells	Lowers blood glucose (sugar) levels

REPRODUCTIVE HORMONES

Hormone	Produced by / in:	Target cell or tissue	Hormonal effects
Androgens (Testosterone)	Interstitial cells in Testes	Most body cells	Secondary sex characteristics, promotes spermatogenesis, sex drive, growth in adolescence
Estrogens (Estradiol)	Follicles in Ovary	Most body cells, uterus	Secondary sex characteristics, develop uterine lining
Progestins (Progesterone)	Corpus luteum in Ovary	Uterus, breast	Develop uterine lining, promotes breast development

Other tissues in the body can make a few hormones, but are not considered a true endocrine gland. For example: the placenta, the skin, the kidney, the heart, and adipose tissue. Please see next page for a sample of some of these hormones.

HORMONES PRODUCED BY ORGANS IN OTHER SYSTEMS

Hormone	Produced by / in:	Target cell or tissue	Hormonal effects
Calcitrol	Kidney	Intestines, bone, kidney	Stimulate calcium and phosphate ion absorption in digestive tract, stimulate osteoclasts, stimulate calcium reabsorption in kidneys
Erythropoietin (EPO)	Kidney	Red bone marrow	Increases red blood cell production
Renin	Kidney	Proteins in blood, adrenal cortex	Triggers renin-angiotensin mechanism (discussed in urinary system chapter)
Natriuretic peptides	Heart	Kidney, hypothalamus, adrenal gland	Increased H_2O loss and sodium loss in the kidneys, decreased thirst, decreased ADH, decreased aldosterone (can help to lower blood pressure and blood volume)
Thymosins	Thymus	Lymphocytes	Maturation of T lymphocytes
Leptin	Adipose	Hypothalamus	Control of appetite, sense of satiation, female reproduction
Resistin	Adipose	Body cells	Decreased insulin sensitivity
Secretin, Gastrin, Cholecystokinin	Intestines	Digestive system organs	These hormones help to coordinate digestive activities
Estrogen and Progesterone	Placenta	Uterus, breast tissue	Assists in the growth and development of the fetus, preparation of breast tissue for lactation
Relaxin	Placenta	Joint tissues	Loosens joint supporting structures

Physical Examination of the Endocrine System

1. Inspect thyroid gland (shape, edema, redness)
2. Palpate thyroid gland for size, shape and consistency

Most endocrine glands are not easily accessible through a physical examination. Hormonal blood laboratory studies are most commonly done to explore endocrine pathologies.

Advanced Imaging and Diagnostic Tests of the Endocrine System
(Abnormal findings should be referred to the patients PCP or an endocrinologist)

Biopsy- Removal of tissue samples from affected area. Tissue samples are then analyzed, usually under a microscope for abnormalities. Doctors take biopsies of areas that look abnormal and use them to detect cancer, precancerous cells, infections, and other conditions. For some biopsies, the doctor inserts a needle into the skin and draws out a sample; in other cases, tissue is removed during a surgical procedure. This could be done, for example, if an unusual growth was detected on the thyroid gland.

Computed Tomography (CT scan) - CT scans are a specialized x-ray machine. The machine circles the body and scans an area from every angle within that circle. The machine measures how much the x-ray beams change as they pass through the body. It then relays that information to a computer, which generates a collection of black-and-white pictures, each showing a slightly different "slice" or cross-section of your internal organs. Because these "slices" are spaced only about a quarter-inch apart, they give a very good representation of your internal organs and other structures. Doctors use CT scans to evaluate all major parts of the body, including the abdomen, back, chest, and head. Often, a technician or other health care professional inserts an IV and injects contrast dye through it. This dye outlines blood vessels and soft tissue to help them show up clearly on the pictures. A CT scan takes about 30–45 minutes.

Magnetic Resonance Imaging (MRI) - MRI is a noninvasive technique for visualizing many different body tissues. Unlike x-rays or a CT scan, MRI does not use any radiation. Instead, it uses radio waves, a large magnet, and a computer to create images. Each MRI picture shows a different "slice," or cross-section, of the area being viewed. Because these slices usually are spaced about a quarter-inch apart, the doctor can get a detailed representation of a particular area. MRI can be used on nearly any body part and is often used to look for structural abnormalities.

Ultrasonography- using sound waves (ultrasound) to detect structural or functional abnormalities. This procedure can be done on many organs of the body.

Pathologies of the Endocrine System

For additional infectious diseases that may affect this system, please refer to the Communicable/Infectious Disease Chart in Chapter 10.

Acromegaly- hypersecretion of GH (growth hormone) in adults (after long bone growth has ended). Usual age of onset is between the ages of 30-50. The person will be of normal height, but facial bones, hands and feet will enlarge. Usually caused by a pituitary tumor. Treatment may include surgery, radiation therapy and growth hormone blocking medications.

Addison's Disease- hyposecretion of adrenal cortex hormones. Is most commonly caused by an autoimmune disease or cancer. Symptoms include a bronze tone to the skin, decreased ability to cope with stress, fatigue and hypoglycemia. Glucocorticoid medications are given for treatment (example: hydrocortisone, prednisone)

Cretinism- hyposecretion of thyroid hormone in babies/children. Body proportions are distorted (head and trunk are 1 1/2 times the length of the legs). The tongue may thicken and stick out. Mental retardation can also occur. Cretinism is often due to an improperly formed thyroid gland. Treatment usually involves the patient taking thyroxine. If the condition is caught within the first month after birth, it can be treated before permanent mental retardation and growth abnormalities occur. If it is not treated in a timely manner, these changes can be permanent.

Cushing's Syndrome- hypersecretion of the hormone cortisol. Usually caused by a tumor. Diagnosed by blood tests measuring cortisol levels. Then, a MRI or CT scan will be done to look for the presence of a tumor in the adrenal gland or pituitary gland. Symptoms include "*moon face*" (swelling in facial region) and "*buffalo hump*" (fat deposition around the cervicothoracic region). The patient may feel tired, bruise easily, and experience muscle weakness. Surgery or radiation can be used to treat the tumor.

Diabetes Insipidus- Hyposecretion of ADH (antidiuretic hormone), which causes excessive urine output (*polyuria*). In response to this fluid loss, the person will become very thirsty and drink excessive amounts of fluids (*polydypsia*). Blood sugar levels and insulin in this individual are NORMAL. Treatment of central diabetes insipidus may involve the medication Desmopressin.

Diabetes Mellitus- hyposecretion of insulin or as a result of defective insulin receptors. Without insulin, glucose cannot be removed from the blood and placed into the tissue cells. This causes glucose levels in the blood ("blood sugar") to climb higher and higher. The signs of diabetes are: *Polyuria-* excessive urine output to flush out the excess blood glucose. *Polydypsia-* excessive thirst due to the dehydration from urinating. *Polyphagia-* excessive hunger due to the tissue cells starving for glucose. There are two forms of diabetes mellitus: **IDDM Type I (juvenile) diabetes** (insulin dependent diabetes mellitus), and **NIDDM Type II (adult onset) diabetes** (non-insulin dependent diabetes mellitus). Diagnosis is done by clinical signs, a fasting blood glucose test, or a glucose challenge test. Treatment involves diet modification, multiple insulin injections during the day, or the use of an insulin pump. If uncorrected, the blood becomes very acidic. The body will desperately try to burn fats for energy since it is unable to access any of the blood sugar. Ketones (a metabolic waste product of utilizing fats for energy) accumulate in the blood, and coma or death can occur. Other complications can develop from diabetes: peripheral neuropathies (decreased sensation and motor control due to progressive nerve damage), decreased immune response, vision difficulties (due to blood vessel damage in the retina of their eyes), kidney damage and possible progressive failure, ulcerations of the skin, and poor circulation- including the extremities. Diabetes raises the risk of developing many cardiovascular diseases, also.

Gigantism- hypersecretion of GH (growth hormone) in childhood. The patient will be an extremely tall individual, but with normal body proportions (tall torso, long arms, and long legs). Usually caused by a pituitary tumor. Treatment may include surgery, radiation therapy and growth hormone blocking medications.

Goiter- an enlargement of the thyroid gland, often due to a lack of iodine in the diet. Iodine is needed to make thyroid hormones. Other causes can include autoimmune diseases and a goiter can be seen in hyperthyroidism (commonly) and in some cases of hypothyroidism.

Graves' Disease- a type of hyperthyroidism. This is an autoimmune disease in which the immune system attacks the thyroid and causes the thyroid to produce excess thyroxine. This results in an abnormally high basal metabolic rate (BMR). Symptoms are weight loss, anxiety, goiter, sweating, increased body temperature. *Exophthalmoses* (protrusion of the eyeballs from the eye socket) may also occur. Diagnosis is commonly done with a thyroid panel blood test. Treatment may include radioactive iodine, surgery, or anti-thyroid medications.

Hashimoto's Thyroiditis- an autoimmune disease which damages the thyroid, causing it to decrease in function and performance. This is the most common cause of hypothyroidism in the United States. Symptoms of hypothyroidism: goiter, low basal metabolic rate (BMR), weight gain, a feeling of sluggishness/fatigue, and decreased body temperature (always feels chilled). This is usually diagnosed by blood tests (thyroid panel). Treatment may include thyroid medications, such as Synthroid.

Hyperglycemia- excess glucose in the blood (high blood sugar). Some of this excess glucose will be stored in the liver; the rest of it will be converted into fat and stored in our adipose tissue. Long term or pathological hyperglycemia could be an indicator of a glucose metabolic disease, such as diabetes mellitus.

Hypoglycemia- low blood sugar. Can be caused by fasting, improper doses of diabetes medications, or a pancreatic tumor, Symptoms often begin after the blood sugar levels fall below 60 mg/dl. Sweating, nervousness, palpitations, faintness and a headache may be some symptoms of hypoglycemia. Treatment usually involves consuming some form of sugar.

Hyperparathyroidism- increased secretion of PTH in which massive bone destruction occurs. Bones become very fragile and fracture easily. Bones look "moth eaten" on x-ray. Blood calcium levels will be abnormally high during blood tests.

Hypoparathyroidism- decreased secretion of PTH, which allows blood calcium levels to fall too low (hypocalcemia). Muscles may go into uncontrollable spasms (tetany). Deep tendon reflexes may be increased and Chvostek's sign (facial muscle spasms when the facial nerve is tapped) may be seen.

Pituitary Dwarfism- hyposecretion of GH (growth hormone) in childhood. Body proportions are normal, but the person is at a maximum of 4 feet tall. Treatment involves injections of growth hormone. The earlier the treatment begins, the more growth will be stimulated and the closer the child may end up having normal height as an adult.

Practice Study and Test Questions:

1) Which hormone is not produced by the anterior pituitary?
     A) growth hormone
     B) aldosterone
     C) thyroid stimulating hormone
     D) prolactin

2) What diagnostic test is most commonly done initially if a physician is concerned with a hormonal imbalance?
      A) culposcopy
      B) biopsy
      C) laboratory blood tests
      D) endoscopy

3) Which hormone is produced by the heart?
      A) epinephrine
      B) luteinizing hormone
      C) androgens
      D) natriuretic peptides

4) A patient complains of feeling sluggish, having weight gain and always feels chilled. This patient could be suffering from
      A) Hashimoto's thyroiditis
      B) Cushing's syndrome
      C) diabetes mellitus
      D) gigantism

5) Which hormone has the nephron as its target tissue/cell?
      A) secretin
      B) parathyroid hormone
      C) aldosterone
      D) Answers B and C
      E) All of the above

6) This condition is commonly caused by a tumor of the adrenal gland
      A) Cushing's syndrome
      B) Gigantism
      C) Graves' disease
      D) goiter

7) A lack of _____ may be one of the causes of a goiter
      A) iodine
      B) calcium
      C) iron
      D) Vitamin C

8) Mental retardation may be a result of
      A) cretinism
      B) acromegaly
      C) hypoparathyroidism
      D) Type 2 Diabetes Mellitus

9) Polydypsia, polyuria and polyphagia may be signs of
      A) Diabetes insipidus
      B) Addison's disease
      C) Diabetes mellitus
      D) hyperparathyroidism

10) The hormone which increases red blood cell production is called
    A) oxytocin
    B) resistin
    C) erythropoietin

11) Which of the following conditions are found in children only?
    A) goiter
    B) pituitary dwarfism
    C) acromegaly
    D) gigantism

12) Increased risk of bone fractures may be seen in
    A) Graves' disease
    B) hypoglycemia
    C) hyperparathyroidism
    D) diabetes insipidus

13) Which hormone helps the body cope with stress?
    A) gastrin
    B) calcitonin
    C) cortisol
    D) relaxin

14) Which of the following pathologies may commonly be a result of an autoimmune disease?
    A) Hashimoto's thyroiditis
    B) Graves' disease
    C) Addison's disease
    D) all of the above

15) Which of the following hormones is a glucocorticoid?
    A) aldosterone
    B) cortisol
    C) thyroxine
    D) renin

16) Which pathology is a result of a hypersecretion of growth hormone?
    A) gigantism
    B) Graves' disease
    C) acromegaly
    D) both A and C

17) Thyroxine may be used as a treatment in
    A) cretinism
    B) acromegaly
    C) Addison's disease
    D) pituitary dwarfism

18) Which gland produces glucagon?
    A) pineal
    B) parathyroid
    C) adrenal glands
    D) pancreas

Answers: 1) B 2) C 3) D 4) A 5) D 6) A 7) A 8) A 9) C 10) C 11) B 12) C 13) C 14) D 15) B 16) D 17) A 18) D

CHAPTER 9: THE CARDIOVASCULAR SYSTEM

Blood

Blood is a liquid connective tissue. It is roughly 38 degrees Celsius (100.4 degrees Fahrenheit) and has a pH of 7.35-7.45 (slightly basic/alkaline). The average male body contains 5-6 liters of blood, whereas the average female contains 4-5 liters. Blood has many functions. It is the main medium of transportation of dissolved gases, nutrients, hormones, and metabolic wastes. It plays a role in the regulation of the pH and ion composition of interstitial fluids. It causes restriction of fluid losses at an injury site (via clotting) and defends against toxins and pathogens. It also assists in stabilization of body temperature.

Blood is formed by two main components: plasma and the formed elements. **Plasma** is the liquid matrix of the blood. Plasma composes 46-63% of whole blood. The other main component is the **formed elements-** the blood cells and cell fragments that float in the plasma (37-54% of whole blood). The formed elements are the *Red Blood Cells*, *White Blood Cells,* and *Platelets.*

Plasma:

Plasma is composed mostly of water (92%). It also contains plasma proteins (7%) and other solutes (1%). Plasma proteins include albumins, globulins, fibrinogen and peptide hormones. These proteins assist in maintaining blood pressure, helping the immune system, and working with the platelets during blood clotting. Solutes in the plasma are things like electrolytes ($Na+$, $K+$), organic nutrients (glucose), and organic wastes (uric acid, ammonia, lactic acid).

Formed Elements: Red Blood Cells /Erythrocytes (RBC's):

RBC's compose 99.9% of formed elements and function to transport oxygen in the blood. Each drop of blood contains on average 260 million RBC's, and the average adult has approximately 25 trillion RBC's. The shape of a red blood cell can be described as a biconcave disc. RBC's have no nuclei, ribosomes, or mitochondria-therefore they lack the ability to repair themselves. Life expectancy is only 100-120 days.

What allows red blood cells to carry oxygen is the fact they contain **hemoglobin (Hb).** Hemoglobin is composed of four **heme** molecules (a pigment complex), and each heme molecule contains iron. *Oxyhemoglobin* is hemoglobin carrying 4 oxygen molecules. *Deoxyhemoglobin* is hemoglobin with no oxygen bound to it. If carbon dioxide is bound to the hemoglobin, it is called *carbaminohemoglobin.*

Red blood cells are formed in the red bone marrow. This process is called *erythropoiesis* and is stimulated by the hormone called erythropoietin (EPO). During the formation and the maturation of the RBC in the bone marrow, the nucleus is ejected from the cell. With no nucleus, RBC's have no ability to repair themselves and only live 100-120 days. As the RBC reaches the end of its life span, it will be removed from the bloodstream by the spleen, liver, bone marrow or kidney. Many of the components of the old RBC's will be recycled and re-used in the body (globular proteins, heme, iron).

Blood Typing: There are four types of red blood cells- Type A, B, AB and O. These blood types differ from one another due to the presence or absence of protein markers on the plasma membrane. These protein markers are called *surface antigens/agglutinogens*. Blood typing in a medical setting is important, especially if a transfusion is needed. To avoid transfusion reactions, the donor and recipient must have compatible blood types.
- *Type A-* RBC's have the A antigen on surface, the patient's immune system produces anti-B antibodies.

- *Type B-* RBC's have the B antigen on surface, and the immune system produces anti-A antibodies.
- *Type AB-* RBC's have both the A and B antigen on surface, and the immune system produces no anti-A or anti-B antibodies (universal recipient).
- *Type O-* RBC's have neither A or B antigen on surface; and the immune system produces both Anti-A and Anti-B antibodies (universal donor). This patient can donate blood to most anyone, yet can only receive a transfusion of Type O blood.
- *Rh positive-* Rh antigen present on surface of RBC. *Rh negative-* Rh antigen absent on surface RBC.

Formed Elements: White Blood Cells (WBC) / Leukocytes:

White blood cells compose less than 0.1% of the formed elements. They contain nuclei and organelles, but no hemoglobin. Their function is to clean and detoxify the body, protect against infection, and they remove dead or damaged cells. WBC's are normally outnumbered by RBC's by about 1000:1.

There are five types of White Blood Cells. A pneumonic you can use is Never Let My Engine Blow- **N**eutrophils, **L**ymphocytes, **M**onocytes, **E**osinophils, and **B**asophils.

- **Neutrophils** (50-70% of WBC's) - act as first responders to acute injury or illness, and are phagocytes. (A *phagocyte* is a cell that will kill invaders or dispose of toxins by "eating" them- kind of like "Pac-Man" cells)
- **Lymphocytes** (20-30% of circulating WBC's) - offer better long term immunity to diseases. There are two main types of lymphocytes: T lymphocytes (T cells) and B lymphocytes (B cells). These lymphocytes will be discussed more in the Lymphatic/Immune System chapter.
- **Monocytes** (2-8% of WBC) are also called "tissue macrophages". Tissue macrophages are vigorous phagocytes and can also stimulate fibroblasts, which can lead to scar tissue. These cells may be present in chronic injuries or illnesses.
- **Eosinophils** (2-4% of WBC's) are prominent cells involved in response to infection with multicellular parasites (parasitic worms and flukes) and will also respond during allergic reactions.
- **Basophils** (Less than 1% of WBC's) respond to areas of injury and release histamine and heparin, which increases inflammation and will support the chemical activity of mast cells at an injured area.

Formed Elements: Platelets:

Platelets are less than 0.1% of formed elements and function to clot the blood. They are not a complete cell, but actually a cell fragment. They circulate for 9-12 days before being disposed of by phagocytes in the spleen. Platelets are produced in the bone marrow (**thrombocytopoiesis**) by cells called megakaryocytes.

During hemostasis (cessation of bleeding) three steps occur. **The Vascular Phase** (begins within a few seconds of injury and lasts about 30 minutes) involves vasoconstriction of the blood vessel in the injured area (vascular spasm), The endothelium (the inner lining of the injured blood vessel) becomes sticky. **The Platelet Phase** (begins within 15 seconds of injury) has platelets adhering to the sticky endothelium (*platelet adhesion*). The platelets stick on top of one another (*platelet aggregation*) and form a growing mass called a *platelet plug.* **The Coagulation Phase** (begins after at least 30 seconds of injury) is when blood clotting occurs. A blood clot is a mass of platelets, blood cells (RBC and WBC), and fibrinogen (protein fibers found in the blood plasma). Proper clotting depends on *clotting factors* or *procoagulants*. These clotting factors will create a cascade- with one factor triggering the activity of another, and so on. After the clot has formed, it will undergo **clot retraction** (*syneresis*), which pulls the edges of the injury closer together. This decreases bleeding, stabilizes the injury, and makes it easier for repair of the area.

The Heart:

The human heart beats 100,000 times each day, and pumps 8000 liters each day. It is located in the mediastinum portion of the chest, beneath the ribs, slightly to the left of midline. The heart extends from the third costal cartilage to the fifth intercostal space.

The heart does not look *exactly* like the heart you see drawn on Valentine's Day cards, but slightly resembles it. It has a wide *base* at the superior portion and tapers inferiorly to the *apex*. The heart is enclosed by a double walled serous membrane called the *pericardial sac*. This sac reduces friction as the heart is pumping in the chest.

The heart wall is composed of three layers. The outermost layer, the *epicardium*, is actually part of the pericardial sac. The middle layer, the *myocardium*, is the thickest layer and is composed of cardiac muscle. And, the innermost layer is called the *endocardium*. This lines the inner chambers of the heart.

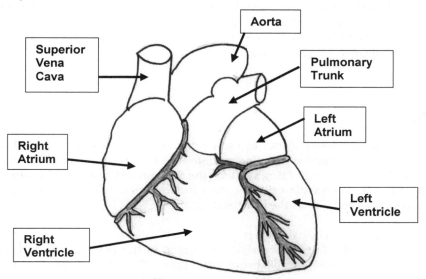

Internal Structure of the Heart:

The heart essentially encloses two pumps- one on the right side of the heart, and the other on the left. Internally, the heart contains four chambers. The **right atrium** is the upper chamber on right side of the heart and collects blood returning from the body tissues. It receives blood from the *superior* and *inferior vena cava*. The **right ventricle** is the lower chamber on the right side of the heart, and ejects deoxygenated blood out to the lungs via the pulmonary trunk and arteries. The **left atrium** is the upper chamber on left side and receives oxygenated blood from the pulmonary veins of the lungs. The **left ventricle** is the lower chamber on the left side and pumps blood out to the body tissues through the aorta. A muscular septum acts as a wall and separates the right side of the heart from the left (preventing mixing of the deoxygenated blood and oxygenated blood).

It is critical that blood flows through the heart in only one direction. To ensure this, the heart has four valves internally to provide proper direction of blood flow. Separating the right atrium and right ventricle and preventing backflow of blood is the **Right Atrioventricular Valve (AV)** - aka *tricuspid valve*. The **Pulmonary Valve**- aka *Pulmonary Semilunar Valve* is a one way valve which prevents backflow of blood between the right ventricle and pulmonary trunk. The **Left Atrioventricular Valve (AV)** - aka *bicuspid valve* or *mitral valve* prevents backflow of blood between the left atrium and left ventricle. The **Aortic Valve**- aka *Aortic Semilunar Valve* is a one way valve which prevents backflow of blood between the left ventricle and ascending aorta. The AV valves are anchored by bands of tissue called the *chordae tendinae*. The heart sounds you hear when you listen to a heartbeat ("lub-dub") are sounds made when valves close. The "Lub" sound (the first heart sound in a heartbeat) occurs when the AV valves are closing. The "Dub" sound occurs when the semilunar valves are closing.

Circulation Pathway of Blood:

Pulmonary Circulation is the circulation pathway of the blood beginning in the right ventricle of the heart, flowing out of the right side of the heart to the lungs, and then back to the left atrium. The *Systemic Circulation* is circulation between the left ventricle of the heart, out to the systemic (body) tissue, and back to the right atrium. *Cardiac (Coronary) Circulation* is the circulation path that nourishes the heart tissue.

Following is the circulation pathway of the blood as it travels through the body (including both the pulmonary circulation and the systemic circulation pathways):

Right Atrium→ Right AV valve (Tricuspid)→ Right Ventricle→ Pulmonary Semilunar Valve→ Pulmonary trunk → Pulmonary Arteries → Lung tissue → Pulmonary Veins → Left Atrium → Left AV Valve (Mitral/Bicuspid) → Left Ventricle → Aortic Semilunar Valve → Aorta → Systemic Arteries → Systemic (body) tissue → Systemic Veins → Superior and Inferior Vena Cava → Right Atrium

The Heartbeat

The conducting system of the heart works to ensure that all of the contractile cardiac muscle cells are working together to create an effective pumping motion. The structures involved in generating a heartbeat are the **contractile cells** and the **conducting system (the SA node, AV node, AV bundle, Bundle branches, and Purkinje fibers).** The contractile cells are the cardiac muscle cells which pump the blood, and the conducting system regulates and directs the heartbeat.

The steps involved in generating a heartbeat are:
1. **Sinoatrial Node (SA node)** "the *pacemaker*"- is located in the posterior wall of the right atrium. It contains *Pacemaker cells* which establish the heart rate. The SA node generates an action potential (similar to a nervous system action potential) approximately 80-100 times per minute, which can be modified by the parasympathetic nervous system. This action potential will eventually trigger the cardiac muscle cells to contract. The cardiac muscle cells in the left and right atrium will first receive the action potential from the SA node and will begin to contract. The action potential will move though the atrial muscle tissue and head towards the AV node.
2. **Atrioventricular Node (AV node)** is located in the floor of the right atrium. The AV node is responsible for taking the action potential as it is traveling through the atrial muscle tissue and then delaying it for about 100 msec before passing the action potential into the ventricles. This delay is necessary to have the atria finish contracting before the ventricles begin to contract. This ensures proper blow of the blood through the heart.
3. **AV Bundle** is connected to the AV node by an electrical connection called the *bundle of His.* The AV bundle carries the action potential from the AV node to the interventricular septum, where it is passed to the bundle branches.
4. **Bundle Branches-** the *Left Bundle Branch-* carries the action potential to the apex of the left ventricle. The *Right Bundle Branch-* carries the action potential to the apex of the right ventricle. The bundle branches will deliver the action potential to both ventricles.
5. **Purkinje Fibers** are located in the apex region of the heart in both the left and right ventricles. They receive action potentials from the left and right bundle branches and distribute the action potential to all of the contractile cardiac muscle cells in both ventricles. This will then trigger ventricular contraction.

The cardiac cycle is composed of two phases. **Systole** is when the heart chambers are contracting and ejecting blood. If taking a blood pressure, the top number of the blood pressure reading is measuring the *systolic* *pressure*. **Diastole** is when the heart chambers are relaxing and re-filling. When taking a blood pressure, the *diastolic pressure* is the bottom number in the blood pressure reading. **Stroke Volume** is the amount of blood ejected by the heart in one cardiac cycle (one heart contraction).

The **Cardiac Output** measures the amount of blood ejected from the ventricles in one minute. Cardiac output can vary throughout the day. When we are at rest, the cardiac output will be less than when we are doing intense activity. The difference between resting and maximal cardiac output volumes is called the *cardiac reserve*. The amount of cardiac output can be influenced by things that alter the heart rate and/or stroke volume (such as autonomic innervation, venous return, hormones, or cardiac reflexes).

The Electrocardiogram (ECG or EKG)

An electrocardiogram is a machine which measures the electrical activity of the heart. Electrodes are placed on the surface of the chest in specific locations to detect electrical activity, and these readings are then displayed on a monitor. The ECG is especially useful in assessing a myocardial infarction or arrhythmia.

This is a typical ECG pattern for a healthy heart contraction.

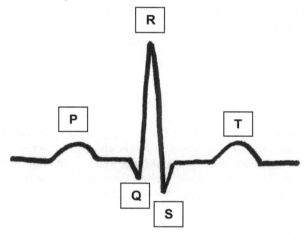

- **P wave:** indicates depolarization of the atria
- **QRS complex**: indicates depolarization of the ventricles. The ventricles begin contracting shortly after the peak of the R wave
- **T wave:** indicates ventricular repolarization
- **P-R interval**: the time from the beginning of the P wave to the beginning of the QRS complex. An increased P-R interval can indicate damage to the AV node
- **Q-T interval:** the time needed for the ventricles to undergo a single cycle of depolarization and repolarization.
- *Atrial repolarization* is hidden by the larger QRS complex

Blood Vessels:

Blood vessels are responsible for transporting blood throughout the body. There are three main categories of blood vessels- *arteries, veins* and *capillaries*. These vessels are very small hose-like structures carrying blood. At any given moment, 64% of our blood is found inside of the systemic veins (whereas the heart only is holding 7% and arteries have only 13%). The walls of arteries and veins have three layers: the **tunica intima** (internal), **tunica media** (middle muscular layer), and **tunica externa** (external). Arteries have a thicker tunica media (muscular layer) than veins. Veins collapse and distend, where arteries can maintain their shape easier due to the thicker walls. Capillaries have a very thin wall consisting of only the tunica intima (no tunica media or externa in a capillary).

Arteries:

Arteries are vessels which carry blood *away from the heart.* With a thicker muscular wall, they are able to perform **vasoconstriction** and **vasodilation.** The change in blood vessel diameter allows the body to be able to alter the afterload on the heart, blood pressure levels, and vary capillary blood flow to various organs in the body. *Elastic arteries* are the largest size of arteries (for example: the aorta). *Muscular arteries* are medium sized, and *arterioles* are the smallest sized arteries.

Capillaries:

Capillaries are the only blood vessels where gas and nutrient exchange can take place between blood and tissue fluids. Capillaries are microscopic, barely wider than a red blood cell. The wall of a capillary consists of an endothelium and very delicate basal lamina, but no tunica media or externa. This thin wall allows the exchange of nutrients and wastes. Arterioles bring blood into the capillaries, and venules carry blood out of the capillaries.

Veins:

Veins carry blood *towards the heart.* Veins come in a variety of sizes: *large veins, medium sized veins*, and *venules* (smallest sized). Blood pressure in veins is lower than in arteries. To keep blood moving in the proper direction and prevent backflow, medium and large sized veins contain *valves. Venous return* is the amount of blood returned to the heart and is assisted by valves and the contraction of skeletal muscles (which help to put pressure on the veins and help "pump" blood back to the heart).

Cardiovascular Physiology

There are a few basic ideas when it comes to blood flow. Ideally body tissues should have an adequate amount of blood flow delivered to them at all times. Blood flow is usually equal to cardiac output- meaning the amount of blood leaving the heart every minute should be equal to the amount of blood that reaches the body tissues. When cardiac output increases, more blood moves into the capillaries and reaches body tissues.

As the blood leaves the heart, the **flow (F)** of blood is dependent upon two main criteria: First, is **Pressure (P)** - this is the amount of force the heart has to push with to overcome any resistance in the blood vessels. Usually if pressure increases, blood flow increases. The second criteria is **Resistance** (R)- this is the resistance to flow that the blood vessels cause. Resistance tends to slow down and decrease blood flow. Things like vasoconstriction or atherosclerosis of the blood vessels (which narrow or block the blood vessels) can increase resistance.

Blood Pressure **(BP)** (also called *arterial blood pressure)* is the pressure pushing blood through the arteries. Blood pressure in the arteries is under the highest level of pressure in the body (for example 100 mmHg). *Capillary Hydrostatic Pressure* **(CHP)** is the pressure of blood in the capillaries. As blood flows through the arteries and enters the capillaries, the pressure will drop. Capillary pressure usually ranges between 18-35mmHg. This pressure dictates capillary exchange (exchange of nutrients from the blood and wastes from the tissues). The **Net Hydrostatic Pressure** pushes water and solutes out of capillaries and into the interstitial fluid (the fluid surrounding the tissue cells). This movement will supply tissue cells with nutrients from the bloodstream. **Net Colloid Osmotic Pressure** tends to pull water and solutes into a capillary from the interstitial fluid in body tissues. This movement will allow waste products to be removed from the body tissue and placed into the bloodstream. **Net Filtration Pressure (NFP)** is the difference between the net hydrostatic pressure and the net colloid osmotic pressure.

Resistance to blood flow:

Resistance to blood flow (in some cases) can be detrimental to our health by causing our heart to have to work harder to overcome this added resistance. There are things that can add resistance and slow blood flow through our vessels. *Vessel Length-* Increasing the length of a blood vessel will increase the amount of friction placed on the blood, causing resistance (for example: for each pound of fat you gain, your body must grow extra *miles* of vessels to serve those newly enlarged fat cells). *Vessel Diameter-* the narrower the diameter of the vessel, the higher the resistance within the blood vessel. Vessel diameter can change during vasoconstriction and vasodilation- or as a result of fatty plaques partially blocking the vessels (atherosclerosis). *Viscosity-* the composition of the blood can affect resistance. Blood composition is usually 5 times the viscosity of water, but diseases that affect the hematocrit can change blood viscosity and make the blood more viscous (thicker)- creating more resistance. *Turbulence-* like a river, turbulence is swirling and erratic movement of blood flow. This is often caused by high flow rates, rough or irregular inner blood vessel surfaces (from atherosclerosis), or sudden changes in blood vessel size. The more turbulent the flow of blood, the more resistance is present.

Exercise and the Cardiovascular System

Light exercise causes vasodilation of vessels, which increases blood flow to body tissues. Venous return increases during exercise and cardiac output rises. Heavy exercise causes sympathetic nervous system stimulation (and will increase heart rate). A well trained athlete will have a heart that has developed with training to have a higher stroke volume for increased efficiency (the athlete's heart will be able to pump more blood each time their heart contracts, compared to a sedentary person). This allows, at rest, the heart rate to decrease and be slower in an athlete when compared to a non-athlete. Moderate exercise can lower blood cholesterol. Exercise, along with proper diet, stress maintenance, no smoking, and weight control can all increase cardiovascular health.

Physical Examination of the Cardiovascular System

Inspection of the Cardiovascular System

1. Inspect skin color, temperature, turgor, evidence of pitting edema in the body trunk or extremities
2. Inspect for any varicosities in blood vessels of the body
3. Inspect for clubbing in the fingers
4. Inspect the neck for carotid artery and jugular vein pulsations
5. Inspect the chest for pulsations, symmetry of movement, heaves
6. Inspect for the presence of the apical impulse (located at the 5th intercostal space on the left side of the chest, at the midclavicular line)

Palpation of Blood Vessels

1. Palpate the radial pulse and measure pulse rate.
2. Palpate other pulses in the body (carotid, brachial, femoral, popliteal, dorsalis pedis) and compare them bilaterally for rate and rhythm. Rate the strength of the pulses as:
   - 0 = absent
   - 1+ = weak
   - 2+ = normal
   - 3+ = increased
   - 4+ = bounding
3. Perform Homan's Test/Sign (for deep vein thrombosis)- this test has been classically performed for DVT in the past, but is not often performed currently due to lack of strong diagnostic data.

Palpation of the Chest/Heart

1. Palpate the apical impulse in the chest (same area as you observed) for any heaves or thrills
2. Palpate for abnormal pulsations (normally no pulsations should be felt)
   - Sternoclavicular area (area where sternum meets clavicle),
   - Aortic Valve (right side of sternal border in the 2nd intercostal space)
   - Pulmonic Valve (left side of sternal border in the 2nd intercostal space)
   - Tricuspid Valve (left side of sternal border in the 5th intercostal space)
   - Mitral Valve (left side of chest at the midclavicular line, in the 5th intercostal space)

Percussion of the Heart

1. Percuss in the left 5th intercostal space, moving laterally to medial.

Auscultation of the Heart Sounds

1. Auscultate the four heart valves (in the same location where they were palpated) and Erb's Point (third intercostal space at the left sternal border). This should be done while the patient is breathing normally and again while holding breath. Listening for:
   - rate and rhythm of heartbeat
   - S1 (first heart sound- LUB)
   - S2 (second heart sound- DUB)
   - S3- "ventricular gallop" and/or S4 "atrial gallop".
   - extra heart sounds (usually abnormal- snaps, clicks, friction rubs, and murmurs)
2. Auscultate murmurs, if present, for timing, pitch, intensity, pattern, quality, location, radiation and respiratory phase variation

Grade	Heart Murmur Intensity
1	Barely heard with stethoscope and may not be heard in all positions or heard intermittently
2	Quiet, but easily heard with a stethoscope and heard consistently with every beat
3	Relatively loud when using a stethoscope; no thrill
4	Loud when using a stethoscope; with a thrill present
5	Very loud, can be heard with stethoscope partially off of the chest; palpable thrill present
6	Very loud, can be heard with no contact between stethoscope and chest; palpable thrill

Auscultation of Blood Vessels

1. Auscultate carotid, temporal, abdominal aorta, renal and femoral arteries for bruits
2. Perform a Blood Pressure examination on the patient (if not already recorded with the vital signs). Equipment used: *sphygmomanometer* and *stethoscope*, and the sounds heard while taking a blood pressure are called *Korotkoff's sounds*.
    ➢ Optimal blood pressure is Systolic 100-119 mmHg and Diastolic 60-79 mmHg.
    ➢ Prehypertension is Systolic 120-139 mmHg or Diastolic 80-89 mmHg
    ➢ Stage 1 Hypertension is Systolic 140-159 mmHg or a Diastolic of 90-99 mmHg
    ➢ Stage 2 Hypertension is Systolic greater than 160 mmHg or Diastolic greater than 100 mmHg.
    ➢ Hypertensive Crisis is Systolic greater than 180 or Diastolic greater than 120 mmHg

Abnormal Findings of the Cardiovascular System

Abnormal findings, if necessary, should be referred to patients PCP, hematologist, or a cardiologist. If this is a life threatening emergency- call 911.

Chest Pain- may occur suddenly or gradually, and there are many different types. Some chest pain is heart related, other chest pains can be caused by different organs
- Aching, squeezing pressure, heaviness, and burning pain which usually resolves in 10 minutes. Location is substernal, may radiate to arms, neck, jaw, back- is usually *angina pectoris*
- Tightness or pressure, burning aching pain, shortness of breath, weakness, anxiety, nausea, sudden onset, and can last for 30 minutes to 2 hours. Location is across chest, may radiate to jaw, neck, arms, back- often indicates an *acute myocardial infarction*
- Sharp and continuous pain, may be accompanied with a friction rub, sudden onset. Location is substernal may radiate to neck or left arm- may indicate *pericarditis*
- Excruciating, tearing pain, may be accompanied by blood pressure difference between right and left arm, sudden onset. Location is retrosternal, upper abdominal, or epigastric, may radiate to back, neck, shoulders- often indicates *dissecting abdominal aortic aneurysm*
- Sudden stabbing pain, may be accompanied by cyanosis, dyspnea, or cough with hemoptysis. Location is over the lungs- often is a *pulmonary embolus*
- Dull or stabbing pain usually accompanied by hyperventilation or breathlessness, sudden onset, lasting as short as one minute to several days. Location could be anywhere in the chest- usually indicates *acute anxiety*.

Abnormal pulsations: depending on location, could indicate various pathologies.
- A displaced apical impulse could indicate an enlarged left ventricle (caused by heart failure or hypertension)
- A forceful apical impulse could indicate increased cardiac output
- An epigastric or sternoclavicular pulsation could indicate an abdominal aortic aneurysm

Weak pulse: may indicate decreased cardiac output, or increased peripheral resistance- usually caused by atherosclerotic diseases

Strong or "bounding" pulse- occurs with patients with hypertension, anemia, hypoxia. Also can be a result of exercise or anxiety.

Bruit- murmur-like sound over blood vessels in the body. Can indicate arteriosclerosis or atherosclerosis, and can sometimes be seen in hyperthyroidism

Thrill- a palpable vibration, usually indicating a valve dysfunction (murmur)

Heave- a lifting of the chest wall felt during palpation.
- If felt on the left sternal border, could indicate right ventricular hypertrophy
- If felt over the left ventricular area, could indicate a ventricular aneurysm

Palpitations- usually a sensation reported by patient. A "pounding, fluttering, flopping, or missing beats" sensation. Can be fast or slow, regular or irregular, sustained or transient. May be a result of stress, caffeine intake, tobacco use, other medication or drug use, hypoglycemia, fatigue or a cardiac disorder (arrhythmia).

Pitting edema- may be seen (most often in the extremities) in patients with heart failure. On palpation of a swollen area, if the indentation in the skin from the palpation remains- this is pitting edema

Syncope- "fainting" the transient loss of consciousness and muscle tone

Aneurysm – a weak bulge in a blood vessel wall that is at risk to rupture. If it ruptures, it may be fatal in a very short period of time. Ultrasound, MRI can be commonly used as diagnostic tests. The most common place for developing an aneurysm is in the aorta, and they can also be seen in the brain (although any vessel could potentially develop an aneurysm).

Murmurs- abnormal sounds heard while assessing S1 and S2
- Low pitched murmur- occurs with aortic valve stenosis, and is usually harsh sounding and heard mid systolic. Shifts from crescendo (increasing intensity) to decrescendo (decreasing intensity). Caused by turbulent blood flow through a stiffened valve
- Medium pitched murmur- occurs with pulmonic valve stenosis. Is harsh and systolic. Shifts from crescendo to decrescendo and back
- High pitched murmur- occurs with aortic or pulmonic insufficiency (where blood is flowing backwards over the valve). Characterized as blowing, decrescendo and diastolic. With pulmonic valve insufficiency, it can be heard at Erb's point (left sternal border of third intercostal space). For aortic valve insufficiency, it can be heard from the aortic valve area to the left sternal border.
- Rumbling murmur- occurs with mitral valve stenosis (mitral valve calcifies and impedes blood leaving the left atrium). Characterized as low pitched and rumbling in the mitral valve area.
- Blowing murmur- occurs with mitral valve insufficiency (leakage)- where blood is flowing backwards past the mitral valve. High pitched and blowing throughout systole. Sound heard best at mitral valve area on the chest and apex of heart.
- Low rumbling murmur- occurs with tricuspid stenosis. Is crescendo-decrescendo in the tricuspid valve area.
- High pitched, blowing murmur- occurs with tricuspid insufficiency. Occurs throughout systole in the tricuspid area and gets louder when the client inhales.

Other abnormal heart sounds:
- Accentuated S1- could indicate mitral stenosis or fever
- Diminished S1- could indicate mitral insufficiency or heart block
- Accentuated S2- could indicate pulmonary or systemic hypertension
- Diminished or inaudible S2- could indicate pulmonic or aortic stenosis
- Persistent S2 split- could indicate delayed closure of the pulmonic valve
- S3 (ventricular gallop)- could indicate mitral insufficiency or ventricular failure in an adult. (Please note, this may be a normal heart sound heard in children and young adults)
- S4 (atrial gallop)- could indicate hypertension, left ventricular hypertrophy

Arrhythmias – irregular rhythm of heart beats. Examples include fibrillations (extremely rapid, uncoordinated shuddering of heart muscle), heart block (damage to the AV node), tachycardia (rapid heart rate), and bradycardia (substantially slower heart rate). ECG studies and auscultation can be used for diagnosis.

Hypertension – high blood pressure, defined as 140/90 or higher.

Raynaud's phenomenon- Skin in the area changes color as blood flow is disrupted. First it becomes pale, and then turns blue. Eventually it will turn red once blood flow returns.

Thrombophlebitis – an inflammation of a vein (phlebitis) that results when a clot forms in a vessel with poor circulation. A common consequence is clot detachment and a resulting pulmonary embolism, which is life-threatening.

Thrombus- A blood clot attached to the inside of a blood vessel wall. Begins when platelets begin attaching to the roughened wall of a blood vessel. The blood vessel can be roughened and damaged by plaques (fat) and residues from cigarette smoke. The clot may grow to the point where it completely obstructs the blood vessel. Thrombolytic drugs and anticoagulant drugs may be given to dissolve the clot and prevent further formation (Coumadin, Warfarin, aspirin, tissue plasminogen activator)

Varicose veins – purple, snakelike, twisted, dilated veins in the feet and legs due to blood pooling because of inefficient venous return. Most often, inactivity or pressure on the veins causes the venous valves to fail. People who stand for long periods of time and obese (or pregnant) people are most at risk.

Homan's Test/Sign- Dorsiflex patient's foot, with the knee extended. Pain in calf could indicate possible DVT (*deep vein thrombosis*). (Please note, not a very accurate test- ultrasound is a much better diagnostic tool for DVT)

Adson's sign- an orthopedic test. Adson's sign is seen when the examiner moves the patient's arm into abduction and external rotation of the arm at the shoulder. A positive sign is when there is a loss of the radial pulse in the arm when performing the movement. It can be a sign of *thoracic outlet syndrome.*

Levine's Sign- is a clenched fist held over the chest when the patient is describing their chest pain symptoms. It is usually seen in patients with a *myocardial infarction (MI)*

Advanced Imaging and Diagnostic Tests of the Cardiovascular System

Arteriography (Angiography) - used to assess the condition of the cerebral arteries in the brain or carotid arteries in the neck commonly, but can be used to assess any artery. A radioopaque dye is injected into the bloodstream, and time is given for the dye to disperse. Then, an X-ray is taken of the arteries of interest. The dye allows arteries narrowed by arteriosclerosis to be localized. It is also used to look for a blockage or arterial defect. This is commonly ordered for individuals that have suffered a myocardial infarction, stroke, or transient ischemic attacks.

Chest x ray. A chest x ray takes an x-ray of the organs and structures inside your chest. These include your heart, lungs, and blood vessels. Useful in measuring heart size (often when looking for enlargement.)

Computed Tomography (CT scan) - CT scans are a specialized x-ray machine which creates 1/4" slices of the body.

Cardiac catheterization. A thin flexible tube (catheter) is passed through an artery in the groin (upper leg) or arm to reach the coronary arteries. Instruments can be inserted onto the tip of the catheter to measure blood pressure, gather tissue and blood samples, view the inside of blood vessels or the heart, etc.

Coronary angiography. This test is done during cardiac catheterization. A radioopaque dye that can be seen by X ray is injected through the catheter into the coronary arteries. The physician can see the flow of blood through the heart and the location of blockages.

Echocardiogram. Ultrasonography of the heart. This test uses sound waves to create a picture of the heart. The picture is more detailed than an x-ray image. The test shows how well the heart chambers fill with blood and pump it to the rest of the body. An echocardiogram also can help identify areas of poor blood flow to the heart, areas of heart muscle that are not contracting normally, and previous injury to the heart muscle caused by poor blood flow. An echocardiogram can also be used with a stress test.

Electrocardiography (ECG or EKG) - Study of the heart's electrical activity. Electrodes are placed on the patient's chest, and they measure the electrical current as it flows through the cardiac muscle. Assists in detecting defects, myocardial infarction, arrhythmia, angina, etc.

Exercise stress test. Some heart problems are easier to diagnose when the heart is working hard and beating fast. During stress testing, a patient exercises (or is given medicine) to make the heart work harder and beat fast while heart tests are performed. During exercise stress testing, blood pressure and ECG/EKG readings are monitored while the patient runs on a treadmill or pedals a bicycle.

Holter Monitor- This is a portable monitor, usually with four chest leads attached to the patient. It is used for patients that have episodes of palpitations, arrhythmias, or syncope that may not be present when the patient is at an appointment in the physician's office. Often it is worn for 24 hours, and will continuously record heart activity, and then the information recorded is evaluated by the physician.

Nuclear heart scan- This test shows blood flow to the heart and any damage to the heart muscle. A radioactive dye (technetium or thallium) is injected into the bloodstream. A special camera can see the dye and find areas where blood flow is reduced. Nuclear heart scans are often taken while the patient is at rest and again after exercise. If the patient cannot exercise, a medicine is given to increase the workload of the heart. The before-and-after exercise scans are compared.

Pulse oximetry- measures the amount of oxygen in the blood and provides an early warning sign of a low level of oxygen in the blood. Often done when monitoring a heart attack victim. This can be measured with a device which rests on the patient's fingertips.

Swan Ganz Catheter- This catheter is introduced through the femoral vein (usually) and is then fed to the right side of the heart. It measures pressure of the movement of blood in the right side of the heart. Can be used in diagnosis or monitoring of patients with heart attack, congenital heart diseases, valve regurgitation (leaky valves), and pulmonary hypertension.

Ultrasonography- using sound waves (ultrasound) to detect structural or functional abnormalities. This procedure can be done on many organs of the body. Can be used to diagnose DVT (deep vein thrombosis).

Venography- X-ray study to detect a blockage of the veins

Blood Lab Panels can be ordered also to assess cardiovascular health

Pathologies of the Cardiovascular System

For additional infectious diseases that may affect this system, please refer to the Communicable/Infectious Disease Chart in Chapter 10.

Anemia – the blood has an abnormally low oxygen-carrying capacity, leading to fatigue. The skin may be pale. This is caused by either a lower-than-normal number of RBCs, or abnormal or deficient hemoglobin within the RBCs. There are several different types, including: **iron-deficiency anemia (lack of iron), pernicious anemia (lack of Vitamin B12 or folate), hemolytic anemia (rupturing of RBC's),** and **sickle-cell anemia (abnormally shaped RBC's).**

Aneurysm – a weak bulge in a blood vessel wall that is at risk to rupture. If it ruptures, it may be fatal in a very short period of time. Ultrasound or MRI can be commonly used as diagnostic tests. The most common place for developing an aneurysm is in the aorta, and they can also be seen in the brain (although any vessel could potentially develop an aneurysm). Aneurysms often grow slowly, so symptoms can be non-existent or develop slowly. *Red flag symptoms of an aortic aneurysm are: a throbbing feeling in the abdomen (felt by the patient or by the physician on physical exam) and pain in the abdomen or back. If the aneurysm ruptures, severe pain will occur.* Risk factors of an aortic aneurysm are: being male, smoking, family history of aneurysm, high blood pressure and atherosclerosis. *Red flag symptoms of a brain aneurysm are: vision difficulties, pain in the eye, numbness or drooping on one side of the face, or a dilated pupil. If the aneurysm ruptures, a sudden horribly severe headache will occur.* Risk factors of a brain aneurysm are: being a woman (especially post-menopausal), having head trauma, smoking, high blood pressure, atherosclerosis, drug abuse, and alcohol abuse.

Angina Pectoris- temporary lack of oxygen to the cardiac muscle. *Red Flag symptoms: can be chest pain and discomfort in the upper middle to 1/3 of the sternum, and may radiate to the left jaw, neck and arm. Pain usually follows exertion, eating meals, or during periods of stress. It is usually relieved by rest.* Treatment can involve the medication nitroglycerine.

Arrhythmias – irregular heart beat rhythm. *Red flag symptoms can include: patient feeling fluttering, flopping, racing heartbeat in chest; acute dizziness; chest pain; shortness of breath; hypotension; and/or abnormal pulse (too fast, too slow or irregular).* ECG studies and auscultation can be used for diagnosis. Depending on the type of arrhythmia and the severity of it, treatment can range from simply monitoring the condition, medications (such as antidysrhythmics), or sinoatrial node replacement (a "pacemaker"). Examples include:

- *Fibrillations-* extremely rapid, uncoordinated shuddering of heart muscle. *Atrial fibrillation (A-fib; AF)* involves irregular contractions of the atrial muscle tissue. It is the most common type of irregular heartbeat. *Ventricular fibrillation (V-fib; VF)* involves irregular contractions of the ventricular muscle tissue.
- *Premature Ventricular Contraction (PVC)* - create an extra contraction of the ventricular muscle prior to its normal contraction. Patients often report a sensation of a skipped beat or a "flip-flopping" sensation in their chest.
- *Heart block* - damage to the AV node, creating a longer gap between heart sounds.
- *Tachycardia-* rapid heart rate. Patients often report that they feel their heart racing or beating very fast, even though they are not exerting themselves at the time.
- *Bradycardia-* substantially slower heart rate.

Atherosclerosis – thickened, hardened blood vessel walls. It is thought that microscopic damage to the inner lining of the walls triggers the deposit of fats and cholesterol, which occlude the vessel and eventually lead to **arteriosclerosis**, the formation of scar tissue and the additional deposit of calcium salts. If this takes place in the coronary arteries which serve the heart, this condition is called *Coronary Artery Disease* (discussed later). If these changes occur in any other arteries in the body (outside of the heart or brain), the condition may be called *Peripheral Vascular Disease* (discussed later).

Bleeding disorders – decreased clotting ability. Commonly called having "thin blood," bleeding disorders most often result from an insufficient amount of circulating platelets (thrombocytopenia) or the chemicals and clotting factors that are necessary to trigger hemostasis. **Hemophilia** refers to bleeding disorders that are hereditary.

Buerger's Disease (also known as **Thromboangitis obliterans**) - an inflammatory disease that affects the blood vessels in the arms and legs. It can cause clots in the extremities. Tobacco use (smoking or chewing) has been strongly linked to this disease. Symptoms are pain in the arms or legs at rest or in movement (*claudication*), numbness, tingling, and burning (paresthesia) in the hands and feet. Hand and feet can be cool and mildly swollen.

Carditis- inflammation of the heart. Can be caused by cardiac infections (for example: endocarditis and myocarditis).

Coronary Artery Disease CAD (sometimes called **Coronary Heart Disease**) - CAD is atherosclerosis in the arteries of the heart. This can compromise blood flow to the myocardium of the heart and negatively impact the heart's functioning. CAD can lead to angina or a myocardial infarction (heart attack). Tests used to diagnose coronary artery disease include: coronary angiography with cardiac catheterization, ECG, exercise stress tests, or an echocardiogram. Treatments can include lifestyle changes (more exercise, quit smoking, increase exercise, dietary changes- low fat, low sodium), medications (antihyperlipidemic, antihypertensives, diuretics), or surgical procedures (angioplasty or cardiac artery bypass surgery).

Deep Vein Thrombosis- this is a blood clot in one of the deep veins of the body- commonly the leg. *Red Flag symptoms: swelling in ankle or lower leg (if clot is in the leg), a cramp-like pain in the calf, increased warmth in the area, or color changes of the skin in the area (may turn red or blue). But, many cases of DVT have no symptoms.* Main concern is that the clot will detach and move elsewhere in the body and become lodged in another vessel. Often if this occurs, the clot will detach and get stuck in the vessels feeding the lungs- causing a pulmonary embolism (a potentially life threatening condition). Diagnosis is often done with an ultrasound. Treatments involve thrombolytic drugs or anticoagulant medications.

Embolus- A drifting blood clot in the bloodstream. Can lead to other complications like pulmonary embolism, strokes, and myocardial infarctions.

Endocarditis- Infection which damages the innermost lining of the heart. It is especially damaging to the chordae tendinae and the heart valves. Mortality rate can be 21-35%. Blood clots may form as a result of the damage, and these clots can then break free causing myocardial infarctions, pulmonary embolisms, kidney damage, and strokes. Heart valves will also gradually become destroyed. Treatment- antibiotic therapy usually administered via IV.

Erythrocytosis- an increased number of RBC's. This is usually due to an increase in release of the hormone erythropoietin. Can be due to trauma to kidneys, or lack of oxygen to kidneys. High elevations can cause body to produce more erythropoietin. Also can be a result of "blood doping"- sometimes seen done by athletes. This causes thicker than normal blood, which may stress the cardiovascular system.

Heart Failure (also called **congestive heart failure- CHF**) - This is not a specific disease, but is usually the end result of other disease processes which have weakened the heart. This makes the heart less effective in pumping blood. Often it is a result of atherosclerosis of the coronary arteries, high blood pressure, and/or a heart attack (myocardial infarction). Left sided heart failure may cause fluid to build up in the lungs, causing breathing difficulties. Right sided heart failure may cause fluid (edema) to build up in the extremities or abdomen. *Red Flag symptoms: fatigue, shortness of breath (especially when lying down), swelling in legs/ankles/feet/abdomen, weight gain, persistent cough (especially if cough produces pink frothy mucus), wheezing, and/or irregular heartbeats.* Once heart failure begins, it is hard to reverse- so prevention is the best key. Exercise, dietary changes (low fat, low sodium), losing weight and quitting smoking all improve cardiovascular health and may help decrease the risk of heart failure.

Hemochromatosis- a genetic disorder that causes too much iron in the blood. Treatment may involve eating a low iron diet, no iron supplementation (so reading multivitamin labels and buying ones without iron), or removal of blood on a regular basis to lower iron levels.

Hemophilia- an inherited blood clotting disorder, causing inadequate production of clotting factors (protiens which help the platelets clot the blood). 80-90% of the time present in males. Transfusions of clotting factors are a common treatment. There are 2 main types of hemophilia. *Hemophelia A* has low levels of clotting factor VIII, and is the most common type (80% of hemophelia patients have this type). *Hemophelia B* is the second most common type, and has low levels of clotting factor IX.

Hyperlipidemia- elevated levels of lipids in the blood. Most commonly cholesterol levels and triglyceride levels are measured in the blood. Please see the Lipid Profile section in the Laboratory Test chapter for more information about triglycerides, total cholesterol levels, HDL cholesterol and LDL cholesterol. Treatment for hyperlipidemia involves dietary changes (low fat, low cholesterol, no trans-fats, and increased fiber), losing weight, increase in exercise and possibly medications (statins- the antihyperlipidemic medications).

Hypertension – high blood pressure, defined as 140/90 or higher. Although it may be asymptomatic for the first 10-20 years (its nickname is the "silent killer"), chronic hypertension slowly strains the heart and damages the arteries. Factors that contribute to high blood pressure include diet (high cholesterol, saturated fat, and sodium intakes), obesity, age, race, heredity, stress, smoking, or occasionally problems with the kidneys or the endocrine system. *Red flag symptoms: It is often asymptomatic; few individuals might have symptoms of headache, nocturia (nighttime urination) and nosebleeds.* Treatment will include lifestyle changes: dietary changes (low fat, low sodium- the DASH diet), increasing exercise levels, losing weight (if needed), and quitting smoking (if needed). Medications may be prescribed as treatment: diuretics, antihypertensives, and/or antihyperlipidemic medications.

Hypertensive Crisis/Emergency- very high blood pressure. 180/120 or higher. This extremely high level of blood pressure can damage blood vessels. *Red Flag Symptoms of emergency hypertensive crisis: blood pressure over 180/120, severe headache, confusion, blurred vision, severe chest pain, seizures, nausea and vomiting, shortness of breath, and/or unresponsiveness.* This is an emergency situation and 911 should be called. This can be fatal.

Hypertrophic cardiomyopathy- inherited condition, where walls of left ventricle thicken to the point where it has trouble pumping blood. Can also cause a fatal arrhythmia. A pacemaker may be implanted to correct arrhythmias.

Hypotension- low blood pressure. Sometimes defined as a blood pressure less than 90/60. Often, hypotension is not a problem- and in a healthy person can be a sign of good cardiovascular fitness. But, it can also be caused by dehydration (most common), heat exhaustion, hypothyroidism, as a result of significant blood loss, side effects of other medications, or as a complication of surgery. People with hypotension may have no symptoms. But, sometimes, hypotension can have symptoms which may be problematic. *Red flag symptoms: dizziness, fainting, lightheadedness, cold skin and extremities, nausea, and blurry vision. These symptoms should be of special concern in an elderly patient.* **Postural hypotension** (sometimes called **orthostatic hypotension**) can cause dizziness, lightheadedness or even fainting when the patient goes from sitting to standing or from lying to sitting. For patients with low blood pressure, it should be stressed to them that they need to take their time when sitting or standing immediately after an acupuncture session to minimize dizziness, falling, or fainting. Treatment could include administering fluids if the patient is dehydrated, wearing compression stockings, increasing salt intake or taking medications to treat postural hypotension.

Leukemia- abnormal (cancerous) blood condition involving the WBC's, causing extremely increased WBC counts. **Myeloid Leukemia-** presence of abnormal cells in the bone marrow (more common in adults). **Lymphoid leukemia-** presence of abnormal lymphocytes (often seen in children).

Murmurs – abnormal heart sounds that usually indicate valve problems, such as incompetent/insufficient valves that do not close tightly, or stenosed (narrowed and thickened) valves. See discussion in the Abnormal Examination Findings section for more information.

Myocardial infarction (MI) – commonly called a *"heart attack,"* an MI occurs when the myocardium is deprived of oxygen (*ischemia*), leading to crushing chest pain and the eventual death of the ischemic cells. MI does not respond to nitroglycerine (whereas angina will respond to nitroglycerine). *Red Flag symptoms of a heart attack are: pain in the chest that lasts more than a few minutes (it may come and go), pressure or squeezing sensation in the chest, shortness of breath, pain that radiates into the arm, neck jaw or back.* This is a medical emergency and 911 should be called right away.

Myocarditis- inflammation of heart muscle, caused by bacteria, viruses, fungi, protozoans. Heart rate may rise due to the damage. Abnormal contractions may occur, and over time the heart muscle will weaken. Treatment depends on what is causing the myocarditis.

Peripheral Vascular Disease (sometimes called *Peripheral Artery Disease- PAD*) - is atherosclerosis in any artery which is not in the heart or brain. This condition will decrease blood flow through the affected artery and reduce blood supply to the tissue or organ that the damaged artery serves. This, in turn, will cause that organ or tissue to perform poorly due to lack of oxygen and nutrients. Risk factors include being over the age of 50, smoking, being overweight, high cholesterol and diabetes. Symptoms will vary, depending on which arteries and body parts are affected. Many people are asymptomatic. A classic symptom of peripheral vascular disease is *intermittent claudication* (pain in the legs with walking, which improves with rest). An angiography/arteriography can be used to diagnose peripheral vascular disease.

Polycythemia Vera- results from an increase in all blood cell numbers, while blood volume remains the same. This causes all of the blood cells to become massively crowded in the bloodstream. RBC's begin to get stuck in and block smaller vessels, thus impairing blood and oxygen flow to tissues. Usual onset ages 60-80. Cause is unknown; treatment will keep disease under control but not cure it.

Pulmonary Embolism- this is a clot in one of the blood vessels in the lungs. Most often, this clot is formed elsewhere in the body (often in the legs as a deep vein thrombosis). If the clot breaks free from the area in which it formed, this moving clot is called an embolism. When the embolism circulates through the blood vessels, it can get stuck in the blood vessels supplying the lungs- a pulmonary embolism. Symptoms may involve pain in the chest, shortness of breath, coughing- sometimes coughing up blood. Untreated pulmonary embolisms can be fatal.

Raynaud's disease- most commonly affects women. Sympathetic nervous system causes excessive constriction of small arteries in the hands, feet, ears, and nose. Often triggered by exposure to the cold. Skin in the area changes color as blood flow is disrupted. First it becomes pale, and then turns blue. Eventually the skin will turn red once blood flow returns.

Rheumatic Heart Disease (RHD) - A complication of rheumatic fever. Rheumatic fever often attacks children ages 5-15, and is a result of an untreated infection by streptococcal bacteria. Fever, joint pain, stiffness, full body rash are symptoms. Carditis can develop, leading to scar tissue forming in the myocardium and valves. The valves become narrowed and thicker making them unable to shut and heal properly. Most commonly affects the mitral and aortic valves (mitral stenosis and aortic stenosis).

Temporal Arteritis- inflammation of the blood vessels bringing blood to the head- most often the temporal arteries. The vessels become inflamed and distended and are more visibly noticeable on observation during the physical exam and are tender upon palpation. Etiology is unknown. Treatment may involve corticosteroids (glucocorticoids) to reduce inflammation and prevent permanent damage.

Thalassemia- an inherited condition which causes an inability to produce hemoglobin, therefore RBC numbers drop. And the RBC's that are produced are very fragile and do not survive well. Treatment- blood transfusions.

Thrombophlebitis – an inflammation of a vein (phlebitis) that results when a clot forms in a vessel with poor circulation. A common consequence is clot detachment and a resulting ***pulmonary embolism***, which is life-threatening.

Thrombus- A blood clot attached to the inside of a blood vessel wall. Begins when platelets begin attaching to the roughened wall of a blood vessel. The blood vessel can be roughened and damaged by plaques (fat) and residue from cigarette smoke. The clot may grow to the point where it completely obstructs the blood vessel. Thrombolytic drugs and anticoagulant drugs may be given to dissolve the clot and prevent further formation (Coumadin, Warfarin, aspirin, tissue plasminogen activator)

Varicose veins – purple, snakelike, twisted, dilated veins in the feet and legs due to blood pooling because of inefficient venous return. Most often, inactivity or pressure on the veins causes the venous valves to fail. People who stand for long periods of time and obese (or pregnant) people are most at risk.

Practice Study and Test Questions:

1) A diagnostic test which may be useful in detecting and visualizing blockages of the coronary arteries is
    A) venography
    B) pulse oximetry
    C) coronary angiography
    D) chest x-ray

2) A patient has episodes of chest pain which radiates into the left arm and jaw. The patient states that the pain is worsened by stress and exertion, but is relieved by rest. This can indicate
    A) bradycardia
    B) myocardial infarction
    C) angina pectoris
    D) deep vein thrombosis

3) A patient reports a skipped beat or flip-flopping sensation in the chest. This can indicate
    A) erythrocytosis
    B) deep vein thrombosis (DVT)
    C) Buergers' disease
    D) preventricular contractions (PVC's)

4) A patient presents to your office with blood pressure over 180/120, severe headache, confusion and severe chest pain. You should
    A) call 911 immediately
    B) call a friend or family member to come pick up the patient after the treatment has concluded
    C) refer the patient to their PCP within 48 hours
    D) treat the patient, but strictly follow the protocol of elevating the patient's legs 6-12 inches

5) A patient reports that their fingers turn pale ("white"), then blue and then finally red whenever they go outside on a cold winter day. This could indicate
    A) hypertensive crisis
    B) a heart murmur
    C) myocardial infarction
    D) Raynaud's disease

6) Which diagnostic tool is a portable monitor which the patient can wear at home? It is usually used for 24 hours and measures the electrical activity of the heart.
        A) Coronary angiography
        B) Swan Ganz catheter
        C) Holter monitor

7) The valve located between the left atrium and left ventricle is the
        A) aortic valve
        B) pulmonic valve
        C) tricuspid valve
        D) mitral valve

8) A Western physical examination will document a weak pulse as
        A) 3+
        B) 4+
        C) 1+

9) Smoking is a risk factor in potentially developing
        A) hypertension
        B) thromboangitis obliterans
        C) atherosclerosis of the coronary and peripheral arteries
        D) all of the above

10) Pain in the legs with walking, which improves with rest is often a symptom of
        A) peripheral artery disease
        B) erythrocytosis
        C) congestive heart failure

11) To auscultate the aortic valve, the physician would place the stethoscope at the
        A) left side of the sternal border in the 2nd intercostal space
        B) left side of the sternal border in the 5th intercostal space
        C) left side of the chest at the midclavicular line in the 5th intercostal space
        D) right side of the sternal border in the 2nd intercostal space

12) The _____ receives blood from the _____ and ejects blood to the _____
        A) left atrium; left ventricle; body tissues
        B) right atrium; right ventricle; body tissues
        C) right ventricle; right atrium; lungs

13) The pacemaker of the heart is the
        A) sinoatrial node
        B) left ventricle
        C) atrioventicular node

14) An epigastric pulsation could indicate
        A) mitral valve murmur
        B) Raynaud's phenomenon
        C) myocardial infarction
        D) abdominal aortic aneurysm

15) The most abundant of the formed elements in the blood are the
        A) White blood cells
        B) Red blood cells
        C) Platelets

Answers: 1) C 2) C 3) D 4) A 5) D 6) C 7) D 8) C 9) D 10) A 11) D 12) C 13) A 14) D 15) B

CHAPTER 10: THE LYMPHATIC SYSTEM, IMMUNE SYSTEM AND COMMUNICABLE/INFECTIOUS DISEASES

The Lymphatic System

The lymphatic system is a main component of our bodies cleaning and defense system. It produces, maintains, and distributes lymphocytes throughout the body. It also serves as a way to circulate and return interstitial fluid back into the bloodstream. The main components of the lymphatic system are: lymph vessels (lymphatics), lymphoid tissues, lymphoid organs, and lymph.

Lymph and Lymph Vessels

Lymph is a fluid, extracted from blood plasma, but has a lower amount of suspended proteins than plasma. In the body tissues, it circulates around tissue cells carrying nutrients and flushing wastes and toxins. While in the tissue, this fluid is technically called *interstitial fluid*. Once drained into the lymph capillaries and lymph vessels, its name changes to *lymph*. An overabundance of interstitial fluid in a tissue is commonly called edema. The lymph, once collected from the tissues by the lymphatic vessels, will be cleansed by the lymph nodes. The lymph will then be returned into the bloodstream and recirculated back out to the body tissues.

In the cardiovascular system, blood flows through blood vessels. In the lymphatic system, lymph flows through *lymphatic vessels*. *Lymphatic capillaries* are the smallest lymphatic vessel, and drain lymph from the tissue. Lymphatic capillaries then pass the lymph into *small lymphatic vessels*. The small lymphatic vessels are similar to smaller veins and will carry the lymph towards the heart. The small lymphatic vessels will drain the lymph into major lymph collecting vessels- the **thoracic duct** and **right lymphatic duct**. The thoracic duct collects lymph from the lymph vessels on the left side of the head, left arm and chest, and both legs. The right lymphatic duct collects lymph from the lymph vessels of the right side of the head, right arm and right chest. The thoracic duct will then empty the lymph into the left subclavian vein, returning the lymph to the bloodstream. The right lymphatic duct will empty its contents into the right subclavian vein.

Lymphoid Tissues and Organs:

Lymphoid tissues are connective tissues dominated by lymphocytes. In a **lymphoid nodule**, it is built as a small area with many lymphocytes packed into areolar tissue. This small mass is *not* surrounded by a fibrous capsule. There is usually a germinal center located in each nodule, which contains dividing lymphocytes. There are two types of lymphoid nodules: *MALT (Mucosa associated lymphoid tissue)* and the *Tonsils*.

Lymphoid organs have a fibrous capsule which surrounds them. Here are a few examples: lymph nodes, thymus and spleen. *Lymph nodes* are cleaning and filtering station for lymph. They are filled with reticular connective tissue (a mesh-like tissue which allows filtering). Living inside of the lymph nodes are macrophages and lymphocytes, which dispose of debris and pathogens in the lymph nodes. Lymph nodes are widespread in location, but large clusters of nodes can be found in the inguinal, axillary, cervical, abdominal, and popliteal areas. The *spleen* is a blood rich organ, located in the left upper abdominal region. It functions to cleanse blood, remove old RBC, and store WBC's. The *thymus* is located beneath the sternum. It is the site of maturation of T-lymphocytes.

Immunity:

There are two main categories of body defenses we will be discussing:

1. **Non-specific defenses-** do not distinguish one threat from another- they do not care what they are attacking, and do not change their method of attack.

2. **Specific Defenses-** protect against a particular threat and will be very specific in their modes of attack. This is primarily accomplished by B and T lymphocytes (B cells and T cells).

Non-Specific Defenses:

Non-specific defenses are our first line of defense against an invading pathogen. There are many examples of non-specific defenses in our body. *Surface Membrane Barriers* (unbroken skin, mucus membranes)- provide a physical barrier and produce secretions which kill pathogens. *Phagocytes* are white blood cells which eat (phagocytize) pathogens. *Natural Killer Cells (NK Cells)* detect pathogens in a body tissue and release cytotoxic chemicals to kill them. *Inflammation* reduces the spread of pathogens and stimulates the immune response. *Interferons* are antimicrobial chemicals released from infected body cells. They function to warn nearby healthy body cells and instruct those cells to increase their defenses and fight off attack from the invading organism. *Complement* are another category of antimicrobial chemicals which agglutinates (stick) onto a pathogen, making it difficult for the pathogen to spread (and making it easier for phagocytes to attack it). *Fever* will stimulate immune cell response and increase internal temperature to make the pathogen uncomfortable in body.

Specific Defense System:

The specific defense system recognizes and destroys specific foreign molecules in our body. It is also known as the **Immune System.**

How are invaders recognized in our body? The answer is **Antigens**. Antigens are substances on the surface of cell membranes that can provoke an immune response. They can be composed of proteins, nucleic acids, and/or carbohydrates. Antigens are found on the surface of most substances and cells. Our immune system (T-lymphocytes and B lymphocytes) are trained to analyze and recognize antigens.

Self-Antigens are antigens found on the surface of our body cells. They are genetically determined protein markers and identify our cells as "self"- belonging to us. These antigens are recognized by our immune system cells and do not provoke an immune response in our body. But, self-antigens can be strongly antigenic to others and cause organ transplant rejections if a proper "match" of antigens between donor and recipient is not found. **Foreign Antigens** are antigens not normally found in our body. They are found on the surface of viruses, bacteria, pollen, mold, fungi, etc. These antigens can provoke an immune response.

Main cells of the Specific Defense System (Immune Response)

Three main cells are involved in an immune response:

1. **Macrophages (Antigen Presenting Cells/APC's)** are phagocytic WBC's. They engulf (eat) foreign particles and place fragments of these particles on their own cell surface to signal immunocompetent T- cells.

2. **T-Lymphocytes (T-cells)** originate in red bone marrow and then become *immunocompetent* in the thymus. The protective action of the T-cells is called the *cell mediated immune response*. There are two major classes of T-Cells. **Helper T-Cells (CD4 cells)** act as "directors"/"managers" of the immune response. Once the Helper T-cell is activated by an antigen presenting macrophage they: stimulate B-cells and killer T-cells to divide and do their jobs; attract other types of WBC's to the area; and stimulate macrophages to become voracious phagocytes. **Killer/Cytotoxic T-Cells (CDB cells)** are specialized killers which directly attack and kill cancer cells, infected cells, and foreign graft cells. They kill by injecting toxic chemicals into the target cell membranes.

A T cell can encounter a foreign antigen (antigen presentation) in two ways:
- *Class I MHC proteins* (major histocompatibility complex)- these proteins are embedded in the membrane of an invading cell or a body cell that has been taken over by a pathogen. When a T-cell encounters a cell with this class of proteins, it recognizes the cell as an invader and destroys it.
- *Class II MHC proteins*- these proteins are found only on the surface of some supporting cells of our immune system (antigen presenting cells and lymphocytes). As APC's are eating an invading cell, the APC's will take the foreign antigens and place them in their outer membrane. The APC can then come in contact with a T-cell, who "reads" the foreign antigens embedded in the APC's membrane. This lets the T-cell know we are under attack, and it begins to hunt any other foreign cells in our body.

Memory T cells are one of the components of our specific defense system that give us immunity from catching an illness a second time. Memory cells do not differentiate (become specialized and active) on the first exposure, but on the second exposure they will immediately differentiate into Cytotoxic T cells. What this means, is that the first time a memory T cell is exposed to the antigen (the first time you get infected) it will not react. But, if that same virus tries to attack you a second time, this T cell will immediately react to that second exposure and wipe out the infection before it has a chance to begin.

3. **B-Lymphocytes (B-cells)** originate in red bone marrow and also will become immunocompetent in red bone marrow. B cells behave differently than T cells. While T cells (Cytotoxic T cells especially) directly attack an invading or infected cell, B cells do not directly engage the attacker. B cells, once sensitized and activated, will produce and release **antibodies** (also called **immunoglobulins)** to destroy the pathogen. Antibodies are capable of binding to specific antigens on foreign cells to inactivate them. The protective action of antibodies is called the *humoral or antibody-mediated immune response*.

Once a pathogen has been encountered by a B cell, the B cell becomes sensitized. If the sensitized B cell comes in contact with a stimulated Helper T cell, the B cell becomes fully activated. An activated B cell immediately starts dividing. It will divide into:
- **Plasma Cells-** these cells are antibody factories and they begin to produce and secrete large amounts of antibodies which are designed to attack the foreign antigen
- **Memory B Cells-** these cells do not attack on a first exposure, but are on guard for a second exposure to the pathogen (much like memory T cells). On a second exposure, these memory cells immediately differentiate into plasma cells and begin secreting mass amounts of antibodies.

There are five antibody classes produced by the B cells:
1. **IgG-** the largest and most diverse class- 80% of all antibodies
2. **IgE-** often involved in allergic reactions
3. **IgD-** intensifies B cell activation
4. **IgM-** first antibody on the scene, holds down the bad guy until IgG's get there; and can also specialize in attacking some bacteria that IgG's can't handle
5. **IgA-** found primarily in saliva, tears and mucus- can be passed from mom to baby when breastfeeding

<u>Primary and Secondary Responses to Antigen Exposure:</u>

These primary and secondary responses are found in both B cells and T cells.

Primary Response is the initial response to exposure to a foreign antigen. For B cells, this response takes time. This is due to the fact that both *sensitization* and then *activation* must take place. Once activation occurs, plasma cells are gradually formed, and antibody levels gradually rise. *Antibody Titer* is the level of antibody activity. It peaks one to two weeks after exposure to the pathogen in the primary response, and then declines. IgM is the first antibody to arrive in the case of infections, and then IgG levels will gradually increase and take over the battle. Memory B cells and Memory T cells are created as a result of this primary exposure and response.

Secondary Response is the exposure of the body to a foreign antigen for the second time (getting infected months or years later with the exact same virus or bacteria). Memory B cells and T cells handle this second exposure. Because they were both sensitized during the primary response, they will immediately activate and begin responding. Memory T cells become Cytotoxic T-cells and start attacking. Memory B cells quickly start differentiating into plasma cells, and these plasma cells start secreting massive amounts of antibodies. Antibody titers rise more rapidly and much higher than in the primary response, thus extinguishing the pathogen before it has a chance to cause symptomatic illness.

Immunizations:

The theory behind an immunization is that the physician will inject a foreign antigen of a virus (the vaccine) into the body, tricking the B cells into thinking that the body is under attack. The B cells then produce antibodies and create Memory cells- thus giving the individual immunity to any future exposures. **Active immunizations** are given before a person becomes exposed to the pathogen (for example, the childhood immunizations). Active immunizations used as a preventative measure and will give the patient lasting immunity from contracting the illness. **Passive immunizations** are given once a person has already been exposed to a pathogen, and are often used to give the immune system a "boost" in its battle with the pathogen. These passive immunizations contain antibodies to fight the infection, but do not give immunity afterwards.

Active immunizations come in a few forms:
• *Attenuated vaccines*- live viruses or bacteria are injected, but are weakened before administering them. This allows the immune system to encounter the viral or bacterial antigens, but hopefully the virus/bacteria is weakened enough that it is unable to create an infection. Examples: Polio (oral form), chicken pox, rubella, mumps, measles, small pox, yellow fever, tuberculosis.
• *Inactivated vaccines*- "killed" vaccines- only consist of the outer coat of the virus or bacteria. May not stimulate as strong immunity as the attenuated vaccines, so may require booster shots. Examples: Hepatitis A and B, Polio (injected form), Influenza A and B, Streptococcal pneumonia, typhoid fever, tetanus, diphtheria.

Passive immunizations can include serum injections. Examples of serum injections are: *anti-venom injections* (used to treat a patient bitten by a venomous snake) and rabies shots that a patient receives after being bitten by a suspected rabid animal. Passive type immunization also includes *breast milk*. When a mother breast feeds her baby, she passes on her antibodies to her baby. This offers the baby some temporary protection from some illnesses as the baby's immune system develops and matures.

Communicable Diseases (Infectious Diseases):

Types of Infectious Pathogens

Bacteria- are one celled organisms. Many bacteria can be classified as **Gram Positive** *(gram positive cocci or gram positive bacilli)* or **Gram Negative** *(gram negative cocci or gram negative bacilli)* bacteria. Gram positive bacteria are bacteria with no outer membrane. Gram negative bacteria have an outer membrane present. Bacteria usually do not contain a nucleus. Most bacterial infections can be treated with different forms of antibiotics. *Bactericidal* substances kill bacteria, while *bacteriostatic* substances prevent bacterial growth.

Viruses- are one celled organisms, and physically smaller than bacteria. Viruses enjoy living inside of the host's body cells, not merely attacking and killing them. The virus uses the host cell as a breeding environment. The immune system of the host has a more difficult time attacking viruses, due the fact the virus will live inside the host cells. This makes treating viral infections a little more difficult. Viral infections cannot be treated with antibiotics. A few viral infections can be treated with anti-viral medications. Vaccines are often used as a preventative mechanism to prevent some viral infections from developing.

Fungi (mycoses)- Fungi can be a single celled organism or a multicellular organism. Yeast infections (for example: *candida*) are a type of fungal infections. Fungal infections can be classified according to their location on the body, route of acquisition, and strength of virulence. The different location classifications are: *superficial* (stratum corneum only), *cutaneous* (all layers of the skin or infections of the skin appendages), *subcutaneous* (infection of the subcutaneous tissues*) or *systemic/deep* (can infect internal organs such as the lungs, bones, central nervous system, etc.). Fungal infections can be acquired in one of two ways: *exogenous* (coming from a source outside the patient- airborne, cutaneous contact, etc.) or *endogenous* (internal colonization of normal flora or reactivation of a previous infection). Lastly, the strength of virulence can be classified as either a *primary pathogen* (infection can be developed in a normal healthy patient) or *opportunistic pathogen* (infection is usually only present in patients with a weakened immune system). Fungal infections might be treated with anti-fungal medications.

Parasite- a living organism that lives inside of a host (*endoparasite*) or on the surface of a host (*ectoparasite*). This parasite will obtain food and nutrients from the host. The parasite may directly harm the host or may produce toxins that in turn damage the host's cell structure and function

Prions- are non-living proteins which can cause changes in the brain of infected people and animals. Prions are implicated as the cause of spongiform encephalopathies, such as Mad Cow Disease (bovine spongiform encephalopathy), Chronic Wasting Disease (also in cows), and Creutzfeldt - Jakob disease (CJD) in humans.

Methods of Infectious Disease Transmission:

Autogenous infections are infections caused by an organism already living inside the host (example: E. coli from the digestive tract causing a UTI). **Cross-infections** are illnesses spread from another person or the environment. Infectious pathogens causing cross infections can be spread through many methods:
- **Droplet contact:** through aerosolized droplets spread by sneezing, coughing, talking.
- **Airborne:** smaller particulates (than in droplet contact) spread in the air. Pathogens can survive longer in the air without drying out (chickenpox, tuberculosis)
- **Oral-fecal:** fecal material comes in contact with something that is ingested orally (food, water)
- **Bodily fluids:** coming in contact with bodily fluids that harbor the pathogen (semen, vaginal secretions, blood, lymph, saliva, sweat)
- **Vector:** another organism carries the pathogen. It may be mechanical or biological. *Mechanical vector*- where the vector carries the pathogen on the outside of its body and transmits it. *Biological vector*- the pathogen enters the vector and then is spread by the vector usually through a bite (for example: a mosquito spreading West Nile Virus)
- **Indirect contact:** touching a contaminated surface (door knob, telephone, computer keypad etc.),

Physical Examination of the Lymphatic System

There are many individual lymph nodes which are widely spread throughout the body. There are also areas where there are larger clusters of lymph nodes aggregated together. The three regions described here are the clusters which commonly show enlargement. But, be aware that lymph nodes can be examined in other areas of the body in addition to the ones described here.

Head and Neck Lymph Nodes:

1. Inspect arms, legs and abdomen for any fluid retention/edema
2. Inspect the lymph nodes of the head and neck for any signs of swelling, redness and inflammation. Compare nodes bilaterally
3. Palpate the lymph nodes in the neck. Assess nodes for size, shape, mobility, consistency, temperature and tenderness. Compare nodes bilaterally

Lymph Nodes of the Axillae and Chest

1. Inspect the lymph nodes in the axillae and observe for any signs of swelling, redness and inflammation
2. Palpate the lymph nodes in the axillae. Assess nodes for size, shape, mobility, consistency, temperature and tenderness.
3. Palpate the clavicular nodes

Lymph Nodes of the Inguinal Region

1. Inspect the lymph nodes in the inguinal region and observe for any signs of swelling, redness and inflammation
2. Palpate the inguinal lymph nodes

General Abnormal Findings of Lymphatic System and Lymph Nodes

Abnormal findings, if necessary, should be referred to patients PCP or an immunologist

Lymphangitis- inflammation of one or more lymphatic vessels. It is often seen in a physical exam as red streaks following the course of a lymphatic vessel. There may also be pain, malaise, fever, and signs of inflammation or infection distal to the lymphatic vessel

Lymphedema- fluid build-up (edema) in various parts of the body. Hard to distinguish this type of edema from other forms- often must look at entire case history to help with diagnosis.

Tender nodes- often suggest inflammation

Hard or fixed nodes (non-painful)- often suggest malignancy

Advanced Imaging and Diagnostic Tests of the Lymphatic System and Lymph Nodes

Biopsy- Removal of tissue samples from affected area. Tissue samples are then analyzed, usually under a microscope for abnormalities. Doctors take biopsies of areas that look abnormal and use them to detect cancer, precancerous cells, infections, and other conditions. This can be done as a ***fine needle aspiration*** (inserting a needle into the node and withdrawing some tissue) or an ***excisional biopsy*** (surgically removing all or part of the lymph node for examination)

Chest x ray. A chest x ray takes an x-ray of the organs and structures inside your chest and around the chest wall (axillary and clavicular nodes).

Enzyme linked immunoabsorbent assay (ELISA)- Blood is drawn, and is mixed with a sample of allergens or microorganisms to test for the presence of specific antibodies. This test is usually done to help diagnose HIV infection.

Gram Staining (Gram's Method)- a procedure used to test and identify bacteria. It is performed on body fluid or tissue samples that are potentially infected. Stain is applied to the fluid or tissue sample, and results are much faster than using a culture. **Gram Positive bacteria** include Staphylococcus, Streptococcus, Listeria, and Bacillus. **Gram Negative bacteria** include the gut bacteria (proteobacteria), spirochetes, and cyanobacteria.

Pathologies of the Lymphatic and Immune Systems

AIDS (acquired immune deficiency syndrome)- caused by infection with the *Human Immunodeficiency Virus (HIV)*. Initial symptoms of HIV infection may be flu-like illness, fever, swollen lymph nodes. Then, often a recovery with no other symptoms for 5-10 years. HIV selectively attacks and kills Helper T cells (CD4/T4 cells). When analyzing a blood sample and counting Helper T cells, if the level of T cells is below 200 per µl (microliter), a person is said to be in late stage or advanced HIV disease (AIDS). HIV is spread by contact with infected bodily fluids. Four main methods of transmission- sexual transmission, IV drug use, blood transfusions with infected product, and prenatal exposure/breastfeeding. Treatments involve drugs to slow the progression of Helper T cell destruction- but there is no cure at this time.

Allergies (hypersensitivities) – an abnormally vigorous immune response. This occurs when the immune system causes tissue damage as it fights off a perceived "threat" that would otherwise be harmless to the body. These "threats" or *allergens* can include pet dander, pollen, dust, etc. The immune system will release histamine as it fights and destroys the allergen. The histamine release can cause the symptoms of the allergic response. Symptoms in the head and neck typically include a runny nose, watery eyes, swollen eyes, and itching, reddened skin. If the allergen is inhaled, symptoms of asthma may appear. Scratch tests (see integumentary system) may be done for diagnosis. Treatment may include over the counter or prescription allergy medications (Benadryl, Claritin, Flonase, Nasonex). For an anaphylaxic reaction (a rare but life threatening allergic reaction), epinephrine may be administered- usually in an injectable form ("EPI-pen"). Anaphylaxis can cause throat swelling, narrowing of airways, and a dramatic drop in blood pressure.

Autoimmune diseases – the immune system loses the ability to tolerate self-antigens while still recognizing and attacking foreign antigens. As a result, the body generates immune responses against its own tissues, causing significant damage. Some examples include *multiple sclerosis (MS), myasthenia gravis, Graves' disease, juvenile (type 1) diabetes mellitus, rheumatoid arthritis*, and others. There appear to be several possible triggers that may lead to autoimmune diseases. One is *inefficient lymphocyte programming*- this means that the lymphocytes have been trained to attack healthy normal body tissue cells instead of foreign invading cells. Another trigger may be *the creation and appearance of new self-antigens that were not previously exposed to the immune system*- some tissues in the body are normally isolated from contact with the immune system (for example: some cells in the internal eye). If damage occurs to the eye, which causes those cells to be exposed and encountered by the immune system, the immune system may not recognize them and attack them. The last possible trigger is *a cross-reaction of antibodies designed to attack foreign antigens with similar self-antigens*- this means that the antigen on the surface of a virus or bacteria is really similar in shape to a self-antigen (a marker found on healthy body cells). The immune system gets confused and accidentally starts attacking the healthy body cells- mistaking them for the invader.

Hodgkin's Disease (Hodgkin's Lymphoma)- is the cause of only 13% of lymphomas. Lymphoma is a cancer of the lymphocytes or lymphocytic stem cells. A key step in Hodgkin's disease involves the development of abnormally large cancerous B cells, called *Reed-Sternberg cells*. Instead of undergoing the normal cell cycle of life and death, these Reed-Sternberg cells don't die, and they continue to produce abnormal B cells in a malignant process. It usually affects people ages 15-35 or over the age of 50. Enlarged painless lymph nodes are a common symptom. Can progress to night sweats, fevers, gastrointestinal problems, weight loss. Physicians are unsure of the cause of Hodgkin's Disease, but some think it could possibly be from exposure to a virus. Treatment with radiation can produce a remission of symptoms for 10 years or more in 90% of patients. Success increases further if radiation is combined with chemotherapy. Chemotherapy drug cocktails (multiple chemotherapy medications combined) are often used.

Influenza *(the "flu")-* Most flu cases in the U.S. are caused by *Influenza A* virus. *Red Flag symptoms are: having a sudden onset of fever, cough, sore throat, headaches, body aches, chills, and possibly nausea/vomiting.* The common cold may have similar symptoms, but comes on more gradually. Very severe symptoms are most often seen in infants and young children, adults over age 65 and pregnant women. Antiviral medications can be administered for treatment. A seasonal flu vaccine is available each year. This flu vaccine offers protection against the three predicted strains that may be most common that flu season.

Leukemia- abnormal (cancerous) blood condition involving the WBC's, causing extremely increased WBC counts. Symptoms can be fatigue, fever, weakened immune response, swollen lymph nodes, and unexplained weight loss. Diagnosis be done with blood tests (looking for increased WBC counts) and a bone marrow biopsy. Treatment may include chemotherapy, radiation, and/or stem cell/ bone marrow transplants.
- ***Myeloid Leukemia-*** presence of abnormal cells in the bone marrow (more common in adults).
- ***Lymphoid Leukemia-*** presence of abnormal lymphocytes (often seen in children).

Lymphangitis- red streaks on the skin due to inflammation of superficial lymph vessels. Commonly occurs on the limbs, starting at an infected site and progressing proximally up the extremity towards the trunk. Lymph nodes in the region may be swollen. Often this can be caused by a Streptococcal infection. Diagnosis may be confirmed by a biopsy and culture of tissue from the area to determine the pathogen present. Treatment will usually include the appropriate type of antibiotic for the pathogen. The concern with lymphangitis is that the infection may spread into the bloodstream.

Lymphedema- accumulation of fluid within a tissue due to inadequate lymph drainage. Could be a result of damage to the lymphatic system or lymph nodes- which can cause scar tissue to form, impeding lymph flow. Could be due to removal of lymph nodes (often due to surgery). Also could be due to an infection by a parasitic roundworm (filiarisis)

Mononucleosis- (also called ***infectious mononucleosis***, ***"mono"*** or ***"kissing disease"***)- affects the spleen, causing enlargement (splenomegaly). This is usually caused by infection with the Epstein Barr Virus. *Red Flag symptoms may include swelling of spleen (splenomegaly) sore throat, swelling of lymph nodes, fatigue, fever. These symptoms may last for weeks.* Usually affects people age 15-25. No treatment available for this virus.

Non-Hodgkin's Lymphoma- Non-Hodgkin's lymphoma is made up of many different types of lymphomas. For this reason, Non-Hodgkin's lymphoma accounts for the majority of lymphoma cases. Non-Hodgkin's lymphoma has been one of the most rapidly increasing types of cancer in the U.S (more than doubled in incidence since the 1970s). In non-Hodgkin's lymphoma, the body produces abnormal lymphocytes (usually B cells) that continue to divide and grow uncontrollably. This oversupply of lymphocytes crowds into the lymph nodes, causing them to swell. In addition, these B cells are usually not functional- so immune system function will decline. Diagnosis is done with blood tests (to look for increased WBC numbers) and is confirmed with a biopsy of a lymph node. Lymphoma cancer can spread to other body areas. Treatment often involves chemotherapy, radiation, and/or stem cell transplant.

Systemic Lupus Erythematosus (SLE)- Symptoms- butterfly shaped rash over the nose and cheeks. In addition to the skin rash, kidney damage, arthritis, anemia, vascular inflammation and CNS deficits can result. Affects women nine times more often than men. Immune system antigen recognition breaks down and the immune system produces *autoantibodies*. Autoantibodies attack normal healthy body cells instead of invading pathogens. This is a widespread autoimmune disease causing vast amount of damage to tissues like the clotting factors, RBC's, platelets, and lymphocytes. Treatment: administering drugs to depress the immune system and/or corticosteroids.

COMMUNICABLE DISEASES / INFECTIOUS DISEASE CHART

Pathogen	Disease Name	Pathogen Type	Infection Information
Candida albicans	Candidiasis In mouth, can be called "thrush"; in vagina can be called "vaginitis"	Fungi	Most common opportunistic fungal infection. May be superficial (affecting skin or mucous membranes of the mouth, vagina, bladder, intestines) or deep (kidney, liver, spleen, brain). In babies, can be a cause of diaper rash.
Coccidiodes species	Coccidioidomycosis, "Valley Fever"	Fungi	Found most often in Arizona or California. Spores of the fungi are inhaled, leading to pulmonary infections, influenza like symptoms. Can progress to meningitis.
Tinea Pedis	Athlete's Foot	Fungi	Causes dry, itchy cracked skin on the feet. Can commonly be seen in the skin in-between the toes, on the soles, or top of the foot. Deep cracks in the skin can lead to bleeding. Can be treated with antifungal creams.
Tinea Cruris	Jock Itch	Fungi	Skin fungal infection in the groin area. Can lead to itching and redness of the skin. Can be treated with antifungal creams.
Tinea Ungulum	Nail fungus	Fungi	Fungal infection of the nails. Can affect the hands or feet- but more commonly the toenails. Antifungal medications can be prescribed.
Entamoeba histolytica	Amebiasis "Amebic dysentery"	Parasite	Spread by contact with feces, food or water contaminated with E. histolytica. Stomach pain and cramping, diarrhea, and fever can be symptoms. Antibiotics can be used to treat this.
Toxoplasmosis gondii	Toxoplasmosis	Parasite	Many infected people have no obvious symptoms. People with compromised immune systems (pregnancy, illness, etc.) can develop serious "flu"-like symptoms (aches and pains that can last for months). Can be spread as a foodborne illness or as a result of contact with fecal material from animals (such as cats).
Pediculus humanis	Pediculosis "Body Lice"	Parasite	Live and lay eggs (called nits) in clothing/ bedding/ upholstery, and move to the surface of the body to feed. Symptoms can be itching and rash on the skin in the areas of the lice bites. Spread through close physical contact with the infected person or the infected clothing/bedding/upholstery. Treatment involves thorough cleaning of the infected linens in hot water and dryer and, if needed, the use of a pediculicide medication.

Pathogen	Disease Name	Pathogen Type	Infection Information
Pediculus humanus capitis	Head lice	Parasite	Found on head, eyebrows and eyelashes of people. They live close to the scalp, lay their eggs (nits) on the human body and feed off of the blood of the human host many times a day. Symptoms can be tickling, or itching on the head- especially at night. Spread by physical (head to head) contact or sharing clothing/hats/helmets, etc. Treatment can involve cleaning of bedding in hot water and dryer. Careful removal of ALL nits or a pediculicide medication can be used.
Phthirus Pubis	Pubic lice "Crabs"	Parasite	They live in pubic region and lay their eggs (nits) on the shaft of the pubic hair. The adults feed off of human blood. Commonly spread during intimate sexual contact. Symptoms can be itching in the genital area. Treatment involves washing clothing and bedding in hot water and dryer and use of a pediculicide medication.
Sarcoptes Scabii	Scabies	Parasite	This parasite burrows into the upper layer of the skin and lays its eggs there. Symptoms are intense itching and rash in the affected areas. Can be spread by direct contact. Scabicides are prescription medications that can kill scabies. Bedding and clothing should be washed and dried at high heat
Trichomonal vaginalis	"Trich"	Parasite	The most common curable STD/STI. May show unusual vaginal or penile discharge- or no symptoms at all (70 % of the cases). Treatment: Antibiotics (metronidazole or tinidazole) are used.
Cryptosporidium	"Crypto"	Parasite	Parasite found in fecal material of humans or animals which can enter the drinking water. One of the most frequent causes of waterborne disease in the U.S. This parasite is very resistant to chlorine treatment of water. Symptoms are diarrhea and abdominal discomfort. Treatment: Notazoxanide
Giardia intestinalis	Giardia "Beaver fever"	Parasite	Parasite found in fecal material of humans or animals which can enter the drinking water; or found on object surfaces which have come in contact with fecal material (bathroom surfaces, changing tables). Causes diarrhea symptoms and abdominal discomfort. Prescription medications are available for treatment.
Anciostoma duodenale and *Necator americanus*	Hookworm	Parasite	Intestinal parasite spread through feces. If infected fecal material is placed on the soil, the eggs will hatch. The hatched larvae can attach and penetrate human skin to create the infection (for example, after walking barefoot, gardening, children playing in the dirt). Itching and rash at the site of infection are often first symptoms, followed by abdominal pain and diarrhea. Medications are available.

Pathogen	Disease Name	Pathogen Type	Infection Information
Plasmodium	Malaria	Parasite	***BLOODBORNE ILLNESS*** Transmitted by mosquitos. Causes serious symptoms: high fevers, chills, flu like illnesses. Untreated, it can be fatal. Diagnoses in US are usually in people who have travelled to or who are immigrants from affected countries (Sub-Saharan Africa and South Asia). Antimalarial drugs can be used for treatment (although some parasites are becoming resistant) - prevention is the best method (mosquito netting over beds, etc.).
Enterobius vermicularis	Pinworm	Parasite	Spread through contact with fecal material (oral-fecal transmission). Common in all ages, but especially children. Lives in the large intestine of humans. The pinworm will leave the intestine while the person is sleeping and lays its eggs around the outer surface of the anus. The symptoms can be itching around the anus. Medication can be given. Proper cleaning of clothing and bedding is necessary to prevent reinfection.
Taenia **species**	Tapeworm infections	Parasite	Infections can occur by consuming raw or undercooked meat. Symptoms can be mild or non-existent, so many people may not even know they are infected.
CJD Prion	Creutzfeldt Jacob Disease, Mad Cow Disease	Prion (an infectious protein)	Is transmitted by consuming contaminated meat, or receiving a contaminated tissue during organ transplant. Symptoms are rapidly progressing dementia and muscular clonus.
Flavivirus	West Nile Virus	Virus	A mosquito borne virus. Infection can cause fever, meningitis, encephalitis, flaccid paralysis. This virus can be carried in birds (crows, jays). It is spread to humans when a mosquito bites an infected bird and then bites a human.
Calcivirus	Norwalk Virus Norovirus "Noro"	Virus	Spread via the oral-fecal route. Symptoms include nausea, vomiting, diarrhea, abdominal pain, muscle aches, headaches, fatigue and fever.
Epstein Barr Virus	Mononucleosis "Kissing Disease"	Virus	Mononucleosis affects the spleen, causing enlargement (splenomegaly). Other symptoms may include sore throat, swelling of lymph nodes, fatigue, fever. Usually affects people age 15-25. No treatment available for this virus.
HAV **Hepatits A Virus**	Hepatitis A "Hep A"	Virus	Spread via the fecal-oral route, usually through contaminated food or water. Symptoms can mimic the flu- fever, fatigue, aches, jaundice may be present. Usually does not have a chronic stage or cause permanent liver damage. Vaccine available.
HBV **Hepatitis B Virus**	Hepatitis B "Hep B"	Virus	***BLOODBORNE ILLNESS*** Spread via blood, semen and vaginal fluids. Can cause vomiting, jaundice, cirrhosis. Rarely fatal. Vaccine available.

Pathogen	Disease Name	Pathogen Type	Infection Information
HCV Hepatitis C Virus	Hepatitis C "Hep C"	Virus	***BLOODBORNE ILLNESS*** Most fatal form of Hepatitis. No vaccine available. Usually no symptoms in early infection. Chronic infection can lead to jaundice and cirrhosis of the liver. This can progress to liver failure and be fatal.
H1N1 Influenza	"Swine Flu"	Virus	In 2009 a pandemic was declared due to the H1N1 virus. Flu viruses (including H1N1) are spread mainly from person to person through coughing, sneezing or close contact with infected persons (or touching objects contaminated by infected person). The symptoms of H1N1 flu virus include fever, cough, sore throat, runny or stuffy nose, body aches, headache, chills and fatigue. Severe illnesses and deaths have occurred as a result of illness associated with this virus
Human Papillomavirus (HPV)	Cervical cancer Warts (genital and hand/foot)	Virus	Cervical cancer is the second most common cancer in women and is most often caused by HPV infection (HPV-16 and HPV-18). HPV can be transmitted during sexual intercourse. Other strains of HPV can cause warts: genital= HPV-6 and HPV-11, foot (plantar) warts= HPV-1, and hand warts= HPV-2.
Varicella zoster	Chicken Pox Shingles	Virus	Symptoms include fever and headache. A rash then begins- with small itchy fluid filled blisters forming on the body. The rash begins on the face or trunk and then can spread to other areas. These blisters are filled with a clear fluid which contains live virus. The blisters will eventually dry and scab- usually leaving no scar. Usually the person recovers with no complications. Shingles is a reoccurrence of the infection later in life, usually only following one dermatome.
Herpes Simplex Virus	Cold sores Genital herpes	Virus	*Herpes simplex virus type 1 (HSV-1)* is the usual cause of cold sores. *Herpes simplex virus type 2 (HSV-2)* is the usual cause of genital herpes. In both cases, painful, blistering lesions can appear on the skin. Live virus is found in the fluid of these lesions and can be transmitted to others. HSV-2 is one of the most common sexually transmitted diseases in the US. The virus lives in the spinal nerves and will cause periodic localized outbreaks of the lesions.
Rubeola virus	Measles	Virus	Highly contagious. Symptoms can include a red rash all over the body, fever, runny nose and a cough. It can also cause ear infections, pneumonia, encephalitis or death (in rare cases). A vaccine (MMR or MMRV) is available for this disease.

Pathogen	Disease Name	Pathogen Type	Infection Information
Mumps virus	Mumps	Virus	Symptoms are fever, headache, muscle aches and fatigue. The salivary glands will then swell (called parotitis). Possible complications are inflammation of the testicles (orchitis) or ovaries (oophoritis), which can lead to sterility. Inflammation of the brain (encephalitis) or meningitis can occur. Vaccine (MMR or MMRV) is available.
Variola major and *Variola minor*	Small Pox	Virus	After a two week incubation period symptoms arise, such as: fever, headache, fatigue. A flat, red rash then appears, first on face and arms, then spreading to trunk. The rash first appears red and then forms blistering lesions (the blisters often have a dimpled appearance). The fluid in the blisters is first clear and then turns to pus. The blisters eventually dry and scab, and will leave deep permanent pitted scars. Blisters can also form in the nose, mouth and throat. Blindness and death can occur.
Rhinoviruses and *Coronaviruses*	Common Cold	Virus	Many different viruses cause what we call the "common cold". Symptoms can include coughing, sore throat, runny nose, sneezing, and fever.
Human Immunodeficiency Virus (HIV)	HIV AIDS (acquired immune deficiency syndrome)	Virus	***BLOODBORNE ILLNESS*** Initial symptoms of HIV infection may be flu-like illness, fever, swollen lymph nodes. Then, often a recovery with no other symptoms for 5-10 years. HIV selectively attacks and kills Helper T cells (CD4/T4 cells). Spread by contact with infected bodily fluids. Four main methods of transmission- sexual transmission, IV drug use, blood transfusions with infected product, and prenatal exposure/breastfeeding. Treatments involve drugs to slow the progression of Helper T cell destruction- but there is no cure. AIDS is diagnosed when the level of T cells is below 200 per µl (microliter).
Orthomyxoviridae family	Influenza	Virus	This large family of viruses has the Influenza A, Influenza B, Influenza C viruses (of which Influenza A is most commonly responsible in human illnesses). Bird flu and swine flu are variants of Influenza A (H1N1 "Swine Flu", H5N1"bird flu", H3N2). Vaccinations are available for some strains of Influenza A and B.
Cocksakie A virus	Hand, foot and mouth disease (HFMD)	Virus	HFMD usually affects infants and children. Usually spread via contact with saliva, mucus or fecal material. Symptoms of HFMD include: fever, sore throat, rash (which may blister) on the hands, feet and sometimes lips.

Pathogen	Disease Name	Pathogen Type	Infection Information
Ebolavirus	Ebola	Virus	***BLOODBORNE ILLNESS*** This is a type of viral hemorrhagic fever seen primarily in Africa. Symptoms are fatigue, chills, muscle pain, nausea, diarrhea, and rashes on the skin. Internally, bleeding (hemorrhage) occurs. Ultimately internal organs fail and death occurs. Spread via contact with fluids such as diarrhea, vomit, blood, and direct contact. Dead bodies may also still transmit disease, so strict burial practices must be followed.
Poliovirus	Polio Poliomyelitis	Virus	In 95% of infected people, the virus causes no effects. In 5% of the people, symptoms will occur. In some people the infection presents as a mild flu, from which they recover. In the severe cases (paralytic polio), the virus attacks somatic motor neurons (the nerves that carry messages from the brain to your muscles), causing paralysis. If the respiratory muscles are affected, this can be fatal. In individuals who survive paralytic polio, they may suffer from *postpolio syndrome* later in life- where muscles not paralyzed by polio earlier, start to lose their strength. A vaccine is available for prevention of polio.
SARS coronavirus	SARS (Severe Acute Respiratory Syndrome)	Virus	Outbreak in 2002-2003. Now, relatively rare. Symptoms of SARS: fever of over 100.4 with a cough, difficulty breathing.
Rotavirus	Rotavirus infection	Virus	Most common cause of diarrhea in young children. Rotavirus A causes over 90% of the infections. Vaccine available.
Respiratory Syncytial Virus	RSV infection	Virus	Causes lower respiratory tract infections, often in infants and children. Most children will have been infected with RSV by the time they are 2 or 3 years old.
Rabies virus	Rabies	Virus	Initial symptoms may be flu-like, then mental confusion, paranoia, hallucinations and paralysis may set in. Without treatment, death will occur within 2-10 days after initial symptoms.
Staphylococcus	Causes many illnesses	Bacteria	Can cause many illnesses. Some examples are: impetigo, abscesses and boils in skin, osteomyelitis, endocarditis, septicemia, toxic shock syndrome, and gastroenteritis (food poisoning).
MRSA (Methicillian resistant Staphylococcus aureus):	MRSA	Bacteria	Infection caused by a staph bacterium which is resistant to antibiotics normally used to treat staph infections. Most occur in people who have been in a health care setting (hospital, dialysis center, nursing home). Spread through skin to skin contact, cuts, and invasive medical procedures.

Pathogen	Disease Name	Pathogen Type	Infection Information
Group A Streptococcus (GAS)	Causes many illnesses	Bacteria	Can cause many illnesses. Some examples are: strep throat, impetigo, septic arthritis, osteomyelitis, meningitis, sinusitis, post-streptococcal glomerulonephritis.
Group B Streptococcus (GBS)	Strep B Newborn GBS disease	Bacteria	Can be found as normal flora in 20-40% of women. But, if the woman is pregnant, GBS could cause infection and death in the baby. Usually a pregnant woman is tested in the 36ᵗʰ week of pregnancy for GBS. If present, IV antibiotics will be administered during delivery.
Streptococcus pneumoniae	Bacterial pneumonia	Bacteria	This bacterium can cause pneumonia, otitis media and bacterial meningitis. Many of these are resistant to penicillin, and may be resistant to some cephalosporins, vancomycin, erythromycin, and tetracycline.
VRE- (Vancomycin resistant Enterococci)	VRE	Bacteria	Enterococci are bacteria normally found in human intestines, female reproductive tract, and in the environment. VRE is a strain which is resistant to the antibiotic normally prescribed for these infections. Most exposure of VRE is in hospitals.
Borrelia burgdorferi	Lyme Disease	Bacteria	Chronic fever, arthritis, rash with a bulls-eye center. Transmitted to humans through a bite from a deer tick. More common on the East coast. Treatment- antibiotics and anti-inflammatory drugs
Mycobacterium leprae and *Mycobacterium lepromatosis*	Hansen's disease- Leprosy	Bacteria	This bacterium destroys cutaneous nerve endings which are sensitive to pain, touch, heat, and cold. Damage to the distal tissues occurs, due to the fact the individual no longer feels pain in the area
Bacillus anthracis	Anthrax	Bacteria	This bacteria forms spores. If the spores are inhaled, it can create a very aggressive pneumonia which can be fatal. Vaccine available. Ciprofloxacin (Cipro) available for treatment if exposure occurs.
Mycobacterium Tuberculosis	Tuberculosis (TB)	Bacteria	Causes a massive inflammatory and immune response, including fibrous or calcified nodules in the lung tissue. Symptoms include fever, night sweats, weight loss, a racking cough, and spitting up blood (blood tinged sputum). It is contagious through the air from actively infected individuals.
Neisseria meningitides and *Streptococcal pneumonia*	Bacterial Meningitis	Bacteria	These two are the most common cause of bacterial meningitis in adults and older children. (Meningitis in newborns is most commonly caused by Group B strep.)

Pathogen	Disease Name	Pathogen Type	Infection Information
Salmonella	Gastroenteritis, "food poisoning" "Typhoid fever" – caused by *S. Typhi*	Bacteria	Common cause of food poisoning, especially in undercooked eggs and poultry. *S. Typhi* is rare in US due to chlorination of drinking water.
Escherichia coli (E. coli)	Gastroenteritis, and urinary tract infections	Bacteria	Common cause of food poisoning, especially in undercooked beef and pork. Also, E. coli is the most common cause of urinary tract infections and pyelonephritis (kidney infections).
Clostridium perfringens	Gastroenteritis and gas gangrene	Bacteria	3rd most common cause of gastroenteritis in US. Also the most common cause of "gas gangrene".
Campylobacter Jejuni	Campylobacteriosis Gastroenteritis	Bacteria	Can be spread via the fecal oral route or through sexual contact. One of the most common causes of gastroenteritis. Post infection (in rare cases)- Guillain Barre Syndrome can develop.
Clostridium botulinum	Botulism	Bacteria	The bacteria produce pathogenic spores. If the spores are consumed via contaminated food or enter through a wound, botulism can develop. Symptoms: muscular weakness and paralysis. Muscles served by the cranial nerve (eye, face, throat) are affected first, then arms and legs. Can be fatal.
Vibrio cholerae	Cholera	Bacteria	Symptoms are diarrhea and vomiting. Spread via fecal contaminated food or water. Dehydration may result, and can be fatal if untreated. Treatment involves rehydration and antibiotics. With proper treatment, survival rate is 99%
Treponema Pallidium	Syphilis	Bacteria	***BLOODBORNE ILLNESS*** A STD/STI spread through sexual contact or from a mother to a fetus. There are 4 stages of illness (primary, secondary, latent, and tertiary). Symptoms depend on the stage, but can include: chancre (painless ulcer – usually in genital region), rash on the hands and feet, and neurological symptoms. Treatment: penicillin or azithromycin.
Chlamydia trachomatis	Chlamydia	Bacteria	One of the most common STD/STI worldwide. Many women infected do not show symptoms, men usually have white penile discharge. Can be treated with azithromycin, erythromycin or doxycycline

Pathogen	Disease Name	Pathogen Type	Infection Information
Neisseria gonorrhoeae	Gonorrhea "The Clap"	Bacteria	A STD/STI. Symptoms in men include penile discharge and painful urination. Females may have no symptoms or vaginal discharge. Treatment with antibiotic cephtriaxone. Often occurs with chlamydia, so treatment may also include antibiotics for chlamydia.
Rickettsia prowazekii and *Rickettsia typhi*	Typhus "Jail fever"	Bacteria	Spread by body lice or fleas. Symptoms include fever, headaches, rash, muscle pain, chills, delirium, and death. Treatment- doxycycline and tetracycline
Clostridium tetani	Tetanus	Bacteria	The bacteria will release a neurotoxin which affects the motor neurons, causing skeletal muscles to go into a sustained powerful muscular contraction. Most common early complaints are headache, muscle stiffness, difficulty in swallowing. Widespread muscle spasms occur 2-3 days after initial symptoms including difficulty opening jaw "lockjaw". 40-60% of severe cases will die. DTaP and Tdap vaccine (Diphtheria, Pertussis, Tetanus) available.
Cornyebacterium diptheriae	Diptheria	Bacteria	Symptoms: sore throat, fever, swelling in neck. DTaP and Tdap vaccine (Diphtheria, Pertussis, Tetanus) available.
Bordatella pertussis	Pertussis "Whooping cough"	Bacteria	Serious condition in infants and in children, can be fatal. Starts with mild cold symptoms, but severe coughing fits begin a few weeks later. During a violent coughing spell, the patient will try to take a big breath of air- the "whooping" sound. DTaP and Tdap vaccine (Diphtheria, Pertussis, Tetanus) available.

Practice Study and Test Questions:

1) Eating food that was contaminated with fecal material is an example of which method of disease transmission?

    A) droplet contact
    B) airborne
    C) oral-fecal
    D) indirect contact

2) Biopsies performed in the lymphatic system can include

    A) fine needle aspiration
    B) excisional biopsy
    C) transdermal biopsy
    D) both A and B

3) Which type of immunization is given before the person has contracted the disease?
    A) passive immunization
    B) active immunization
    C) noxious immunization
    D) humoral immunization

4) Cold sores are commonly caused by
    A) Human papilloma virus
    B) Varicella zoster
    C) Herpes simplex virus type 2
    D) Herpes simplex virus type 1

5) Examples of gram positive bacteria are
    A) Streptococcus and Proteobacteria
    B) Cyanobacteria and Spirochetes
    C) Staphylococcus and Streptococcus
    D) Staphylococcus and Escherichia Coli

6) HIV infection is commonly diagnosed using
    A) fine needle aspiration
    B) Gram staining
    C) enzyme linked immunoabsorbent assay (ELISA)
    D) all of the above

7) A non-living infectious protein which can cause changes in the brain of the infected individual is called a
    A) bacteria
    B) virus
    C) fungi
    D) prion

8) Which of the following is a STD/STI?
    A) Toxoplasmosis gondii
    B) Enterobius vermicularis
    C) Borrelia burgdorferi
    D) Treponema pallidium

9) The presence of Reed Sternberg cells are a diagnostic key for
    A) Lupus
    B) HPV infection
    C) Mononucleosis
    D) Hodgkin's lymphoma

10) If E. coli from a patient's digestive tract is moved into the patient's urinary tract, this can cause
    A) a cross-infection
    B) an autogenous infection
    C) a parasitic infection
    D) an opportunistic infection

11) Sore throat, swelling of the spleen, and fatigue may be signs of
    A) AIDS
    B) lymphangitis
    C) Mononucleosis
    D) Systemic lupus erythematosus

12) The thoracic duct will collect lymph from the
    A) right arm, right side of the head and right side of the chest
    B) left and right leg
    C) entire right side of the body
    D) left and right arm

13) The most common virus family which causes influenza is the
    A) Group A Streptococcus family
    B) Norovirus family
    C) Orthomyxoviridae family
    D) Coccidiodes family

14) B lymphocytes
    A) produce antibodies
    B) are the "managers" of the immune response
    C) directly attack and kill cancer cells
    D) release cytotoxic chemicals to kill pathogens

15) Which of the following is the most common opportunistic fungal infection?
    A) Candida albicans
    B) Tinea pedis
    C) Tinea cruris
    D) Tinea ungulum

16) Which of the following is not an example of a non-specific defense?
    A) Natural Killer Cells
    B) phagocytes
    C) interferons
    D) humoral response

17) Diarrhea and gastrointestinal distress can be symptoms of an infection with
    A) Giardia
    B) Campylobacter jejuni
    C) Clostridium perfringens
    D) All of the above

18) Lymphatic fluid is returned to the bloodstream at the
    A) aorta
    B) right atrium of the heart
    C) subclavian veins
    D) vena cava

Answers: 1) C 2) D 3) B 4) D 5) C 6) C 7) D 8) D 9) D 10) B 11) C 12) B 13) C 14) A 15) A 16) D 17) D 18) C

CHAPTER 11: THE RESPIRATORY SYSTEM

Functions of the Respiratory System:

1. Providing an extensive surface for exchange between air and circulating blood
2. Moving air to and from the exchange surfaces of the lungs along the respiratory passageways.
3. Protecting respiratory surfaces from dehydration, temperature changes, or other environmental variations, and defending the respiratory system from invasion by pathogens.
4. Producing sounds involved in speaking, singing, and other forms of communication
5. Facilitating the detection of olfactory stimuli by olfactory receptors in the superior portions of the nasal cavity

Organization of the Respiratory System:

The respiratory system can also be called the *Pulmonary System*. The respiratory system can be divided into: the **upper respiratory system** (nose, nasal cavity, paranasal sinuses, and pharynx); and the **lower respiratory system** (larynx, trachea, bronchi, bronchioles, and alveoli).

The **nose** is the primary passageway for air entering the respiratory system. It consists of the *external nares, nasal vestibule, nasal septum, the nasal meatuses (superior, middle, and inferior), hard and soft palate*, and *paranasal sinuses*. Lining the nasal cavity is the *nasal mucosa*, which is highly vascularized (to bring nutrients to the mucosa and warm the incoming air). The nasal cavity also has a lot of mucus and goblet cells (for cleaning and adding moisture to the air), and hair (for cleaning and filtering the air).

After leaving the nose, the air enters the **pharynx**. The pharynx (aka the throat) is a muscular tube which carries both air and food/water from the digestive system. There are three parts to the pharynx: *nasopharynx, oropharynx*, and *laryngopharynx*.

Inferior to the pharynx is the **larynx** (the "voice box"). The larynx is composed of many different pieces of cartilage. The largest is the *thyroid cartilage*, which in men is often called the "Adam's apple". The *epiglottis* is found on top of the larynx, and can elevate and lower- covering and uncovering the central passageway (glottis) of the larynx. The epiglottis helps to prevent food from entering the larynx. Located inside the larynx are the *vocal folds* (vocal cords). These folds can vibrate as air passes by- creating the sounds we use for speech. The pitch of our voice depends on the diameter, length and tension of the vocal folds. A vocal fold with a thin diameter and shorter length will give a higher pitch than a thicker, longer vocal cord. The tension on the vocal folds is created by the laryngeal musculature pulling on them. The more tension placed on the folds, the higher the pitch of the voice. The volume of speech is determined by the velocity of air moving the vocal folds. *Phonation* is sound production at the larynx. *Articulation* is the modification of those sounds into intelligible words (often done by the pharynx, lips, and tongue).

Next, the air will pass through the **trachea** (the "windpipe"). The trachea begins at the level of C6 and extends down to approximately T5, where it splits into two branches called the *primary bronchi*. The trachea contains about 15-20 *tracheal cartilages* (C-shaped rings), stacked on top of one another. Mucus and pseudostratified ciliated columnar cells line the inside of the trachea.

At the level of T5, the trachea divides into the **left and right primary bronchi**. The left primary bronchi carries air to the left lung, the right primary bronchi carries air to the right lung. The primary bronchus will enter each lung at the *hilus*- a notched area on the medial surface of the lung. The primary bronchi, nerves, and blood vessels will all enter the lung at this area.

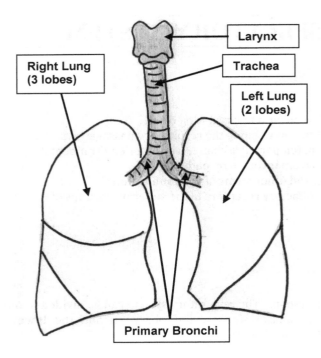

Right Lung (3 lobes)

Larynx

Trachea

Left Lung (2 lobes)

Primary Bronchi

An individual has two **lungs**- a right lung and left lung, located in the chest. The chest cavity is separated into two *pleural cavities* (right and left), and each lung fills a pleural cavity. The pleural cavity is lined with a friction reducing membrane called the *pleura*. The *parietal pleura* covers the inside of the ribcage, and the *visceral pleura* covers and lubricates each lung. The right lung is larger and has three lobes (*superior, middle,* and *inferior lobes*). The left lung is smaller and has two lobes (*superior* and *inferior lobes*).

Within the lungs, the **bronchi** and **bronchioles** extend off of the primary bronchi. This begins the *bronchial tree* in each lung. Each bronchi and bronchiole has thin amounts of cartilage, mucus, cilia cells, and smooth muscle in its inner lining. The primary bronchi, upon entering the lung, divide into *secondary bronchi*. In each lung, a secondary bronchi branch will go to each lobe of the lung (therefore, the right lung has three secondary bronchi and the left lung only has two). The secondary bronchi then divide into smaller *tertiary bronchi* (or *segmental bronchi*). Off of each tertiary bronchi come many smaller branches which are called *bronchioles*. Bronchioles do not have cartilage in their walls, but they do have smooth muscle and mucus. This smooth muscle allows for bronchoconstriction and bronchodilation. Bronchioles will continue to divide and branch into *terminal bronchioles*. Eventually, the terminal bronchioles will branch into very tiny and delicate *respiratory bronchioles*. These little bronchioles deliver the air to the alveolar ducts and alveoli.

Alveolar Ducts and **Alveoli** are located at the end of the respiratory bronchioles within the lungs. *Alveolar ducts* are air passageways which carry air from the bronchioles. The alveolar ducts empty air into the *alveoli*- the microscopic air sacs. It is here in the alveoli, where oxygen and carbon dioxide exchange can occur. There are about 150 million alveoli in each lung. Each alveoli has an extended capillary associated with it. This allows easy diffusion of gases (oxygen and carbon dioxide) between the alveoli of the lungs and the bloodstream. Alveolar epithelium is a delicate layer of simple squamous epithelium. *Alveolar macrophages* try to clean the inside of the alveoli. *Septal cells* produce a secretion called *surfactant*, which decreases the surface tension of the inner lining of the lungs (making them less sticky and less likely to collapse).

The **respiratory membrane** is where gas exchange takes place and is composed of the simple squamous epithelium of the alveoli, the endothelium of the capillary, and the basal lamina which is in between the alveoli and capillary. *Diffusion* allows gases to pass through the respiratory membrane. (Diffusion is when a gas moves from an area of higher concentration/partial pressure to an area of lower concentration/partial pressure). Oxygen will diffuse from the alveoli into the capillary, and carbon dioxide will diffuse from the capillary into the alveoli.

Respiratory Physiology

Respiration involves four main steps: **Pulmonary Ventilation**: the physical act of breathing; **External respiration**: gas exchange (diffusion) between the lungs and blood in the pulmonary capillaries; **Gas transport**: moving oxygen and carbon dioxide through the bloodstream; and **Internal Respiration**: gas exchange (diffusion) between the systemic capillaries and body tissue. Let's discuss these four steps:

Pulmonary Ventilation: The goal of pulmonary ventilation is to move air in and out of the alveoli of the lungs. In order to move air in and out of the lungs, we must change the pressure inside of the lungs as compared to the atmospheric pressure outside of the lungs. **Boyle's Law** states that if you decrease the volume (the container size) of a gas, the pressure the gas is under will rise; if you increase the volume of a gas, the pressure the gas is under will fall. To achieve Boyle's Law, contraction and relaxation of thoracic musculature and the elasticity of the lungs allow the volume of the ribcage to increase on inspiration, and decrease on expiration. During inspiration, muscles contract and increase the volume inside the ribcage. Pressure inside the ribcage will drop and air will rush into the lungs, inflating them (called **inspiration**). As we move into **expiration**, the volume inside the ribcage decreases and air pressure inside the lungs increases-expelling air from the lungs. Muscles involved in the act of inspiration are the contraction of *diaphragm* and *external intercostals*, thus lifting the ribs and creating more volume inside the chest. *SCM, serratus anterior, pectoralis minor* and *scalenes* contract to also elevate the ribs and sternum, creating more volume in the chest during forced breathing. In exhalation, the above muscles simply relax. As they do, the volume inside the ribcage decreases, and this increase in pressure forces air out of the lungs. In forced exhalation (coughing, blowing out candles), other muscles will be recruited to help force the air out: *internal intercostals, tranversus thoracis,* and *abdominal muscles* will be used.

External Respiration: External respiration is the process of gas exchange between the lungs and the bloodstream. The air in the atmosphere is 78.6% nitrogen, 20.9% oxygen, less than .04% is carbon dioxide and about .5% water. While nitrogen is the highest percentage gas in the air we breathe, our body does not utilize it. We simply inhale it and exhale it- without it usually entering our bloodstream. For oxygen and carbon dioxide, those gases WILL exchange in our bloodstream. Oxygen will diffuse from the alveoli into the blood capillary and carbon dioxide will flow from the capillary into the alveoli of the lung.

Gas transport: This is the process of moving the gases within the bloodstream. When oxygen enters the bloodstream from the lungs, 98.5% of it will be bound to *hemoglobin* in the red blood cells. Red blood cells then circulate and transport oxygen to all body tissues. If pH drops in a body tissue, that will cause hemoglobin to release its oxygen more readily- this is called the **Bohr Effect**. One way a tissue can have a drop in pH, is if carbon dioxide levels have risen within the tissue. High carbon dioxide levels will cause an increase in carbonic acid, and this acid lowers the pH in the area. As the tissue becomes more acidic, the blood will release oxygen for use in the tissue. For carbon dioxide, most (70%) is transported as molecules of carbonic acid (H_2CO_3). Carbonic acid is then converted into the bicarbonate ion (HCO^{3-}). The bicarbonate ion then moves into the blood plasma for circulation and eventual removal. 23% of carbon dioxide will bind onto hemoglobin and form carbaminohemoglobin for transport in the blood. The remaining 7% of the carbon dioxide will be carried freely in the blood.

Internal respiration: Internal respiration takes place between the blood and body tissues. Here, oxygen will diffuse from the blood into the tissue and carbon dioxide will diffuse from the tissue into the blood.

Controls of Respiration:

The two main areas of the brain which control respiration are the **medulla oblongata** and **pons**. The medulla oblongata has two groups of regulating cells for the rate of breathing. The *dorsal respiratory group* innervates the diaphragm and external intercostals, triggering inhalation. The *ventral respiratory group* controls the accessory muscles used in forced breathing. **Eupnea**, the normal rate of breathing, is 12-15 breaths per minute.

The pons has 2 nuclei that control the depth of breathing. The *apneustic center* controls the depth of breathing during inspiration and the *pneumotaxic center* inhibits the apneustic center- causing exhalation to begin.

Other factors that can affect respiration: physical activity (talking, coughing, laughing, exercise), increased body temperature, O_2 demand, increase of blood CO_2 (which can cause a decrease in blood pH), conscious control and emotional factors (fear, anger).

Respiratory Rates and Volumes:

MEASUREMENT	DESCRIPTION	NORMAL VALUE
Tidal Volume (TV)	Quantity of air moved into and out of the lungs during a normal breath	500ml
Minute Respiratory Volume (MRV)	Quantity of air moved into and out of the lungs in one minute (MRV= TV X Respiratory Rate) **average resp. rate is 12 breaths/ min**	6000 ml/min
Inspiratory Reserve Volume (IRV)	Quantity of air that can be forcefully inspired after a normal tidal inspiration	3600 ml male and 1900ml female
Expiratory Reserve Volume (ERV)	Quantity of air that can be forcefully expired after a normal tidal expiration	1200 ml
Vital Capacity (VC)	Maximum quantity of air that can be moved into and out of the lungs (VC= IRV + TV + ERV)	4800 ml male and 3400 ml in female
Residual Volume (RV)	Quantity of air remaining in the lungs after a maximal expiration	1200 ml
Total Lung Capacity (TLC)	Maximum quantity of air the lungs can hold (TLC = VC + RV)	6000 ml male and 4200 ml female
Alveolar Ventilation (V_A)	Amount of air reaching the alveoli each minute (not on graph below) V_A= (Resp. rate) X (TV- anatomic dead space)	4.2 liters/min

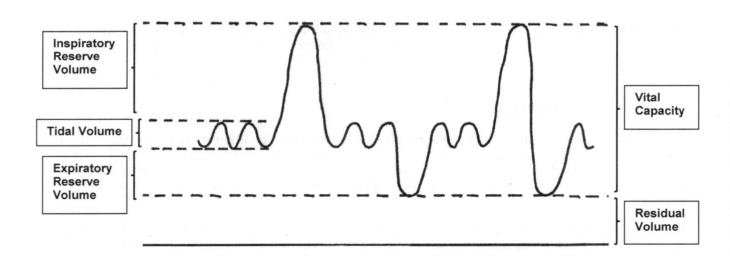

Physical Examination of the Chest and Lung

1. Inspect the chest for scars, trauma, symmetry, chest diameter (from anterior to posterior), and the costal angle
2. Count respiratory rate (if not already done during the vital signs) and observe the inspiration/expiration ratio. The ratio should be 1:2
3. Watch for uneven chest movement while breathing
4. Inspect the trachea for midline position
5. Inspect the skin and oral mucus membranes for cyanosis (indicates poor oxygenation)
6. Inspect the fingers for digital clubbing (indicates long term hypoxia)
7. Palpate the chest for tenderness, alignment, bulging, lumps, masses
8. Palpate for "tactile fremitus"
9. Palpate for chest expansion during breathing
10. Percuss the chest
11. Auscultate the chest and listen for tracheal breath sounds, bronchial breath sounds, bronchovesicular breath sounds, and vesicular breath sounds. Document each sound for: intensity, location, pitch, duration, and if present on inhalation/exhalation/both.
12. Auscultate for vocal fremitus, if abnormal breath sounds have been noted. Utilize the following tests: bronchophony, egophony, and whispered pectoriloquy.

General Abnormal Findings of Chest and Lungs

Abnormal findings, if necessary, should be referred to patients PCP or a pulmonologist

Costal Angle- This is the angle between the ribs and sternum. It should be less than 90° normally. Abnormal finding: costal angle may be larger than 90° in an individual with COPD.

Bronchophony: Instruct patient to say "99" while the health care provider is listening. In normal lung tissue, the words will sound muffled. Over consolidated areas, the words are unusually loud.

Egophony: Ask patient to say "E". In normal lung tissue, the "E" will sound muffled. Over consolidated areas, the "E" will sound like an "A"

Whispered pectoriloquy: Ask patient to whisper "1, 2, 3". In normal lung tissue, the words will not be heard or barely heard. Over consolidated areas, the numbers will be loud and clear

Percussive chest sounds:
*   *Resonant sounds-* are heard over normal ling tissue
*   *Dull sounds-* normally will be heard in the chest over the heart (3rd or 4th intercostal space to the 6th intercostal space on the left side).
*   *Hyperresonant sounds-* indicate increased air in the lung or pleural space (pneumothorax, emphysema, acute asthma)
*   *Abnormal dullness* (noted as "Flat" or "Dull")- indicates areas of decreased air in the lungs (pneumonia, consolidation, tumor)

Tactile Fremitus- palpable vibrations caused by air moving through respiratory air passages
*   *Increased vibration* on one side could indicate pneumonia or tissue consolidation in that lung
*   *Decreased vibration* could indicate emphysema, pneumothorax or pleural effusion

Chest expansion- measured during breathing.
- *Asymmetrical expansion* could indicate pneumonia, pneumothorax, atelectasis
- *Decreased expansion* bilaterally could indicate emphysema, diaphragm paralysis, atelectasis or ascites

Cyanosis- a bluish tinge to the skin or mucosa/gingivae of the mouth. Indicates improper oxygenation of the blood.

Hemoptysis- coughing up blood. Can be a result of an infection (bronchitis, TB), smoking or cancer

Sputum- mucus or pus that is coughed up. Sputum sometimes can be tinged with blood. Color and quantity of sputum can change if infection is present

Cough- The most common symptom of lung disease. Can be productive (cough produces secretions) or dry (no secretions are coughed up).

Barrel Chest- increased front to back chest diameter, commonly seen in COPD (example: emphysema). A normal examination finding is when the chest diameter is half the width of the chest

Funnel Chest- also known as pectus excavatum, is a funnel shaped depression of anterior chest. This may compress the heart or lungs, and may cause murmurs

Pigeon Chest- also called pectus carinatum- refers to a sternum that protrudes out past the abdomen

Atelectasis- partial or complete collapsed lung

Dyspnea- troubled breathing "shortness of breath". Can be graded as:
- **Grade 0**- not troubled by breathlessness, except in strenuous exercise
- **Grade 1**- notices shortness of breath when hurrying on a level path or walking up a slight hill
- **Grade 2**- walks more slowly on a level path than other people their age due to shortness of breath. Or has to stop to breathe while walking on a level path
- **Grade 3**- stops to breathe after walking 100 yards on a level path
- **Grade 4**- breathlessness with dressing or undressing, cannot leave house due to shortness of breath

Orthopnea- shortness of breath when lying down

Trepopnea- patient breathes more comfortably in a side-lying position. May be seen in patients with congestive heart failure.

Paroxysmal nocturnal dyspnea- sudden onset of shortness of breath while sleeping.

Tachypnea- respiratory rate greater than 20 breaths per minute, with shallow breathing. Often seen in patients who may be elderly, have lung disease, in pain, obesity, anxiety, or due to fever.

Bradypnea- respiratory rate below 10 breaths per minute. Typically noted before a period of apnea or respiratory arrest.

Apnea- absence of breathing. May be for a short duration or longer. May occur spontaneously during Cheyne-Stokes respirations, Biot's respirations, and other abnormal respiratory patterns

Hyperpnea- deep rapid breathing. May be seen in patients with anxiety or after exertion. In a comatose person, it may indicate hypoxia or hypoglycemia

Kussmaul's respirations- rapid, deep, sighing, breaths (more than 20 per minute), indicates metabolic acidosis and diabetic ketoacidosis.

Cheyne- Stokes respirations- a regular pattern of deep breaths alternating with periods of apnea (each pattern lasting 30-170 seconds). Occurs in patients with heart failure, kidney failure, or CNS damage.

Biot's respirations- rapid shallow breaths that alternate with abrupt periods of apnea. This type of breathing does not follow a regular pattern. This is a very ominous sign of CNS damage, often to the medulla oblongata.

Abnormal breath sounds: *Abnormal breath sounds in only one lung* could indicate pneumothorax, tumor, pleural effusion. *Diminished but normal breath sounds in both lungs* could indicate emphysema, atelectasis, bronchospasm.

Crackles- abnormal breath sounds (similar to the sound of static), classified as either fine or coarse. Not usually cleared by a cough
  ✓ **Fine crackles**- usually occur in the lung bases, when the patient stops inhaling – often caused by asbestosis, heart failure, pneumonia, pulmonary fibrosis, and silicosis
  ✓ **Coarse crackles**- usually can be heard when the patient starts to inhale, and may also be heard on exhalation. Can be a result of COPD or pulmonary edema

Wheezes- high pitched whistling sounds, heard first when a person exhales. May be the result of asthma, infection, heart failure, infection, airway obstruction from a tumor or foreign body

Rhonchi- Low pitched, snoring, rattling sounds. Occurs usually on exhalation, can change or disappear with coughing. Occurs when fluid partially blocks large airways.

Stridor- Loud, high pitched crowing sound. Usually heard without stethoscope. Caused by an obstruction in the upper airway.

Pleural friction rub- low pitched, grating, rubbing sound. Heard on inhalation and exhalation. This results from pleural inflammation which causes two layers of pleura to rub together. Pain can also be present where rubbing occurs.

Tissue consolidation- occurs when the alveoli air spaces become filled with solid tissue or fluid (instead of air). Can be seen in pneumonia, other lung infections, pulmonary edema, tumors, or lung collapse.

Advanced Imaging and Diagnostic Tests of the Chest and Lungs

Bronchoscopy- involves passing a flexible tube through the nostril, down into the airway (larynx, trachea, bronchi and bronchioles). The airway can be viewed through the bronchoscope, and a biopsy of tissue can be taken. Used to assess a possible tumor or abnormality.

Chest x ray. A chest x ray takes an x-ray of the organs and structures inside your chest. This is the most commonly used diagnostic exam- it is quick and cheap. Masses or consolidation may show up on a chest x-ray as white or hazy objects. Pneumothorax may show up as a darker area on x-ray.

Computed Tomography (CT scan) - CT scans are a specialized x-ray machine. A CT scan generates a collection of black-and-white pictures, each showing a slightly different "slice" or cross-section of your internal organs. These "slices" are spaced only about a quarter-inch apart, and give a very good representation of internal organs and other structures. This can also be performed with a contrast dye injected in the bloodstream. This dye outlines blood vessels and soft tissue to help them show up clearly on the pictures. A CT scan takes about 30–45 minutes. CT scans are more precise than a chest x-ray, but more costly. CT scans are better (than a MRI) for assessing disease that may be near the alveolar sacs.

Magnetic Resonance Imaging (MRI) - MRI is a noninvasive technique for visualizing many different body tissues. Unlike x-rays or a CT scan, MRI does not use any radiation. Instead, it uses radio waves, a large magnet, and a computer to create images. Each MRI picture shows a different "slice," or cross-section, of the area being viewed. Because these slices usually are spaced about a quarter-inch apart, the doctor can get a detailed representation of a particular area. MRI can be used on nearly any body part and is often used to look for structural abnormalities. MRI's are better than a CT scan for assessing pathologies near the hilar region of the lung and mediastinal region.

Pulmonary Angiogram (also called a **Perfusion Scan**)- A radioactive substance is injected into the bloodstream. The scan then shows all areas perfused with blood. Can be used if concerned with a pulmonary embolism.

Ventilation Scan- Xenon gas is inhaled and the scan is performed. This scan shows all areas that can fill with air upon ventilation. May be used to diagnose consolidation diseases (pneumonia, tumors, etc.)

Pulse oximetry- measures the amount of oxygen in the blood and provides an early warning sign of a low level of oxygen in the blood.

Sinus Endoscopy- A flexible viewing tube is inserted into the sinuses to view the internal sinus chamber.

Rapid Strep Test- A throat infection with streptococcus bacteria (strep throat) can be treated with an antibiotic. The traditional test for a strep throat has been a throat culture, which takes two to three days to produce results. Several different types of rapid strep tests, however, can produce results within minutes to hours. A rapid strep test can only detect the presence of Group A strep, the one most likely to cause serious throat infections; it does not detect other kinds of strep or other bacteria. A cotton swab is rubbed against the back of the throat to gather a sample of mucus. This takes only a second or two and makes some people feel a brief gagging or choking sensation. The mucus sample is then tested for a protein that comes from the strep bacteria.

Spirometry- This test measures how fast and how much air can be blown out of the lungs after taking a deep breath. Used to assess the functioning of the lungs. The results will be lower than normal if the airways are inflamed and narrowed, or if the muscles around the airways have tightened up.

Thoracentesis- Insertion of a needle into the chest (thorax) to remove fluid for examination

Pathologies of the Respiratory System

For additional infectious diseases that may affect this system, please refer to the Communicable/Infectious Disease Chart in Chapter 10.

Asthma – an acute inflammation and spasm of the smooth muscle that lines the bronchioles, causing coughing, dyspnea (difficult or labored breathing), wheezing, and chest tightness. Possible triggers include cold air, exercise, and many of the same airborne irritants that cause allergic reactions in some people. Medications can be prescribed to open the airways. These medications can be prescribed on a daily basis, for prevention of attacks, or given in an inhaled form in acute attacks (a "rescue" inhaler).

Allergies- Allergies involving the respiratory system are most often due to allergens being inhaled. Common airborne allergens are: pollen, dust, mold, mildew, and animal dander. These airborne allergens can trigger symptoms such as: watery eyes, itchy nose or throat, runny nose, cough, and/or wheezing.

Bronchitis- is inflammation of the air passageways inside the lung (the bronchi and bronchioles). Acute bronchitis can be caused by infection (viral or bacterial). Chronic bronchitis is most commonly caused by smoking cigarettes. Symptoms can involve coughing, mild fever, mild chills and chest discomfort.

Chronic obstructive pulmonary disease (COPD) – a general category of disorders characterized by history of smoking, dyspnea, coughing, frequent pulmonary infections, and ultimately respiratory failure. One such disease is ***emphysema***, in which chronic inflammation of the lungs causes the alveoli to scar, lose elasticity (making expiration difficult and tiresome), trap air and become permanently enlarged. This creates a "barrel chest" appearance on visual inspection of the patient's chest. Another example of COPD is ***chronic bronchitis***- most commonly caused by smoking.

Cystic fibrosis (CF) – a birth defect that causes oversecretion of thick mucus that clogs respiratory, pancreatic, and gall bladder passages and makes the child more prone to respiratory infections. CF is the most common lethal genetic disease in the U.S for Caucasians.—1 out of every 3,200 white children (of Northern European Origin) are affected.

Lung cancer – accounts for one-third of all cancer deaths in U.S., with over 90% of lung cancer patients having been smokers. It metastasizes (spreads) rapidly and widely, leading to an extremely low cure rate: most people with lung cancer die within 1 year of diagnosis, and the overall 5-year survival rate is about 7%. *Red Flag symptoms: Unfortunately in the early to mid-stages of development, lung cancer usually has no symptoms. When symptoms show, the cancer is advanced. Those symptoms can be a persistent cough which does not go away, unexplained weight loss, wheezing, coughing up blood, shortness of breath, and chest pain.* Diagnosis can be done with an x-ray, CT scan or bronchoscopy (often with a biopsy being completed). Lung cancer spreads easily through the body, so additional tests may be done to determine if that has happened (bone scans, PET scans, etc.). Treatments can include surgery, chemotherapy, radiation and/or targeted drug therapies.

Pneumonia – Is an infectious inflammation of the lungs, in which fluid accumulates in the alveoli. There are over 50 varieties of organisms which cause pneumonia, with most of them caused by a virus (Influenza A, for example) or bacterium (Streptococcus pneumonia, for example). Treatment will vary depending on the cause of the pneumonia. Symptoms may involve cough, fever, chills, fatigue, and shortness of breath.

Pneumothorax- (also called "***collapsed lung***") -   This occurs when air leaks out of the lungs and fills the pleural space (the space within the chest between the outside of the lungs and the ribs. This air in the chest compresses the lung, collapsing it. Usually only part of a lung will collapse, not the whole thing. This can be spontaneous, or as a result of something puncturing the chest and lung (knife, bullet, fractured rib, even acupuncture needle). *Red Flag symptoms: sharp, sudden pain in the area of the chest where the lung has collapsed; and shortness of breath.* Diseased or weak lung tissue (emphysema, lung cancer, cystic fibrosis, tuberculosis, pneumonia, and sarcoidosis) is more likely to suffer pneumothorax than healthy tissue. Pneumothorax is usually diagnosed with a chest x-ray. Small pneumothoraxes will heal on their own (often with the patient on bed rest to avoid exertion); larger ones may require a chest tube inserted or surgical repair.

Pulmonary Embolism- this is a clot in one of the blood vessels in the lungs. Most often, this clot is formed elsewhere in the body (often in the legs as a deep vein thrombosis). If the clot breaks free from the area in which it formed, this moving clot is called an embolism. When the embolism circulates through the blood vessels, it can get stuck in the blood vessels supplying the lungs- a pulmonary embolism. *Red Flag symptoms may involve pain in the chest, shortness of breath, coughing- sometimes coughing up blood.* Untreated pulmonary embolisms can be fatal. Treatment may include medications (anticoagulants or thrombolytic drugs) or surgery.

Sarcoidosis- an inflammatory disease with an unknown cause. Inflammation occurs in the lungs, causing granules to form in the lung tissue. Some patients are asymptomatic, and the condition is discovered on accident (during a chest x-ray for another condition, for example). Others may show symptoms of dry cough, shortness of breath, fatigue, wheezing. The disease may also affect the heart, skin, eyes or liver. Some cases of sarcoidosis may resolve on its own. Other cases may need corticosteroids or other immune modulating medications.

Sinusitis- inflammation of a sinus. Most commonly caused by an infection (bacterial or viral) or allergies. Symptoms can include nasal discharge, post-nasal drip, feeling pressure in the head and/or headache. Sinusitis of the frontal sinuses gives pain in the forehead. Pain in the upper jaw or teeth may indicate sinusitis in the maxillary sinuses. Pain or pressure in the bridge of the nose (between the eyes), may indicate sinusitis of the ethmoid sinus. Sinusitis can last from days (acute) to weeks or months (chronic).

Sleep Apnea- Interruption of air flow to the lungs while sleeping. There are two main forms of sleep apnea. ***Obstructive sleep apnea*** is caused by occlusion of the throat or upper airway. ***Central sleep apnea*** is caused by dysfunction in the respiratory area of the brain. Symptoms may be snoring, dry mouth at night, gasping, choking, and pauses in breathing. Oxygen levels in the blood can plummet while carbon dioxide levels can climb. Drugs, obesity, alcohol use can increase symptoms. Sleep apnea can cause cardiac problems. Often treated with a machine called the CPAP (continuous positive airway pressure).

Strep Throat- an infection caused by *Group A Streptococcus*. Symptoms: a sore throat, redness and swelling in the throat, white patches (pus) may be visible in the throat or on the tonsils, fever, pain with swallowing, swollen lymph nodes in the neck, and sometimes a rash. Having a sore throat does not automatically mean a patient has "strep throat"- a rapid strep test must be done to confirm Group A streptococcal infection (other pathogens, including viruses, can cause a sore throat). Antibiotics can be prescribed, if needed.

Tuberculosis (TB) – a bacterial lung infection caused by *Mycobacterium Tuberculosis*. Causes a massive inflammatory and immune response, including fibrous or calcified nodules in the lung tissue. Symptoms of active tuberculosis (active TB) can include fever, night sweats, weight loss, a racking cough, and spitting up blood (blood tinged sputum). It is contagious through the air from actively infected individuals. Many people have been exposed to TB, but the bacterium is sealed off in their lung tissue by their immune system- this is called Latent TB. Latent TB does not usually harm the patient, nor is it usually transmissible to another person. 90-95% of people with latent TB will never develop active TB. Treatment involves long courses of antibiotic therapy, and unfortunately, some strains are becoming antibiotic resistant.

Practice Study and Test Questions:

1) Strep throat is usually caused by
      A) Group B Streptococcus
      B) Group E Streptococcus
      C) Group C Streptococcus
      D) Group A Streptococcus

2) A barrel chest may be noted during inspection in the physical examination in a patient with
      A) cystic fibrosis
      B) pneumothorax
      C) emphysema
      D) pneumonia

3) The quantity of air moved in and out of the lungs in a normal breath is the
      A) vital capacity
      B) tidal volume
      C) residual volume
      D) expiratory reserve volume

4) External respiration is
      A) gas exchange between the blood and the body tissues
      B) gas exchange between the blood and the lungs
      C) gas exchange between the blood and the heart
      D) gas exchange between the blood and the skin

5) Sudden pain in the chest, shortness of breath, and coughing can be signs of
      A) pulmonary embolism
      B) sarcoidosis
      C) lung cancer
      D) emphysema

6) Breathing is controlled by which regions in the brain?
      A) medulla oblongata and cerebellum
      B) pons and hypothalamus
      C) medulla oblongata and pons
      D) thalamus and hypothalamus

7) If a patient has to stop to breathe after walking 100 yards on a level path, the grade of dyspnea that they have is
      A) Grade 3
      B) Grade 1
      C) Grade 4
      D) Grade 0

8) During auscultation in a physical examination, hearing breath sounds in only one lung could indicate
      A) myocardial infarction
      B) asthma
      C) pneumothorax
      D) tuberculosis

9) The diagnostic test which measures the volume of air exhaled after taking a deep breath is called
     A) perfusion scan
     B) spirometry
     C) pulse oximetry
     D) thoracentesis

10) Treatment for a large pneumothorax could involve
     A) radiation
     B) a chest tube
     C) chemotherapy
     D) Both A and C

11) The most common lethal genetic disease in the U.S. for Caucasians is
     A) asthma
     B) cystic fibrosis
     C) lupus
     D) sarcoidosis

12) A diagnostic test used in diagnosing a pulmonary embolism is
     A) perfusion scan
     B) ventilation scan
     C) pulmonary angiogram
     D) both A and C

13) The area of gas exchange in the lungs are the
     A) tertiary bronchi
     B) alveoli
     C) secondary bronchi
     D) bronchioles

14) During a physical examination, normal sounds heard when percussing the lung tissue in the chest are
     A) egophony sounds
     B) hyperresonant sounds
     C) dull sounds
     D) resonant sounds

15) Symptoms of early stage lung cancer are
     A) coughing up blood
     B) chest pain
     C) collapsed lung
     D) no symptoms felt by the patient

16) A respiratory rate of below 10 breaths per minute can be documented as
     A) normal
     B) tachypnea
     C) bradypnea
     D) apnea

Answers: 1) D 2) C 3) B 4) B 5) A 6) C 7) A 8) C 9) B 10) B 11) B 12) D 13) B 14) D 15) D 16) C

CHAPTER 12: THE DIGESTIVE SYSTEM

Digestive system- provides the body with organic and inorganic molecules needed to keep the body alive. The digestive system is made up of the *digestive tract* (also called the *gastrointestinal tract*) and the *accessory organs*. The digestive tract is composed of the mouth, pharynx, esophagus, stomach, small intestine, and large intestine. The accessory organs are the teeth, tongue, salivary glands, liver and pancreas. Our digestive system can be controlled by our nervous system and hormonal action.

The functions of the digestive system are: ingestion, mechanical processing of food, chemical digestion, secretion, absorption of nutrients, and excretion of wastes. The majority of our digestive organs are located in the abdominopelvic cavity. The area of the abdomen where these organs are positioned is called the **peritoneal cavity**. The peritoneal cavity is lined by a serous membrane. This serous membrane, when lining the abdominal wall, is called the **parietal peritoneum**. This lining also dips into the cavity and covers the digestive organs, and at that time is then called the **visceral peritoneum**. A thin layer of peritoneal fluid fills the space between the parietal and visceral peritoneum, and lubricates the surfaces to reduce friction. The layers of tissue which connect the parietal and visceral peritoneal layers are called the *mesenteries*. The various mesenteries are the lesser and greater omentum of the stomach, the mesocolon and the mesentery proper. Any organ whose mass sits behind the mesenteries is described as being in the *retroperitoneal* position (for example: pancreas, kidney, and rectum)

There are four major layers of tissue making up the walls of the organs in the digestive tract. The **mucosa** is the innermost layer which comes in contact with the food we eat. Underneath the mucosa is the **submucosa**, a layer filled with nerves and blood vessels. Next is the **muscularis externa**, composed of two layers of smooth muscle (three layers in the stomach). The outermost layer is called the **serosa** or **adventitia.** The serosa is found as the outermost layer of tissue for organs in the peritoneal cavity. The adventitia is found in the esophagus.

The Organs of the Digestive System:

The **mouth** (or **buccal cavity**) is composed of the lips, cheeks, gingiva, uvula, and oral mucosa. It functions to add lubrication to the food, mechanical processing, sensory analysis of material before swallowing and limited digestion of carbohydrates.

The **tongue** is located in the oral cavity. The functions of the tongue are mechanical processing, manipulation of food to assist in chewing and swallowing, sensory analysis of food, and secretion of mucins and lingual lipase.

The **salivary glands** are located around the oral cavity, and empty their secretions (saliva) into the oral cavity to mix with the food. There are three pairs of salivary glands: *parotid salivary glands* (25% of production), *sublingual salivary glands* (5% of production) and *submandibular salivary glands* (70% of production). Saliva is composed of 99.4% water, 0.6% electrolytes, buffers, glycoproteins (mucins), antibodies to fight bacteria, enzymes (salivary amylase), and waste products. Saliva keeps the pH of the mouth at 7.0, which helps to inhibit build-up of bacterial by-products. Saliva production is controlled by the ANS, by both the sympathetic and parasympathetic branches. The parasympathetic system does most of the control of the salivary glands. Functions of saliva include: lubricating the mouth and food, dissolving chemicals in the food which can stimulate the taste buds, and initiate digestion of complex carbohydrates (done by salivary amylase).

Teeth are also located in the mouth. Some important components of teeth include the pulp cavity, root canal, periodontal ligament, cementum, and crown. *Dentin* is the bone-like material which makes up the bulk of the tooth. *Enamel* is the hardest substance in the body and coats the outer surface of dentin. There are **32 teeth** in an adult: the *incisors* (4 on top and bottom), the *cuspids* (2 on top and bottom), the *bicuspids/ premolars* (4 on top and bottom) and the *molars* (6 on top and 6 on bottom). In children, there are usually **20 deciduous (primary) teeth**. The main function of teeth is mastication- the mechanical processing (chewing) of food.

After leaving the oral cavity, the food enters the **pharynx**. The pharynx connects the oral cavity to the esophagus. It has three regions: the *nasopharynx, oropharynx* and *laryngopharynx*. In the digestive system, the pharynx functions to act as a common passageway for air, food, and fluids during swallowing.

The **esophagus** connects the pharynx to the stomach. It is a hollow muscular tube about 10 inches long and 2 cm wide. At the inferior end, the *lower esophageal sphincter (*also called the *cardiac sphincter* or the *gastroesophageal sphincter)* connects the esophagus to stomach. If this sphincter is not working correctly, reflux of stomach contents back into the esophagus can occur. The esophagus functions in swallowing. Swallowing occurs in three phases: *the buccal phase, pharyngeal phase,* and *esophageal phase.*

After the food leaves the esophagus, it enters the **stomach**. The stomach is located in the left upper abdominal quadrant. The food (*bolus*) entering from the esophagus will become *chyme* once processed by the stomach and mixed with the gastric secretions. The region of the stomach which attaches to the esophagus is called the *cardia region*. The *fundus* is the upper portion, the *body* is the middle portion and the *pylorus region* is the lower portion of the stomach. The *pyloric sphincter* regulates the passage of food leaving the stomach and entering the small intestine. The stomach has a wrinkled appearance internally- these wrinkles are called *rugae.* In the stomach there are three layers of muscle in its walls: the circular, longitudinal, and oblique layers. The stomach has an extra (third) layer of muscle (compared to the other digestive organs) to assist with the churning and pulverization of food. The stomach has gastric glands in its mucosal lining which produce digestive secretions. **Parietal cells** produce *intrinsic factor* (needed for vitamin B12 absorption) and hydrochloric acid. **Chief cells** produce *pepsinogen, pepsin, rennin* (infants) and *gastric lipase* (infants). **Pyloric glands** produce *mucus* and the hormones *gastrin* and *somatostatin* which help regulate the processing of the chyme. The stomach will begin the preliminary digestion of proteins- done by the enzyme pepsin. The final breakdown of proteins will be finished in the small intestine. The stomach also physically and mechanically breaks down the food from chewed pieces into a milkshake consistency. There is no absorption of nutrients in the stomach, but some drugs (for example, aspirin and alcohol) can be absorbed here.

The **small intestine** connects the stomach and small intestine. It performs most of the chemical digestion and absorption of our foods. This is accomplished by secretions produced by the small intestine AND secretions pumped into the small intestine from accessory organs (liver, gall bladder, and pancreas). The small intestine has 2200 square feet of absorptive surface area (about the size of an average 2 story home). It is on average 19.7 feet long and is 1.6 inches in diameter. It is divided into three main sections. The **duodenum** is the 1st 12 inches. Most of the chemical digestion and absorption is done here. It receives additional digestive enzymes from the liver, gall bladder, and pancreas. The middle section is called the **jejunum** and is 8 feet long. The last section is the **ileum**, which is 12 feet long. *Peyer's patches*, a type of lymphatic tissue, are located at the end of the ileum near the ileocecal valve and function to prevent entry of bacterial flora from the large intestine. The small intestine performs many functions. It has great absorptive capabilities as a result of increased surface area. This increased surface area is due to the following structural modifications which are unique to the small intestine: *circular folds (plicae circularis), villi,* and *microvilli.* All carbohydrates, fats and proteins in a meal will be absorbed here, along with some vitamins, minerals and water. The small intestine will also finish any remaining carbohydrate and protein chemical digestion- in addition to all of the chemical digestion of lipids. The muscular contractions of *segmentation* and *propulsion* assist in the digestion, absorption and movement of food through the small intestine.

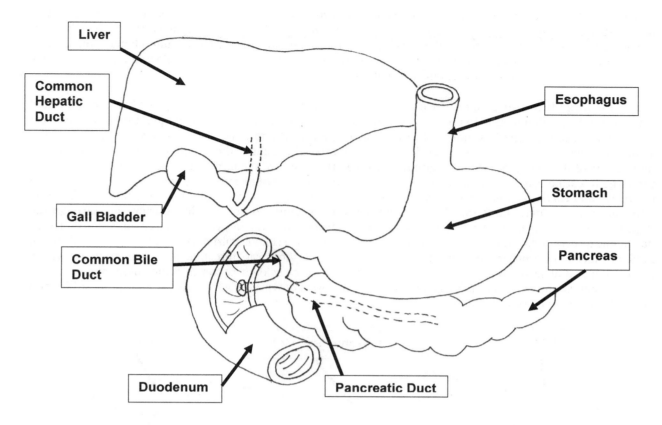

Assisting the small intestine is the **pancreas**. The pancreas does not directly touch or handle food- but makes digestive secretions which it pumps into the duodenum of the small intestine. The pancreas is located behind the stomach, and the head of the pancreas is nestled in the duodenum as it curves around the pancreas. It is composed of three sections- the *head, body* and *tail*. Inside, the cells of the pancreatic acini and pancreatic islets produce secretions. The ***pancreatic islets*** produce the hormone insulin. The ***pancreatic acini*** produce digestive secretions such as: pancreatic lipase, pancreatic alpha-amylase, nucleases, proteolytic enzymes (trypsinogen, chymotrypsinogen, procarboxypeptidase). These digestive enzymes will break down proteins, carbohydrates and lipids. They are carried out of the pancreas and into the duodenum of the small intestine by the *pancreatic duct*.

Another organ which assists the small intestine is the **liver**. The liver is the largest visceral organ in the body, and is located in the right upper abdominal quadrant. It is composed of four lobes (*right, left, caudate, quadrate*). It does not directly touch or handle food, but makes a digestive secretion, ***bile***, which it pumps into the duodenum of the small intestine. It is in the small intestine where the bile interacts with our foods and assists in mechanically breaking down lipids. In addition to assisting the small intestine in digestion, the liver is a very important cleaning and metabolic organ as well. It is the body's major metabolic organ. It detoxifies drugs, alcohol and toxins; degrades proteins, hormones, bacteria; builds new proteins; makes 85% of our body's cholesterol; can store excess levels of blood glucose; and can begin gluconeogenesis (the formation of glucose from fats and proteins). Internally, the liver is composed of ***hepatocytes*** arranged inside *liver lobules*. These hepatocytes are responsible for cleansing the blood and producing bile. Bile is composed of water, bilirubin, cholesterol, and bile salts- and it functions to emulsify fats in the foods we eat. The bile, after being produced in the liver lobule, will be released into the right and left bile ducts. The right and left bile ducts will join together and form the common hepatic duct. The common hepatic duct will then send some of the bile down into the duodenum of the small intestine through the *common bile duct*. The rest of the bile will leave the common hepatic duct and flow through the cystic duct into the gallbladder for storage.

Also involved in the emulsification of fats is the **gall bladder**. The gall bladder is found underneath the liver, behind its right lobe. It does not directly touch or handle food, but it stores and concentrates extra bile from the liver. It then pumps the bile into the duodenum of the small intestine via the common hepatic duct, when needed (usually after consuming fatty meals). It is in the small intestine where the bile will interact with our foods and assist in mechanically breaking down lipids.

Lastly, the **large intestine** ("*colon*") will handle the remnants of our meal. It will carry food products and waste from the small intestine to the outside of the body. It is joined onto the small intestine by the ileocecal valve. The large intestine lies inferior to the stomach and liver, and looks like a picture frame around the small intestine. Multiple pouches, called *haustra*, are located throughout the small intestine. A small band of muscle, called the teniae coli, runs longitudinally down the center of the large intestine. The main sections of the large intestine are: *cecum, ascending colon, hepatic flexure, transverse colon, splenic flexure, descending colon, sigmoid colon, rectum, anal canal* and *sphincters*. Chyme/fecal material will travel through the large intestine in that order. Haustral churning and mass movements propel the chyme remnants through the large intestine. The defecation reflex expels the fecal material out of the body. In the large intestine, there are no chemical secretions which process the food. Instead, bacteria (like E. coli) perform the final breakdown of food products. In addition to defecation, the functions of the large intestine are absorption of water; production and absorption of vitamin K, B5 and biotin by the resident bacteria in the colon; absorption of some urobilins and stercobilins (organic wastes); and breakdown of organic wastes and indigestible food products for removal from the body.

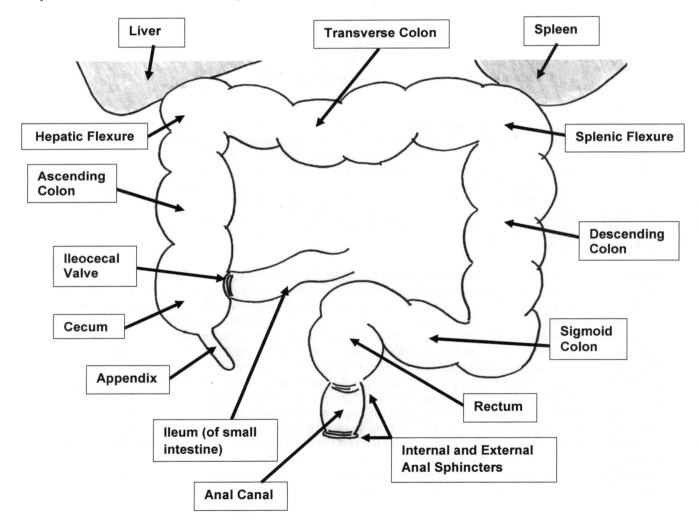

Physical Examination of the Digestive System

Examination of the Mouth and Throat

1. Inspect the mouth: lips, oral mucosa, gums (gingivae), teeth, and tongue.
2. Inspect the throat (oropharynx)
3. Palpate the lips and tongue
4. Elicit gag reflex

Examination of the Abdomen:

1. Inspect the abdomen for: symmetry, bumps, bulges, masses, shape, contour, stretch marks ("striae"), dilated veins, discoloration, Cullen's sign, Grey-Turner's sign and scars.
2. Inspect the umbilicus
3. Observe any pulsations or abdominal movements
4. Auscultate the four abdominal quadrants (Right Upper, Right Lower, Left Upper, Left Lower) for bowel sounds
5. Auscultate for bruits in the aorta, renal arteries, iliac arteries, and femoral arteries.
6. Percuss the four quadrants
7. Percuss the liver and spleen
8. Perform light palpation of the abdomen (1/2 inch deep) in all four quadrants. (If patient has pain in the abdomen, have them describe the quality and location of the pain.)
9. Perform deep palpation of the abdomen (2-3" deep)
10. Palpate McBurney's point and the liver

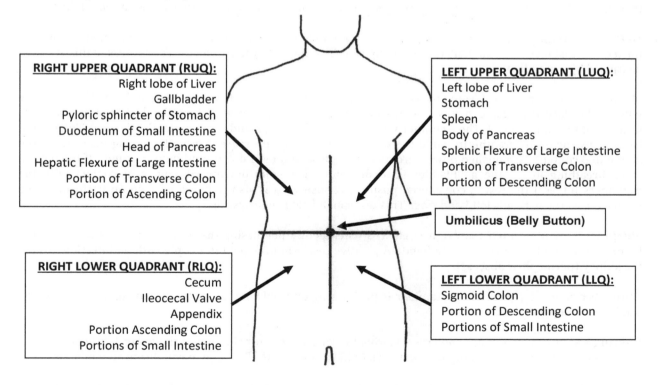

RIGHT UPPER QUADRANT (RUQ):
Right lobe of Liver
Gallbladder
Pyloric sphincter of Stomach
Duodenum of Small Intestine
Head of Pancreas
Hepatic Flexure of Large Intestine
Portion of Transverse Colon
Portion of Ascending Colon

LEFT UPPER QUADRANT (LUQ):
Left lobe of Liver
Stomach
Spleen
Body of Pancreas
Splenic Flexure of Large Intestine
Portion of Transverse Colon
Portion of Descending Colon

Umbilicus (Belly Button)

RIGHT LOWER QUADRANT (RLQ):
Cecum
Ileocecal Valve
Appendix
Portion Ascending Colon
Portions of Small Intestine

LEFT LOWER QUADRANT (LLQ):
Sigmoid Colon
Portion of Descending Colon
Portions of Small Intestine

THE ABDOMINAL QUADRANTS

General Abnormal Findings of the Digestive System

Abnormal findings, if necessary, should be referred to patients PCP or a gastroenterologist

Aaron's sign- is a referred pain felt in the epigastrium (area above the belly button) upon continuous firm pressure over McBurney's point. It is indicative of chronic appendicitis.

Balance/Ballance sign- the presence of a dull percussion note in both flanks, constant on the left side but shifting with change of position on the right. This can indicate a ruptured spleen.

Blumberg's (Rebound) test/sign- The abdominal wall is compressed slowly and then rapidly released. Presence of pain upon release is a positive sign and is indicative of peritonitis.

Cullen's sign is black and blue bruising of the area around the umbilicus (belly button). Ectopic pregnancy and pancreatitis could be a cause.

Dance's sign is retraction in the right lower quadrant of the abdomen, which can be an indication of intussusception (a cause of bowel obstruction where the intestines fold in on themselves).

Grey-Turner sign- bruising of the flank. This can be an indication of pancreatitis or a ruptured ectopic pregnancy.

Kehr's sign is the occurrence of acute pain in the tip of the shoulder when a person is lying down and the legs are elevated. Kehr's sign in the left shoulder is considered a classical symptom of a ruptured spleen. A ruptured ectopic pregnancy can also give a positive Kehr's sign.

Markle test/sign- pain elicited in the abdomen when a patient standing on tip-toes quickly drops down onto their heels. Abdominal pain upon this jarring landing may be indicative of peritonitis and/or appendicitis.

McBurney's point/sign is the name given to the point over the right side of the human abdomen that is one-third of the distance from the ASIS (anterior superior iliac spine) to the umbilicus. Tenderness in this area can be caused by appendicitis.

Murphy's test/sign- Is performed by asking the patient (lying supine) to breathe out and then the examiner will gently place their hand below the ribs on the right side at the mid-clavicular line (the approximate location of the gallbladder). The examiner will push their fingertips under the patient's rib cage. The patient is then instructed to breathe in while the examiner maintains pressure. Normally, during inspiration, the abdominal contents are pushed downward as the diaphragm moves down (and lungs expand). If the patient stops breathing in (as the gallbladder is tender and, in moving downward, comes in contact with the examiners fingers) the test is considered positive. A positive test also requires no pain on performing the maneuver on the patient's left hand side. This test can indicate cholecystitis.

Murphy's/Lewin's punch test/sign is elicited when gently percussing the area of the back overlying the kidney with the ulnar surface of the hand. A positive test produces pain in people with an infection around the kidney (perinephric abscess).

Obturator sign- RLQ pain when examiner is performing internal rotation of the flexed right hip. This sign can indicate appendicitis.

Rovsing's sign is a sign of appendicitis. Positive Rovsing's Sign= if palpation of the lower left quadrant of a person's abdomen results in more pain in the right lower quadrant. This sign may indicate appendicitis.

Psoas/Iliopsoas sign- RLQ pain when the examiner hyperextends the right hip. This sign can indicate appendicitis.

Abdominal pain- abdominal pain may vary in its location and cause. Here are some common conditions and the pain description of them. *RLQ= right lower quadrant, LLQ= left lower quadrant, RUQ= right upper quadrant, LUQ= left upper quadrant*

- **Appendicitis:** Pain often begins initially around umbilicus and later shifts to the RLQ. Pain will often be seen at Mc Burney's point. Nausea, vomiting, and a low grade fever may be seen. Positive Aaron, Rovsing, Markle, and McBurney's signs.
- **Cholecystitis (gall bladder)** - severe unrelenting RUQ pain or epigastric pain. Pain may also be referred to right subscapular area. Positive Murphy sign, vomiting, fever, possible jaundice.
- **Pancreatitis**- sudden, knifelike, excruciating LUQ, epigastric or umbilical pain. Pain may be present in both flanks and also refer to left shoulder. Tenderness, fever, vomiting, and/or shock may occur. Positive Grey Turner sign and Positive Cullen sign- both signs occur 2-3 days after onset.
- **Perforated ulcer**- abrupt RUQ pain, may be referred to shoulders, tenderness in RUQ, rebound tenderness
- **Diverticulitis**- epigastric pain radiating down the left side of abdomen after eating, with flatulence, diarrhea, tenderness on palpation
- **Gall stones (cholelithiasis)** – Episodic, often severe RUQ pain- lasting 15 min to several hours. Pain may be referred to right subscapular area. RUQ tenderness on palpation. Vomiting, and jaundice may also be present
- **Spleen Rupture**- Intense left upper quadrant pain, radiating to left shoulder. May worsen with the foot of bed elevated. Positive Kehr's sign in left shoulder is often a classic sign for this.
- **Peritonitis**- Pain may have sudden onset or gradual, generalized or localized, dull or severe. There may also be unrelenting muscle guarding and pain on deep inspiration. Shallow respiration will be seen in a patient with this. Positive Blumberg (Rebound), Markle signs, Balance signs, reduced bowel sounds, nausea, vomiting, Positive obturator and iliopsoas tests.
- **Hiatal hernia**- Sharp severe pain over lower chest or upper abdomen
- **Peptic Ulcer**- Burning feeling after eating in the epigastric region, sometimes accompanied by hematemesis (vomiting blood) or tarry stools, sudden onset that generally subsides within 15-20 minutes

Descriptions of Abdominal Pain:
- Burning- could indicate peptic ulcer or GERD
- Cramping- could indicate gall bladder inflammation, gallstones, IBS, diarrhea, constipation, flatulence
- Severe Cramping- could indicate appendicitis, Crohn's disease, diverticulosis
- Stabbing- could indicate pancreatitis or cholecystitis

Visible abdominal bumps, bulges, masses- Can be due to cancerous tumors, splenomegaly, hepatomegaly, enlarged gall bladder, uterine fibroids, and gastric distension

Changes in abdominal shape and contour- Distension of the abdomen can be caused by obesity, ascites, and bowel distension (due to gas or liquids)

Abdominal Stretch marks ("striae") - Can be caused by pregnancy, obesity, ascites, Cushing's syndrome

Dilated veins in abdomen- Can be caused by portal hypertension or inferior vena cava obstruction

Umbilical protrusion- can indicate umbilical hernia (also can be present in pregnant women)

Bowel Sounds:
- *Normal*- are high pitched, gurgling noises
- *Borborygmus*- stomach growling
- *Hyperactive*- loud, high pitched, tinkling sounds that can occur frequently (can be due to laxative usage, diarrhea
- *Hypoactive*- sounds are heard infrequently or absent. Could indicate paralytic ileus or peritonitis

Friction rubs- heard when auscultating over liver or spleen. Could indicate a liver tumor or splenic infarction

Abdominal bruits- "swishing" sounds heard over major arteries in the abdomen. Could be caused by aortic aneurysm, or partial obstructions in blood vessels creating turbulent blood flow

Hematochezia- passage of bloody stools. Usually indicates GI bleeding- possibly from anal fissure, colitis, colorectal cancer, Crohn's disease, or hemorrhoids.

Hematemesis- vomiting blood

Dysphagia- Difficulty swallowing, can be due to cranial nerve damage (IX or X), esophageal stenosis or cancer in esophagus

Venous distension/tortuous veins- enlarged and dilated veins visible on abdomen. Can be due to cirrhosis, liver failure or inferior vena cava obstruction

Splenomegaly- spleen enlargement. May be due to mononucleosis, trauma

Hepatomegaly- liver enlargement. May be due to cirrhosis, hepatitis, uncontrolled diabetes, leukemia or lymphoma

Advanced Imaging and Diagnostic Tests of the Digestive System

Barium X-ray Study- Barium is ingested and then x-rays are performed to detect ulcers, tumors, or other abnormalities. Commonly used to evaluate the esophagus, stomach, intestines, and rectum. An *Upper GI Series* is a barium x-ray study used to examine the esophagus, stomach and small intestine. A *Lower GI Series* (also called a *barium enema*) is used to examine the large intestine (colon).

Colonoscopy- Using an endoscope inserted into the colon to view the internal surface of the colon (large intestine). Biopsies can be performed during this procedure, if needed.

Computed Tomography (CT scan) - CT scans are a specialized x-ray machine which are able to take slices of images ¼ inch apart. (see more discussion in the respiratory system section). In the gastrointestinal system, CT scans can be used to diagnose appendicitis, abdominal abscesses, and gallstones

Esophagogastroduodenoscopy (EGD)- an examination of the esophagus, stomach, and upper duodenum by inserting a flexible endoscope down through the throat. Used in cases of abdominal pain, heartburn, vomiting blood, tarry stools, Crohn's disease. Biopsies may be taken during this procedure.

Endoscopic Retrograde Cholangiopancreatography (ERCP) - An endoscope is inserted into the mouth and down the digestive tract into the duodenum. From there, a fine tube is inserted into the bile duct. Radioopaque dye is injected into the bile duct, and then x-rays are performed. Often done to assess gallstones or bile duct blockage

Endoscopy- A flexible viewing tube is inserted into the digestive tract to view the inner lining of the organs of the alimentary canal.

Fluoroscopy- Barium is consumed and the doctor watches it with continuous x-ray (moving pictures) as it continues through the digestive tract. The esophagus and stomach contractions can be monitored, and blockages can be viewed. Often used with patients who have Crohn's disease

Laparoscopy- An endoscope is inserted through an incision in the abdominal wall, often near the umbilicus. The endoscope is used to view the outside of the abdominal organs and abdominal cavity. Corrective procedures can be performed during the laparoscopy.

Magnetic Resonance Imaging (MRI)- MRI scans use radio waves, a large magnet, and a computer to create images. Each MRI picture shows a different "slice," or cross-section, of the area being viewed (1/4 inches apart). Used in the gastrointestinal system to help diagnose aortic aneurysm, iliac artery aneurysm, tumors in the abdomen. MRI is more expensive, and takes longer to perform- but often provides clearer images than a CT scan.

Occult blood test- A stool sample is taken, and is tested for blood in the stool.

Paracentesis- insertion of a needle into the abdominal cavity to remove fluid for further examination.

Percutaneous transhepatic cholangiography- X-ray of liver and biliary tract after injection of radioopaque dye.

Sigmoidoscopy- an endoscope is inserted through the rectum and into the sigmoid colon to observe the inner lining of the sigmoid colon and rectum.

Ultrasonography- using sound waves (ultrasound) to detect structural or functional abnormalities. This procedure can be done to assess liver, pancreas, gallstones, appendicitis, ovarian cysts, and aortic aneurysms

Pathologies of the Digestive System
For additional infectious diseases that may affect this system, please refer to the Communicable/Infectious Disease Chart in Chapter 10.

Appendicitis- Inflammation/infection of the appendix. *Red Flag symptoms: May include pain in the abdomen, first around the belly button, then moving to the lower right area (called McBurney's point). Loss of appetite, nausea, vomiting, constipation or diarrhea, inability to pass gas, low fever that begins after other symptoms, and abdominal swelling can also be reported.* Surgery is often done to remove the appendix before it ruptures. Rupture could cause **peritonitis** (infection in the abdominal cavity) which can be life threatening. Initial diagnosis is often done by physical exam, often followed by a CT scan and blood tests (to check for presence of infection). Here are a few physical exam tests for appendicitis: *"Rebound tenderness"* is when the doctor presses on a part of the abdomen and the patient feels more tenderness when the pressure is released than when it is applied. *"Psoas Sign"* the physician or examiner will perform flexion of the patient's hip and test for pain at Mc Burney's point. *"Obturator Sign"* shows pain at Mc Burney's point on internal rotation of the hip. *"Rovsing's Sign"* has pain on the right side of the abdomen when pressing on the left side of the abdomen.

Celiac Disease- an immune reaction to the consumption of gluten. As gluten moves through the small intestine, the immune system attacks the gluten- and damages the small intestine, as well. This damage will prevent the small intestine from being able to absorb nutrients from food. Examples of gluten: wheat, barley and rye. Symptoms can include: nausea, diarrhea, weight loss, gas, bloating, and fatigue. It can lead to nutritional deficiencies, including iron deficiency anemia. It is usually diagnosed by an endoscopic examination, including a biopsy. Celiac disease is different from a food intolerance/sensitivity. Many people claim to be gluten sensitive, but do not actually have Celiac Disease. Individuals who have a gluten sensitivity may have some similar symptom as Celiac, but do not have actual damage to the lining of the small intestine.

Cholecystitis- Inflammation of the gall bladder- gives upper abdominal pain with referral into the back or shoulder. Nausea, vomiting and a jaundiced color of the skin may be seen.

Cholelithiasis- "gall stones"- right hypochondriac region pain (the hypochondriac regions is a region in the right upper abdominal quadrant)- which especially increases after eating a fatty meal. The patient may also have abdominal bloating, colic, indigestion. Ultrasound is the best diagnostic test for gall stones. Surgery to remove the gallbladder is the most common way to treat symptomatic gallstones.

Cholestasis- "bile duct blockage"- prevents bile from entering the intestine. The bile pigments accumulate in the blood and they will get deposited in the skin- causing a yellow color.

Cirrhosis- Chronic inflammation of the liver due to chronic alcoholism and/or chronic hepatitis. Alcohol and hepatitis damages the hepatocytes (liver cells) creating scar tissue. As a result, the liver becomes fibrous and its activity is decreased. Ascites (abdominal swelling and bloating), distended abdominal veins, spider veins on upper half of body, jaundice, and weight loss may be seen.

Colon Cancer (Colorectal Cancer)- Cancer in the colon or rectum. Risk factors can include family history of colorectal cancer, being over age 50, having colon polyps, smoking, eating a low fiber diet, and having a history of Crohn's disease or Ulcerative Colitis. _Red Flag symptoms are: blood in the fecal material, constipation, abdominal pain or bloating, unexplained weight loss, and fatigue. Early in the growth of the cancer there may be no symptoms._ Diagnosis can be done using a fecal occult blood test, sigmoidoscopy or colonoscopy (with biopsy, if needed), and a digital rectal exam. Treatment may include surgery, chemotherapy and/or radiation.

Colon Polyps- A polyp is extra tissue that grows inside the body. Most are benign, but could turn cancerous over time. As a precaution, doctors usually remove all polyps (often during a colonscopy) and test them. Most are asymptomatic and are found during a regular check-up. If symptoms are present, some symptoms are: anal bleeding, blood in the stool, constipation or diarrhea that lasts more than a week.

Crohn's Disease (aka _ileitis_ or _enteritis_**)-** In Crohn's disease, the large or small intestine may have ulcers forming in the intestinal wall, all layers of the intestine wall may be involved, and normal healthy bowel can be found between sections of diseased bowel. Most commonly, Crohn's disease occurs in the last portion of the small intestine (the ileum). Crohn's disease affects men and women equally and seems to run in some families. Cause not fully known. The most common symptoms of Crohn's disease are abdominal pain, often in the lower right area, and diarrhea. Rectal bleeding, weight loss, arthritis, skin problems, and fever may also occur. The most common complication of Crohn's is blockage of the intestine. The doctor may do an upper GI series (Barium X-rays) to look at the small intestine. The doctor may also do a visual exam of the colon by performing either a sigmoidoscopy or a colonoscopy.

Cystic fibrosis (CF) – a birth defect that causes oversecretion of a thick mucus that clogs respiratory, pancreatic, and gall bladder passages and makes the child more prone to respiratory infections. CF is the most common lethal genetic disease in the U.S.—1 out of every 3,200 white children (of Northern European descent) are affected.

Diverticulosis- occurs when small pouches in the colon form that bulge outward through weak spots in the wall of the colon. Each pouch is called a diverticulum. _Red flag symptoms of diverticulosis: usually there are no symptoms. If symptoms are present, it might include cramping, bloating or constipation. Usually symptoms do not occur until the condition progresses to diverticulitis (when the pouches become inflamed/ infected.)_

Diverticulitis (also called **diverticular disease**)- When the diverticula become infected or inflamed, the condition is called diverticulitis. _Red Flag symptoms: The most common sign is tenderness around the left side of the lower abdomen (which worsens on palpation). If infection is the cause, fever, nausea, vomiting, chills, cramping, bloating and constipation may occur as well._ Diverticulitis can lead to bleeding, infections, perforations or tears, or blockages. Sigmoidoscopy can be used to assess. A common theory of cause is low fiber diets.

Esophageal Carcinoma- cancer of the esophagus. Progressive dysphagia (trouble swallowing), and weight loss may be symptoms. Barium GI study may show narrowing of esophagus.

Esophageal Varicies- Distension of the blood vessels of the esophagus. Commonly seen in patients who abuse alcohol.

Gastric Carcinoma (Stomach cancer). _Red Flag symptoms:_ _weight loss, indigestion, possible tenderness on palpation of left upper quadrant, possible vomiting of bloody materials or materials that look like dark coffee grounds._ Barium x-rays may be used as well as other scans- MRI or CT scan for diagnosis. Endoscopic exam (with biopsy, if needed) may also be done. Men are more likely to develop stomach cancer. Other risk factors involve being over age 70, dietary risk factors (eating diet high in processed foods, high in nitrates, high levels of sodium, low in fruits and vegetables), smoking, alcohol consumption, and a family history of stomach cancer. Treatment involves surgery, chemotherapy and/or radiation.

Gastritis- is inflammation of the stomach mucosa (inner lining) and can be acute or chronic. It may cause pain in the upper abdominal area- but often has no symptoms. The inflammation of the lining can interfere with proper production of stomach secretions (digestive enzymes or mucus). Some forms of gastritis can become erosive (leading to bleeding and ulcers). Most chronic cases of gastritis are caused by an infection with Helicobacter pylori (H. Pylori). Most erosive cases of gastritis are caused by prolonged use of NSAIDs (aspirin, ibuprofen).

Gastroenteritis (often times called "**food poisoning**" or "**stomach flu**")- Usually caused by an infection with a microorganism. Common infectious microorganisms are: _Campylobacter (causing Campylobacteriosis), Salmonella, Escherichia coli, Entamoeba histolytica, Vibrio cholera, Staphylococcus aureus, rotaviruses, Norwalk virus, Giardia_ and _cryptosporidium._ Improper hygiene (not washing hands after going to the bathroom), contaminated drinking water, improperly cooked foods, or contact with animals carrying the pathogen can all spread the infectious organism. Common symptoms are loss of appetite, nausea, vomiting, diarrhea (can be bloody or mucus filled), cramps, fever, and abdominal discomfort. Symptoms can develop quite quickly. Dehydration and electrolyte loss can easily occur and can be a serious complication especially in the very young, elderly, or those with chronic diseases.

Gastroesophageal Reflux Disease (GERD)- - "heartburn" – occurs when the gastroesophageal sphincter doesn't close tightly and gastric juice backs into the esophagus causing a burning sensation. Is sometimes also called **Reflux Esophagitis** or **Acid Reflux.** Symptoms are pain and burning sensation (usually behind the sternum) after eating. A dry cough or difficulty swallowing may also be seen. Ulceration and inflammation of the esophagus may be seen on endoscopic examination, often an esophagogastroduodenoscopy (EGD). Treatment may include dietary changes (small, frequent meals), staying upright at least 3 hours after eating a meal (no meal right before bed, for example), raising the head of the bed 6-8 inches, wearing loose fitting clothing (especially the waistbands of pants), and losing weight (if needed). Treatment can also include medications: antacids (Tums, Maalox, Alka-Seltzer, Rolaids) or H2 blockers (Tagamet, Pepcid AC, Zantac).

Hepatitis - inflammation of the liver, most commonly due to a viral infection. This can impair liver functions- such as removal of toxins from the blood. Can lead to symptoms such as fatigue (malaise), arthralgia (joint pain), weight loss, jaundice. Blood tests may be done to assess liver function. Biopsy of the liver may also be done. There are six forms of the hepatitis virus- the 3 most common are:
- **HBV- Hepatitis B.** Spread via contact with blood or bodily fluid. Vaccine available
- **HAV- Hepatitis A.** Spread via the fecal-oral route, usually through contaminated food or water. Does not have a chronic stage or cause permanent liver damage. Vaccine available
- **HCV- Hepatitis C.** Spread most commonly via blood-blood contact. Most fatal form. No vaccine available.

Hiatal Hernia- occurs when the stomach partially herniates up through the esophageal hiatus in the diaphragm. Could be congenital or as a result of trauma. Most common symptom is heartburn. X-ray is usually done for diagnosis.

Hemorrhoids- are veins in the anus and rectum that are swollen and inflamed. Symptoms are pain on defecating, itching, visible red blood in the stool, swelling or bulges around the anus, or discomfort when sitting. Hemorrhoids can be caused by low fiber diets, straining too hard when defecating, pregnancy, obesity, anal intercourse, and constipation.

Irritable Bowel Syndrome- Irritable bowel syndrome is a disorder characterized most commonly by cramping, abdominal pain, bloating, constipation, and diarrhea. IBS causes a great deal of discomfort and distress, but it does not permanently harm the intestines and does not lead to a serious disease, such as cancer. There is no ulceration in the wall of the intestines, which is different than ulcerative colitis and Crohn's disease. Most people can control their symptoms with diet, stress management, and prescribed medications.

Lactose Intolerance- (also called *lactase deficiency*). This condition is the lack of the digestive enzyme lactase- which is needed to digest milk sugar (lactose). Symptoms often begin 30 min to a few hours after eating dairy products, and can include: gas, bloating, diarrhea, nausea, or abdominal cramps. Treatment involves dietary changes (avoiding or limiting consumption of dairy) and/or using lactase enzyme supplements (such as Lactaid).

Liver Cancer- cancer of the liver. Some of the main causes of liver cancer is infection with Hepatitis B and/or Hepatitis C. *Red Flag symptoms: Pain in right upper abdominal quadrant, jaundice, unexplained weight loss, abdominal swelling, nausea and vomiting.* Diagnosis may be done using a liver blood panel, CT, MRI, or ultrasound. Treatment can involve surgery (to remove part of the liver), liver transplant, ablation, chemotherapy and/or radiation.

Pancreatic Cancer- Cancer of the pancreas. *Red Flag symptoms: pain in the upper abdomen that may radiate into the back (left sided), weight loss, decreased appetite, jaundice and fatigue.* Unfortunately, pancreatic cancer usually has a poor prognosis. Diagnosis may be done with CT, MRI, ultrasound, and ERCP. Treatment may involve surgery, chemotherapy and/or radiation.

Pancreatitis- Inflammation of the pancreas. Can be due to gallstones, alcohol or drug abuse, some viral infections, and digestive enzymes. Gallstones and alcohol abuse account for 80% of hospital admissions for acute pancreatitis. Acute pancreatitis is a sudden inflammation that can be mild or life threatening. *Red Flag symptoms: severe abdominal pain in the upper mid-abdomen and below the sternum. The pain often penetrates into the back. The pain can begin suddenly, and reach maximum intensity in minutes and then remain constant and severe for days.* Blood tests and CT scan may be used for diagnosis.

Peptic Ulcer- It is a crater-like erosion in the mucosa of any part of the GI tract. Most commonly occur in the the first part of the duodenum of the small intestine (*duodenal ulcer*), lower portion of the stomach (*gastric ulcer*), or esophagus. Duodenal ulcers are three times as common as gastric ulcers. Esophageal ulcers are the least common of the three areas. Gastric Juice- a chemical mixture of hydrochloric acid, pepsin (another digestive acid), pepsinogen, and intrinsic factor- will eat away at the lining of the digestive system organ if the protective mucosal lining has been compromised. Common symptom- burning or gnawing pain in the abdomen 1-3 hours after eating. The patient may vomit blood, or pass stools with different coloration. Studies now show that a good number of ulcers may be caused by an acid resistant strain of bacteria: Helicobacter Pylori (*H. pylori*).

Ulcerative Colitis- Ulcerative colitis is a disease that causes inflammation and sores (ulcers) in the superficial lining of the rectum and colon. Ulcers and inflammation cause pus, bleeding, and triggers the colon to empty frequently- causing diarrhea. Crohn's disease differs because it causes inflammation deeper within the intestinal wall and can occur in other parts of the digestive system including the small intestine, mouth, esophagus, and stomach. The most common symptoms of ulcerative colitis are abdominal pain and bloody diarrhea. Patients also may experience: anemia, fatigue, weight loss, loss of appetite, rectal bleeding, loss of body fluids and nutrients, skin lesions, joint pain, and growth failure (specifically in children). A colonoscopy or sigmoidoscopy are the most accurate methods for making a diagnosis of ulcerative colitis and ruling-out other possible conditions, such as Crohn's disease, diverticular disease, or cancer.

Practice Study and Test Questions:

1) The gall bladder is located in the
     A) left lower quadrant
     B) right lower quadrant
     C) left upper quadrant
     D) right upper quadrant

2) The preliminary digestion of proteins in the stomach is done by
     A) gastric lipase
     B) hydrochloric acid
     C) intrinsic factor
     D) pepsin

3) A test that may be done to assist in diagnosing gall stones is
     A) fluoroscopy
     B) esophagogastroduodenoscopy
     C) endoscopic retrograde cholangiopancreatography
     D) sigmoidoscopy

4) A patient has nausea, diarrhea and gas after consuming foods containing wheat, barley and rye. This person might have
     A) gastroenteritis
     B) diverticulosis
     C) appendicitis
     D) celiac disease

5) Which disease is transmitted via contact with blood of an infected individual?
     A) Hepatitis C
     B) Hepatitis A
     C) Crohn's disease
     D) Cholestasis

6) Blood in the fecal material, unexplained weight loss and fatigue may be signs of
     A) colon cancer
     B) GERD
     C) cirrhosis
     D) pancreatic cancer

7) Which test can be used for cholecystitis?
     A) Obturator test
     B) Murphy's test
     C) Markle test
     D) Cullen's test

8) An upper GI series (including barium x-rays) may be used in diagnosing
     A) Crohn's disease
     B) cystic fibrosis
     C) cirrhosis
     D) gastroenteritis

9) A risk factor for pancreatitis is
      A) a diet low in fruits and vegetables
      B) colon polyps
      C) a high fat diet
      D) alcohol abuse

10) The first portion of the small intestine is the
      A) cecum
      B) duodenum
      C) ascending colon
      D) jejunum

11) Tenderness in the lower left side of the abdomen is often a sign of
      A) appendicitis
      B) Crohn's disease
      C) diverticulitis
      D) GERD

12) Which of the following signs can indicate appendicitis?
      A) Aaron's sign
      B) Obturator sign
      C) Rovsing's sign
      D) all of the above

13) Sudden, stabbing, excruciating pain in the left upper quadrant may indicate
      A) pancreatitis
      B) appendicitis
      C) gall stones
      D) perforated ulcer

14) A patient presents with abdominal pain, diarrhea, and bloating. On further examination, no ulcerations are detected. This patient may have
      A) diverticulosis
      B) Crohn's disease
      C) ulcerative colitis
      D) irritable bowel syndrome

15) The _____ carries bile from the liver and gall bladder into the duodenum
      A) common hepatic duct
      B) common bile duct
      C) pancreatic duct
      D) liver duct

16) The area in the right lower abdomen that is located one third of the distance between the ASIS and umbilicus is called
      A) Rovsing's point
      B) Kehr's sign
      C) Mc Burney's point
      D) Cullen's sign

Answers: 1) D 2) D 3) C 4) D 5) A 6) A 7) B 8) A 9) D 10) B 11) C 12) D 13) A 14) D 15) B 16) C

CHAPTER 13: THE URINARY SYSTEM

The urinary system is composed of the kidneys, ureters, bladder and urethra. The urinary system has some important functions in the body. It serves to excrete and eliminate wastes and help support the liver in its detoxification efforts. It helps to regulate pH, volume and solute concentration of ions in blood plasma (sodium/Na$^+$, potassium/K$^+$, chloride/Cl$^-$) and regulates blood pressure.

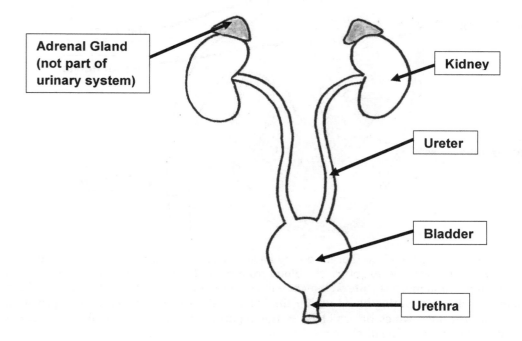

The Kidney

Usually we have 2 kidneys in our abdomen (one on the right side of the spine, one on the left) located between T12 and L3. The left kidney is slightly higher than the right kidney in the abdomen. The adrenal glands sit on top of the kidney. Kidneys are about the size of a bar of soap, and are shaped like a kidney bean that we might eat in a bowl of chili. The notched area of the kidney is called the *hilus/hilum* and faces the midline of the body. The hilum is the area where all blood vessels (renal artery and vein), urinary structures (ureter), and nerves (renal nerves) enter and leave the kidney. The kidney is suspended in place by the *renal fascia* and is protected by a fatty layer which surrounds and cushions it, called the *adipose capsule*.

If we were to cut a kidney longitudinally in cross section, we would see that the kidney is composed of a couple layers of tissue. Covering the kidney, like an outer shell, is the leather-like *renal capsule*. The tissue inside of the kidney has two main layers. The outer layer is called the *renal cortex*. It is lighter in color and will house many of the **nephrons** in the kidney. (A nephron is the microscopic filtering structure within the kidneys, which filters the blood and produces the urine.) The deeper and darker colored layer is called the *renal medulla*. Near the hilum of the kidney is the hollow *renal pelvis*. This hollow pelvis has fingerlike extensions on it- small ones called the *minor calyx* and larger ones called the *major calyx*. The calyces and renal pelvis serve to collect and hold the urine before it drains out of the kidney through the ureters.

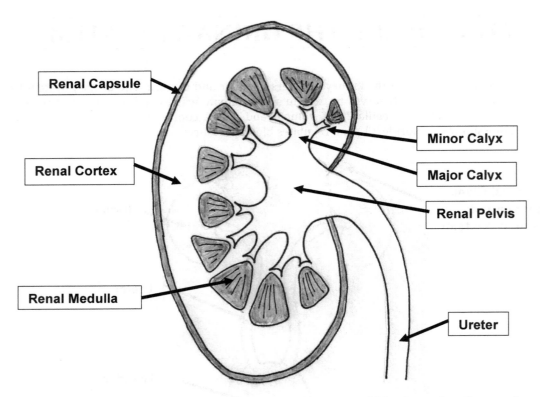

The kidneys filter and clean our blood, so therefore they have a good blood supply. The *renal arteries* bring blood to each kidney, and the *renal veins* return the blood from the kidney back into circulation. Within the kidney, there are millions of nephrons (filters) which will clean the blood. Coming off of the renal arteries are many smaller vessels distributing blood within the kidney. Each nephron has its own private blood supply- called *afferent arterioles* which brings blood to the nephron. The rate of blood flowing through the arterioles can be altered to assist in the filtering mechanism.

The Kidney: The Nephron

Each kidney contains 1.25 million microscopic nephrons. The **nephron** is a tube shaped structure, which has good contact with the bloodstream and blood vessels. The nephron is the main area of filtration, balancing, and processing of the blood in the urinary system. Each nephron, when done processing the blood, will empty their content (which becomes the urine) into one of many collecting ducts. The *collecting ducts* carry fluid away from the nephron, towards the renal pelvis of the kidney. 85% of all nephrons are *cortical nephrons* (with a short loop of Henle), 15% are *juxtaglomerular nephrons* (with long loop of Henle).

There are three general functions of the nephron: **Filtration, Reabsorption,** and **Secretion.** *Filtration* is the process of taking materials (water, electrolytes, vitamins, minerals, toxins, wastes) out of the blood and placing them inside the hollow nephron. After flowing through the full length of the nephron, any materials (called *filtrate*) that remain in the nephron will become the **urine** we expel from our body. After filtration is done, then reabsorption and secretion can take place. *Reabsorption* is the process of taking materials that were just filtered out of the blood and into the nephron, and placing them back into the bloodstream. Reabsorption is done to allow helpful nutrients or water that was filtered out of the blood during filtration to be placed back into the blood (so that the nutrients can be used by the body cells). *Secretion* is the process where materials are moved out of the bloodstream and into the nephron- much like filtration accomplished. Secretion is done later in the nephron and is accomplished with specialized pumps and channels. Secretion allows materials that were too large to be filtered in the initial filtration process to be removed from the bloodstream. It also allows for balancing of ions to regulate pH in the blood. Secretion is not done as often as filtration and reabsorption are. After flowing through the full length of the nephron (and undergoing all of the effects of filtration, reabsorption, and secretion), any materials that remain in the nephron will become the urine which we then expel from our body.

The nephron is a long hollow tube composed of many sections with varying functions. The main parts of the nephron are the **Renal Corpuscle** (made up of the **Bowman's capsule** and **glomerulus**) and the **Renal Tubule** (made up of the *Proximal Convoluted Tubule*, *Loop of Henle*, and *Distal Convoluted Tubule*). Surrounding the renal tubule are two types of blood capillaries called the *peritubular capillaries* and the *vasa recta*.

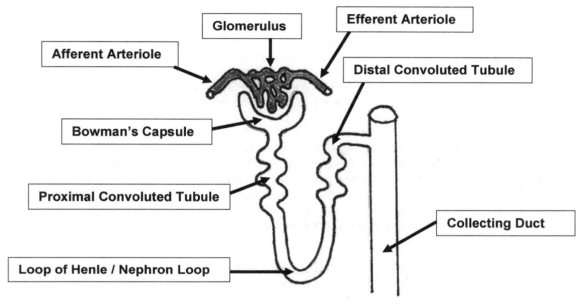

THE NEPHRON

In the **renal corpuscle**, there are two main components- the **glomerulus** and the **Bowman's Capsule.** The glomerulus is also known as the *glomerular capillary*, and is a blood vessel which receives blood from the afferent arteriole. The glomerulus brings blood to the nephron so that the blood can be filtered and processed. Surrounding the glomerulus is a cup- shaped structure, called Bowman's capsule. Bowman's capsule is the beginning of the tube shaped structure that will form the rest of the nephron. The Bowman's capsule is composed of cells called *podocytes.* These podocytes have small gaps between them called *filtration slits.* These filtration slits serve as a filtering membrane. Blood in the glomerulus is under high levels of pressure. As blood flows through the glomerulus and along the wall of the Bowman's capsule, materials in the blood can be pushed through the filtration slits- thus leaving the bloodstream and entering the nephron. Materials that can be filtered through Bowman's capsule are relatively small things, such as: water, electrolytes (Na^+, K^+), glucose, vitamins, minerals, and some wastes and toxins. Larger structures in the blood, like blood cells, some proteins, and some types of wastes and toxins are usually too large to fit through the filtration slits and will remain in the bloodstream (to be processed later). The materials and fluid that can be filtered out of the blood and into Bowman's capsule are called **filtrate**.

The rate of filtrate production per minute is called the Glomerular Filtration Rate (GFR) and is about 125mL per minute. In a 24 hour period, the glomerulus will produce around 50 gallons of filtrate. The GFR can be influenced by:
- The *blood pressure* in the glomerular capillary. If blood pressure in the glomerular capillary goes up, filtrate production goes up. If blood pressure in the glomerular capillary goes down, the filtrate production goes down- example: dehydration. If filtrate production drops, then the blood will not be thoroughly cleansed, and wastes and toxins can accumulate in the body.

- GFR can also be regulated by *Autoregulation* (changing the diameter of the capillaries leading into and out of the glomerulus). For example, if the blood pressure drops, the afferent arteriole will dilate, the glomerular capillary will dilate, and the efferent arteriole will constrict. This will try to boost the blood pressure to ensure proper filtration
- GFR can be regulated by *hormones produced in the kidney*. A drop in blood pressure can stimulate the juxtaglomerular apparatus (JGA) and trigger the **renin-angiotensin system** (also called the **renin-angiotensin mechanism)**. This causes the JGA to produce the hormone renin. Renin will in turn stimulate production of angiotensin I. Angiotensin I is converted into Angiotensin II by Angiotensin Converting Enzyme (ACE). Angiotensin II will then cause constriction of the efferent glomerulus-raising glomerular blood pressure and increasing filtration rates. Angiotensin II will also stimulate the release of aldosterone, antidiuretic hormone, and increase the thirst sensation.
- GFR can also be regulated by the *sympathetic nervous system*. Sympathetic stimulation to the kidney will cause vasoconstriction of the afferent arteriole. This will decrease the GFR and decreases filtrate production.

We mention these different means of influencing GFR because some medications that patients take will influence the function of the nephron at this level- either as its primary effect or as a side effect of the medication usage (ex: ACE inhibitors).

After the Bowman's capsule, the filtrate will enter the **Renal Tubule** portion of the nephron. This tube-like section of the nephron can be divided into different areas: the ***Proximal Convoluted Tubule, Loop of Henle / Nephron Loop,*** and ***Distal Convoluted Tubule***. The filtrate will flow through those areas in the order listed above. Along the way, materials will be pulled out of the filtrate and returned back into the bloodstream (reabsorption) or materials still trapped in the bloodstream can be pumped into the filtrate of the nephron for eventual removal from the body (secretion). Let's look at each of these sections of the renal tubule and their respective functions.

The **Proximal Convoluted Tubule (PCT)** is the first segment of the renal tubule. It receives tubular fluid and filtrate from Bowman's capsule. Reabsorption is the main function of the PCT. So much reabsorption is done here that 60-70% of the filtrate materials filtered and produced in Bowman's capsule are reabsorbed back into the bloodstream here in the PCT. Let's think about this for a moment. We said earlier that during filtration at Bowman's capsule, 50 gallons of filtrate are produced each day. This filtrate contains toxins and wastes, but the majority of it also contains a lot of helpful and needed nutrients. Filtrate, if left untouched becomes your urine. *Do you urinate 50 gallons of fluid a day?* No, of course not. Therefore, the majority of the filtrate produced at Bowman's capsule must be returned back into the bloodstream. Hence, the large amount of reabsorption done here in the PCT. The PCT will reabsorb (put back into the bloodstream): 60-70% of the water that was just filtered out in Bowman's Capsule. Things that will be reabsorbed back into the bloodstream in the PCT are: 99-100% of organic substances (like glucose, small amino acids); 60-70% of sodium and chloride ions; 90% of bicarbonate ions, and potassium, magnesium, phosphate, and sulfate ions. Wastes and toxins will NOT be reabsorbed, and will remain in the filtrate as it continues its movement through the rest of the renal tubule.

The **Loop of Henle** (**Nephron Loop**) is formed by a *descending limb* and *ascending limb*. In the descending limb (which travels down from the PCT to the bottom of the loop), water is reabsorbed. In the ascending limb, sodium and chloride ions will be reabsorbed. The ***Vasa Recta*** is the name of the blood vessel that surrounds the Loop of Henle and reabsorbs ions and water back into the bloodstream.

The **Distal Convoluted Tubule (DCT)** receives the remaining tubular fluid from the ascending limb of the Loop of Henle. By this time, only about 15-20% of the tubular fluid produced by the glomerulus remains. The DCT will reabsorb Na+ (sodium) ions via the Na+ /K+ pump. During the action of this pump, K+ (potassium) will be secreted as a result- K+ is literally traded for Na+. The DCT also does secretion. If the body and blood are becoming acidic (the pH drops), this can be toxic. The intercalated cells of the DCT will secrete H+ ions out of the blood and into the tubule for removal from the body. This makes our blood pH less acidic and more neutral- healthier for all of our body tissues. Ammonia, a toxin, will be secreted from the blood into the tubular fluid, while the bicarbonate ion will be reabsorbed into the bloodstream. Other toxins, wastes, creatinine, and some types of drugs will also be secreted into the tubular fluid.

The Kidney: The Collecting System and Renal Pelvis

The **collecting ducts** will receive (collect) tubular fluid/filtrate from many nephrons out in the cortex of the kidney. Collecting ducts are larger than the tubules in the nephron. This size difference is because they collect fluid from many nephrons and begin to carry the fluid towards the renal pelvis and eventually out of the kidney. The collecting ducts are influenced by the hormones aldosterone and ADH and will perform reabsorption and secretion. The tubular fluid that travels through the collecting duct is the urine which we release from our body when we urinate.

Urine then drains into the **renal pelvis** from the collecting ducts. The composition of urine can no longer be changed once the urine enters the renal pelvis. The collecting ducts will carry urine from the nephrons into the *minor calyces* of the renal pelvis. The minor calyces will drain into larger *major calyces*. The major calyces open up and become the renal pelvis. The renal pelvis will fill with urine, and the urine will then flow out of the kidney and into our next organ- the ureter.

The Ureters:

The ureters are a pair of muscular tubes. These organs are retroperitoneal in location. Ureters are composed of three layers of tissue. The inner layer is a *mucosa*, the middle layer is composed of *smooth muscle*, and the outer layer is composed of *connective tissue*. The smooth muscle in the ureter contracts in peristaltic waves to propel the urine toward the bladder. Each kidney will have one ureter exiting it and the ureter will function to carry urine to the bladder. The ureters will join onto the bladder wall at an oblique angle. The opening of the ureter into the bladder is a slit-like shape and narrow. This helps prevent backflow of urine from the bladder back into the ureter.

The Bladder:

The bladder is a hollow, muscular organ that can hold urine until the time to urinate. A full bladder can hold, on average, 500-600 milliliters (about 2.5 cups) of urine. The bladder is supported and held in place by the middle umbilical ligament and the lateral umbilical ligaments on its superior surface. The inner surface of the bladder appears folded and rippled- these folds are called *rugae*. As the bladder fills, these folds will flatten and disappear. The innermost layer of the bladder wall is called the *mucosa*. This mucus layer helps urine pass through easily and also helps to trap bacteria and prevent infections. The *muscularis layer* is composed of three smooth muscle layers. These layers of muscle are called the **detrusor muscle**. The area of the bladder between the urethral opening and the ureter openings is called the **trigone**. At the most inferior area of the bladder, the urethra will attach and drain urine from the bladder. At the opening of the urethra is a band of muscle called the *internal urethral sphincter*. This sphincter is under involuntary control.

The Urethra:

The urethra is a hollow tube which carries urine from the bladder to the outside of the body. The male urethra and female urethra are slightly different lengths. The male urethra is about 7-8 inches in length and is composed of three portions: *prostatic urethra, membranous urethra,* and *spongy urethra*. The external opening of the urethra at the tip of the penis is called the external urethral orifice. The urethra in a male carries urine and semen out of the male body. The female urethra is much shorter (only 1-2 inches in length) and only carries urine. In both sexes the urethra has an inner mucus lining, passes through the urogenital diaphragm, and has an *external urethral sphincter*. This sphincter is under voluntary control.

Composition of Urine:

Out of the 50 gallons of filtrate produced by the glomerulus each day, about 99% of it is reabsorbed back into the bloodstream. The remaining 1% (about 1-1.8 liters per day) will become urine. Normally urine is clear, pale yellow, and without a strong odor. Materials normally found in urine are: water (composes 93-97% of urine), electrolytes (sodium, potassium, calcium, chloride, and magnesium), nitrogenous wastes (urea, creatinine, ammonia, uric acid, hippuric acid, urobilin, and bilirubin), and excess amino acids. Materials NOT normally found in urine are things like: excess amounts of red blood cells and white blood cells (pus), bacteria, excess amounts of glucose and large proteins. Due to the consistent nature of the composition of urine, it can be used as a bodily fluid to be tested in a medical setting. A physician will look for the presence of the normal materials (at appropriate levels) and also screen for the presence of anything abnormal. In some cases, urinalysis can allow for a diagnosis of a medical disease.

Micturition Reflex and Urination

The **Micturition Reflex** coordinates the activities of urination. The steps of the micturition reflex are as follows:
1. The ureters continuously drip urine into the bladder.
2. As the bladder fills to 200 ml, the stretch receptors in the bladder wall send messages to the spinal cord- this triggers the beginning of micturition.
3. The spinal cord then sends parasympathetic messages back to the bladder causing the detrusor muscle in the bladder to rhythmically contract. While the spinal cord is making the detrusor muscle contract, another set of messages move up the spinal cord, through the thalamus, and into the cerebral cortex- this gives you the conscious "urge" that you need to urinate.
4. As the contractions of the detrusor muscle increases, pressure in the bladder will increase.
5. The lower external urethral sphincter is voluntarily controlled, so we can consciously decide to hold or excrete the urine. If we decide to urinate, we consciously relax the external urethral sphincter. When the external sphincter relaxes, the internal sphincter will automatically relax as well.
6. If the time is not appropriate to urinate and the external sphincter is kept closed, the reflex contractions of the detrusor muscle will stop and the urge to urinate will often cease.
7. Urine will continue to drip into the bladder. After around an hour of additional filling (or another 100-200 ml of urine empty into the bladder), the micturition reflex begins again- this time with stronger contractions.
8. If volume in the bladder exceeds 500 ml, the detrusor contractions may overpower the internal sphincter. When the internal sphincter is forced open, the external sphincter will automatically open as well. Unfortunately, urination is not able to be consciously controlled at this point.

Physical Examination of the Urinary System:

Due to the close proximity of the organs of the urinary and reproductive system, they are often examined at the same time on a physical examination. Please see the examination discussion at the end of the Reproductive System chapter for the examination and abnormal findings of the **Genitourinary System** (reproductive and urinary systems).

Pathologies of the Urinary System

For additional infectious diseases that may affect this system, please refer to the Communicable/Infectious Disease Chart in Chapter 10.

Cystitis- "bladder infection"- a urinary tract infection located in the bladder. See more information under Urinary Tract Infection.

Glomerulonephritis- inflammation of the glomeruli- often due to the streptococci bacteria. Symptoms may be hematuria (blood in the urine), proteinuria (protein in the urine), edema, and hypertension. If it progresses to a chronic state, the kidneys will start to fail which can cause pH levels in the blood to become abnormal and bleeding disorders can occur.

Incontinence- the loss of control of the ability to urinate. A person is unable to voluntarily control the external urethral sphincter.

Interstitial cystitis *("Painful bladder syndrome")*- Patient experiences pain in the bladder, or in the lower abdominal/pubic area- and pain descriptions differ from patient to patient. Symptoms can include increased urinary frequency, increased urinary urgency, or both. Pain may occur and change intensity as the bladder fills or as it is being emptied. Symptoms may increase during menstruation or during intercourse. Interstitial cystitis is more common in women (usually over the age of 40) than in men. The cause is still relatively unknown, although a defect with the bladder lining may be one cause. Cystoscopy and biopsy may be done after other causes of bladder pain are ruled out (such as urinary tract infection).

Nephrosis- the glomerulus of the nephron becomes damaged and allows the passage of large proteins into the urine (*proteinuria*). This can be seen as a result of some respiratory infections, after some prophylactic childhood immunizations, or as a result of an autoimmune process.

Nocturia- nighttime urination- usually waking up more than once in the middle of the night to urinate. This can be a normal occurrence as we age, or a sign of another condition. Causes can be high fluid intake in the evening or before bed, untreated diabetes mellitus (both type I and II), diabetes insipidus, gestational diabetes, pregnancy, medications (such as diuretics, lithium, cardiac glycosides, etc.), urinary tract infection, bladder cancer, prostate cancer, or benign prostatic hyperplasia (BPH).

Polycystic Kidney- a degenerative condition that appears to run in families (a congenital abnormality). The kidneys become enlarged and contain many blister-like urine filled sacs. These sacs can impede and prevent proper urine drainage from the kidney. Infections can occur as a secondary effect, and renal failure is the eventual outcome. Kidney transplants are performed to improve chances for survival.

Pyelonephritis "kidney infection" - inflammation of the kidney pelvis and surrounding kidney tissues. Is often caused by a urinary tract infection involving *Escherichia Coli* (a bacteria normally found in the intestines), which goes untreated and then spreads into the kidney. *Red Flag symptoms: Fever, pain, increased frequency of urination, and painful urination may be seen. There may be referred lumbar pain.* Pyelonephritis could cause permanent damage to the nephrons, so treatment (usually antibiotics) is administered to try to avoid or minimize nephron damage.

Renal Calculi- "Kidney Stones"- If urine is allowed to accumulate in the renal pelvis and concentrate, solutes in the urine (such as uric acid salts and minerals) may start to coagulate and form larger crystals. As these crystals move from the larger renal pelvis and begin to descend down the narrow ureters, excruciating pain will occur. *Red Flag symptoms: Sharp intense pain in the abdomen or low back, pain with urinating, and/or blood in the urine.* Treatment for small stones can involve just letting the stone pass (the patient will usually be given pain medications and be encouraged to drink a lot of fluids). Larger stones may need more aggressive treatment such as ureteroscopy or shock wave lithotripsy.

Renal Failure "Kidney failure"- occurs when the number of functioning nephrons becomes too low to carry out normal kidney functions. Possible causes are: repeated damaging infections of the kidney, physical trauma to the kidneys, chemical poisoning of the kidneys, and inadequate blood supply to the kidneys. Dialysis and/or kidney transplantation must be done if both kidneys are failing, otherwise death will occur.

Urinary Tract Infection- Usually caused by *E. Coli*- the bacteria naturally found in the colon. In a urinary tract infection, the bacteria get deposited in the urethra or bladder and can cause an infection. _Red Flag Symptoms:_ *Painful, frequent, sometimes blood-tinged or cloudy urination. There may be a fever present. The urine may have a strong, unusual odor (some call it "fishy").* More commonly seen in females due to the location and length of the female urethra. UTI in the urethra is called *urethritis*, UTI in the bladder is called *cystitis* (bladder infection), and UTI in the kidney is called *pyelonephritis* (kidney infection). Urinalysis will be used for diagnosis. If the UTI is in the lower urinary tract, increasing fluid intake may be enough to flush the infection out. Otherwise, antibiotics can be prescribed for treatment.

Urethritis- urinary tract infection in the urethra.

Practice Study and Test Questions:

1) The structure which carries urine from the kidney to the bladder is called the
    A) urethra
    B) collecting duct
    C) ureter
    D) nephron loop

2) Nighttime urination is called
    A) oligouria
    B) anuria
    C) hematouria
    D) nocturia

3) The muscle located in the bladder is called the
    A) detrusor
    B) piriformis
    C) scalene
    D) multifidi

4) A degenerative condition in which the patient's kidney fills with urine filled sacs is called
    A) interstitial cystitis
    B) polycystic kidney
    C) glomerulonephritis
    D) nephrosis

5) 60-70% of the water which was filtered in the Bowman's capsule will be reabsorbed in the
    A) nephron loop
    B) collecting duct
    C) distal convoluted tubule
    D) proximal convoluted tubule

6) Interstitial cystitis is most common in
     A) women ages 20-30
     B) children ages 2-8
     C) women over the age of 40
     D) men over the age of 40

7) Sharp, intense pain in the abdomen or low back may be a sign of
     A) renal failure
     B) cystitis
     C) renal calculi
     D) urethritis

8) Cystitis is
     A) kidney stones
     B) a kidney infection
     C) a genetic defect in the kidney
     D) a bladder infection

9) Glucose is reabsorbed into the bloodstream in the
     A) proximal convoluted tubule
     B) collecting duct
     C) nephron loop
     D) distal convoluted tubule

10) The correct pathway for urine to move through the kidney is
     A) nephron-collecting duct-minor calyx-major calyx-renal pelvis
     B) nephron-collecting duct--major calyx-renal pelvis- minor calyx
     C) renal pelvis-collecting duct-minor calyx-major calyx-nephron
     D) collecting duct-nephron-minor calyx-major calyx-renal pelvis

11) The most common cause of a urinary tract infection is
     A) Escherichia Coli
     B) Staphylococcus Aureus
     C) Group A strep
     D) Herpes simplex

12) The movement of substances out of the blood and into the nephron is called
     A) filtration
     B) reabsorption
     C) secretion
     D) both A and C

13) If blood pressure goes up, GFR will
     A) decrease
     B) increase
     C) not change

14) A streptococcal infection can cause
     A) urethritis
     B) renal calculi
     C) glomerulonephritis
     D) polycystic kidney

15) Which substance is not normally found in urine?
   A) creatinine
   B) bilirubin
   C) red blood cells
   D) uric acid

16) Cloudy urine with a "fishy" odor may be signs of
   A) urinary tract infection
   B) kidney stones
   C) nocturia
   D) benign prostatic hypertrophy

17) _____can lead to renal failure
   A) glomerulonephritis
   B) chemical poisoning of the kidney
   C) polycystic kidney
   D) all of the above

18) Referred lumbar pain, fever and painful urination may be signs of
   A) polycystic kidney
   B) pyelonephritis
   C) glomerulonephritis
   D) nephrosis

19) The internal urethral sphincter is under _____ control
   A) voluntary
   B) involuntary
   C) conscious
   D) both A and C

20) The functional unit of the kidney is the
   A) nephron
   B) renal cortex
   C) renal medulla
   D) renal capsule

Answers: 1) C 2) D 3) A 4) B 5) D 6) C 7) C 8) D 9) A 10) A 11) A 12) D 13) B 14) C 15) C 16) A 17) D 18) B 19) B 20) A

CHAPTER 14: THE REPRODUCTIVE SYSTEM

Male and female reproductive systems each produce genetic material (gametes) that can be used to create a new human being. The male gonads are the *testes*. The testes produce the male gametes called spermatozoa (sperm). The female gonads are the *ovaries*, which produce a gamete called an oocyte (ovum).

Male Reproductive System:

The main organs of the male reproductive system are: testes, epididymis, ductus deferens, ejaculatory duct, seminal vesicles, prostate, bulbourethral glands, ureter, scrotum, and penis.

Testes

The **testes** are the gonads of the male. They are responsible for producing the genetic material (sperm) and male reproductive hormones. There are two testes in the male and they are suspended under the pelvic cavity by the **scrotum**. The scrotum is a fleshy pouch which is divided into two scrotal chambers by the scrotal septum. Each testis resides in one of the chambers. The *dartos* and *cremaster muscle* can elevate and lower the testis for temperature regulation or during sexual arousal.

The testes begin inside the pelvic cavity during embryological and fetal development. The *gubernaculum testis* is a piece of connective tissue that attaches onto the testis at the beginning of development. It holds the testes in place, so as the pelvis of the body grows, the testicles remain attached in the lower portion of the pelvis. During the 7th developmental month, hormones will cause the gubernaculum testis to contract, pulling and descending the testes through the abdominal wall to the outside of the pelvic cavity. The ductus deferens, blood vessels and nerves are also pulled through the abdominal wall with the testes.

The testes are composed of structures called **interstitial cells** and **seminiferous tubules**. The interstitial cells (aka cells of Leydig) produce the male reproductive hormones, called *androgens*. A very important androgen is the hormone testosterone. Androgen production by the testes is regulated by Gonadotropin-releasing hormone (GnRH) and luteinizing hormone (LH). After production, the androgens leave the testes via the bloodstream to then travel throughout the male body.

The seminiferous tubules contain **sustentacular cells** (aka **sertoli cells**). The sustentacular cells perform *spermatogenesis* (the formation of spermatozoa/sperm). Spermatogenesis involves the process of meiosis. **Meiosis** is a type of cell formation in which a cell is created with only half of the chromosomes of a regular body cell. A regular body cell contains 46 chromosomes. Gametes, such as sperm, only contain 23 chromosomes. Sperm production by the testes is regulated by Gonadotropin-releasing hormone (GnRH) and follicle stimulating hormone (FSH).

Sperm, produced by the seminiferous tubules, are composed of the following structures. The **head** is the genetic region. It contains the nucleus (and chromosomes) and an acrosomal cap. The *acrosomal cap* is a helmet-like structure containing hydrolytic enzymes that enable the sperm to penetrate an egg. The **midpiece** of the sperm is the metabolic region. It contains mitochondria. The **tail** is the locomotor region and is composed of a flagellum. The tail propels the sperm as it seeks out an egg to fertilize.

The Epididymis

The **epididymis** is found at the top of the testes. It can be palpated through the scrotum. Immature spermatozoa (nonmotile) from the sustentacular cells of the seminiferous tubules are sent here. They slowly pass through the epididymis, and become motile. The walls of the epididymis are lined with smooth muscle to help propel the sperm into the next organ, the ductus deferens. The epididymis is composed of a head, body and tail region. It functions to store and protect spermatozoa and stimulates their maturation and mobility (capacitation). It monitors and adjusts composition of fluid produced by the seminiferous tubules. During ejaculation, the epididymis contracts, expelling sperm into the ductus deferens.

The Ductus Deferens:

The **ductus (Vas) deferens** is a 16-18 inch long tube which carries sperm from the epididymis to the ejaculatory duct and then into the prostate gland. A *vasectomy* is the cutting and ligating of the ductus deferens, which is a nearly 100% effective form of birth control. Sperm can be stored in the ductus deferens for several months. It contains smooth muscle to help propel the sperm. Just before entering the prostate gland, the ductus deferens widens into the *ampulla*. At the junction of the ampulla and the duct from the seminal vesicles, the ductus deferens becomes the *ejaculatory duct*. The ejaculatory duct is very short (less than 1 inch long) and will carry the sperm and materials from the seminal vesicles into the prostate gland.

Path of travel of the sperm: Seminiferous tubules in testes ➡epididymis ➡spermatic cord ➡inguinal canal➡ ductus deferens➡ejaculatory duct➡prostatic urethra in prostate gland ➡membranous urethra ➡spongy urethra

The Accessory Organs/Glands

The **accessory organs/glands** are responsible for producing the liquid secretions that compose the majority of the fluids in semen. The accessory glands activate the spermatozoa, provide buffers and nutrients for the spermatozoa, and propel fluid and spermatozoa along the reproductive tract. The accessory organs are the seminal vesicles, the prostate and the bulbourethral glands.

The **seminal vesicles** drain its secretions into the beginning of the ejaculatory duct. It is located in the area between the bladder and the rectum. It contributes about 60% of semen volume, and the fluid is alkaline. The fluid from the seminal vesicles contain fructose (fuel for the sperm), prostaglandins (to increase contractions in the reproductive tracts), and fibrinogen (to cause temporary clotting in the vagina).

The **prostate gland** is a small, rounded, doughnut shaped organ which sits underneath the bladder. The urethra will pass through the prostate gland as it leaves the bladder. It produces prostatic fluid, a slightly acidic solution that is about 20-30% of semen. Prostatic fluid contains *seminalplasmin-* an antibiotic which may help prevent urinary tract infections in the male. The prostate also contains smooth muscle to help propel its secretions into the urethra.

The **bulbourethral glands** (aka **Cowper's glands**) are located at the base of the penis. It empties its secretions into the urethra as it enters the penis. The bulbourethral glands produce a thick alkaline mucus secretion, which is used to neutralize any urinary acids in the urethra and lubricate the tip of the penis during intercourse.

Semen is a combination of products from the testis and accessory organs. A typical ejaculation produces 2-5 ml of semen. Semen is composed of sperm, fluid and enzymes. The sperm count ranges from 20 million to 100 million spermatozoa per milliliter of semen. Of the fluid in semen, 60% is from the seminal vesicles, 30% is from the prostate gland, 5% from the sustentacular cells in testis, and 5% from the bulbourethral glands. Semen also contains a variety of enzymes. *Proteases* dissolve mucus in the vagina to allow easier mobility for the sperm. *Seminalplasmin* is a prostatic enzyme used to convert fibrinogen to fibrin for clotting and thickening of the semen in the vagina. This helps keep the semen inside the vagina after intercourse (to allow the sperm more time to begin their journey to the egg). *Fibrinolysin* is an enzyme used to dissolve the clotted semen after 15-30 min.

The Urethra

In the male, the **urethra** is part of both the reproductive system and the urinary system. It conveys both urine and semen (at different times). In the reproductive system, the urethra will begin to receive reproductive fluids as it passes through the prostate. The male urethra has three regions: *prostatic urethra* (in prostate), *membranous urethra* (in urogenital diaphragm), and the *spongy (penile) urethra* (in penis).

The Penis

The **penis** is a tubular organ and houses the spongy portion of the urethra. The urethra will release its contents (either urine or semen) at the tip of the penis. The penis contains sensitive nerve endings which can be aroused during stimulation. The penis consists of the *root* and *shaft* that ends in the *glans penis*. The *prepuce*, or *foreskin* is the cuff of loose skin covering the glans (*circumcision* is the surgical removal of the foreskin). The *crura* is the proximal end of the penis and is surrounded by *ischiocavernosus muscle* (which anchors the penis to the pubic arch). The spongy urethra of the penis is surrounded by three cylindrical bodies of erectile tissue. The *corpus spongiosum* surrounds the urethra and expands to form the glans and bulb. The *corpora cavernosa* are paired dorsal erectile bodies. The corpus spongiosum and corpora cavernosa will fill with blood during erection, causing the penis to enlarge and become rigid.

The Female Reproductive System

The main organs of the female reproductive system are the: ovaries, uterine tubes, uterus, vagina, external genitalia and mammary glands.

Ovaries:

The **ovaries** are the gonads of the female. They are responsible for producing the genetic material (ova) and female reproductive hormones. Ovaries are supported in the pelvic cavity by the broad ligament, mesovarium, ovarian ligament, and suspensory ligament. The broad ligament encloses not only the ovaries, but also the uterine tubes and uterus. There are usually two almond sized ovaries- one located in the right and one in the left lower abdominal quadrants.

Ovaries are covered externally by a fibrous *tunica albuginea*. Internally, there are two poorly defined regions. The *cortex* contains the **ovarian follicles**. The *medulla* is deeper inside of the ovary and contains large blood vessels and nerves. In the cortex, there will be many follicles. A follicle is an immature egg (oocyte) surrounded by follicle cells and protective granulosa cells.

As the egg is developing "ripening", the follicle will proceed through the following stages: *Primordial follicle* ➡*Primary follicle* ➡*Secondary follicle* ➡*Late secondary follicle* ➡ *Vesicular (Graafian) follicle* (this follicle bulges from the ovary surface).

Ovulation is the ejection of the oocyte from the ripening vesicular follicle. After ovulation, the vesicular follicle is called the *corpus luteum*.

The ovary serves two main functions. First, it produces the female reproductive hormones: *estrogen* and the *progestins (progesterone)*. Estrogen production is stimulated by follicle stimulating hormone (FSH) and is the dominant female hormone in the first half of a woman's monthly menstrual (uterine) cycle. The progestins (progesterone) are produced by the corpus luteum of the ovary and are the principal hormone in the luteal phase of the menstrual cycle. Progestin production is triggered by a surge in luteinizing hormone (LH).

The second main function of the ovary is **oogenesis**- the production of eggs (ova). Like the development of sperm, this process will also involve *meiosis* (the formation of a cell with only 23 chromosomes). The oogonia (stem cells of female eggs) are formed while the woman is developing in the womb as a fetus. The primary oocytes will partially mature while the woman is a fetus and will then halt development until puberty. At birth, a female has about 2 million of these primary oocytes. Once puberty has been reached, about 400,000 primary oocytes have survived. After puberty, one primary oocyte per month (approximately) will be stimulated to fully mature and be released from the ovary during ovulation. This continues during her reproductive years, until menopause. During the course of her life, a woman will ovulate only about 500 oocytes.

The Uterine Tubes (aka Fallopian Tubes)

The **uterine tubes** will receive the egg after ovulation. They are hollow muscular tubes about 5 inches long. There are two uterine tubes in the body, each one extending from each ovary to the uterus. The uterine tubes are composed of the following regions: The *ampulla* is the distal expansion (with infundibulum) near the ovary. It is the usual site of fertilization of the oocyte (egg) by the sperm. The *fimbriae* of the infundibulum are "fingerlike" projections which create currents to draw the oocyte into the uterine tube. The *isthmus* is constricted region where the tube joins the uterus. The uterine tubes transport the oocyte or ovum from the ovary to the uterus.

The Uterus

The **uterus** is a pear-shaped muscular organ, about 3 in. long and 2 in. diameter. It is also known as the "womb", because it functions as the developmental site for a fertilized egg as it grows into a fetus. The uterus will then expel the fetus during labor. The uterus is supported by the uterosacral ligaments, round ligaments, broad ligament, lateral (cardinal) ligaments, and muscles of the pelvic floor. It is located in the hypogastric region of the lower pelvis. The parts of the uterus are the *body* (major portion), *fundus* (rounded superior region), *isthmus* (narrowed inferior region) and *cervix* (opening which leads into vaginal canal).

The uterus is a hollow organ. There are three layers of the uterine wall. The *perimetrium* is the outer layer, a serous layer (visceral peritoneum). The *myometrium* is the middle layer, and is made up of interlacing layers of smooth muscle. This layer is used during labor contractions to push the baby out. The *endometrium* is the inner layer. It is a mucosal lining that is richly supplied with blood. The endometrium will be sloughed off during menses.

The Vagina:

The **vagina** is a muscular tube (about 3 inches long) that leads from the uterus to the outside of the body. It is lined with stratified squamous epithelium, and the lining is usually folded into *rugae* in the relaxed state. The vagina serves as the "birth canal" and organ of copulation. The functions of the vagina are: that it serves as a passageway for menstrual fluids, receives the penis and spermatozoa during intercourse, and forms the inferior portion of the birth canal.

External Genitalia:

The **external genitalia** are parts involved with the pelvic female genitalia. The *mons pubis* is a fatty area overlying the pubic symphysis. The *labia majora* are hair-covered, fatty skin folds. The *labia minora* are smaller skin folds lying within the labia majora. The *vestibule* is the recess between the labia minora. The *greater vestibular glands (Bartholin's glands)* are homologous to the bulbourethral glands and release mucus into the vestibule for lubrication. The *clitoris* is the erectile tissue hooded by a prepuce. Lastly, the *perineum* is the diamond-shaped region between the pubic arch and coccyx. In some cases, during childbirth, the woman can experience tearing of this tissue- requiring stitches.

Mammary Glands

The **mammary glands** are modified sweat glands consisting of 15-25 lobes. They function to provide nourishment for a newborn baby. Covering the breast tissue is a layer of fat called the pectoral fat pad. The *areola* is the pigmented skin surrounding the nipple. The nipple is centrally located and contains openings for the milk to be released. *Suspensory ligaments* attach the breast to underlying muscle. Lobules located within lobes contain *alveolar glands/glandular alveoli* that produce milk. Milk production is stimulated by the hormone prolactin. The hormone oxytocin stimulates the mammary glands to release the milk (called milk "let-down" or milk ejection).

Milk will flow through the following structures in the breast: alveolar glands➡lactiferous ducts➡lactiferous sinuses➡ out to the surface of the nipple

The Female Reproductive Cycle

Men are constantly making sperm- 24 hours a day, at a pretty even pace. The female reproductive system is cyclical in nature. There are two main cycles to follow in a female- the **ovarian cycle** and the **uterine (menstrual) cycle**. Both cycles are occurring simultaneously in the female body.

Ovarian Cycle: The ovarian cycle involves one follicle in an ovary maturing and releasing its egg during ovulation. The ovarian cycle consists of two consecutive phases (in an average 28-day cycle). The first phase is called the ***follicular phase*** and is the period of follicle growth (days 1-14). **Ovulation** occurs midcycle- at day 14. The second phase of the ovarian cycle is called the ***luteal phase*** and is the period of corpus luteum activity after ovulation (days 14-28). In the follicular phase, the dominant hormone is estrogen. At around day 14 of the ovarian cycle, estrogen levels peak. This will trigger a massive release of luteinizing hormone (LH) from the pituitary gland- which in turn stimulates ovulation. In the luteal phase, the corpus luteum will secrete progesterone. During this phase, estrogen levels fall and progesterone levels rise. The corpus luteum will produce progesterone for about 12 days after ovulation. Progesterone prepares the uterus for pregnancy. If fertilization does not occur, after 12 days the corpus luteum degenerates, progesterone and estrogen levels drop, and the pituitary will begin secreting follicle stimulating hormone (FSH), triggering a new ovarian cycle.

Uterine Cycle: The other female reproductive cycle, (which is occurring simultaneously in the body along with the ovarian cycle) is called the uterine cycle. The uterine cycle is the cyclic changes of the endometrium in response to ovarian hormones. The uterine cycle (also called the ***menstrual cycle***) averages 28 days in length (but normally ranges between 21 and 35 days) in healthy women. It consists of three phases:
Days 1-5: Menstrual phase- menstrual bleeding is occurring here.
Days 6-14: Proliferative (preovulatory) phase. This phase ends when ovulation occurs.
Days 15-28: Secretory (postovulatory) phase (usually a constant 14-day length)

In the menstrual phase, estrogen and progesterone levels are low. As the woman's body moves into the proliferative phase, estrogen levels rise. At the end of the proliferative phase, LH levels will surge- triggering ovulation. Progesterone becomes the dominant hormone in the secretory phase. If fertilization does not occur during the secretory phase, her body returns to the menstrual phase and the cycle begins again.

Hormones and Basal Body Temperature: Basal body temperature is about 0.3 degrees Celsius lower in the follicular phase than in the luteal phase. Basal body temperature often dips around the time of ovulation, and then surges and increases after ovulation. It will remain elevated until menses begins.

Pregnancy:

Pregnancy is the events that occur from fertilization until the infant is born. The *gestation period*, the time from the last menstrual period until birth, is usually about 280 days. A **zygote** is the fertilized egg which has begun division, during days 1-4. A zygote becomes a *blastocyst* during days 4-5. The blastocyst will implant into the uterine wall. The term **embryo** is used from implantation of the blastocyst through week 8 of development. After week 8, we use the term *fetus* to describe the development from week 9 through birth.

The oocyte (egg) is viable for 12 to 24 hours after ovulation. Sperm is viable 28-72 hours within the female body. For fertilization to occur, intercourse must occur two days before ovulation and/or 24 hours after ovulation. Fertilization is when the sperm's chromosomes combine with those of an oocyte to form a fertilized egg (zygote). In determining the gender of the offspring, the sex chromosomes (X and Y) are utilized. An egg always contains an X chromosome. Sperm can contain either an X or a Y chromosome (about 50% of sperm contain the X chromosome, 50% contain Y chromosome). Therefore, it is the type of sperm which will determine the gender of the offspring.
- If an X egg is fertilized by an X sperm ➡ XX (female offspring) will result.
- If an X egg is fertilized by a Y sperm ➡XY (male offspring) occurs.

Fertilization:

When a male ejaculates during intercourse, about 200-300 million sperm are deposited in the vagina. The sperm are fully engaged for fertilization when exposed to the female reproductive tract. The sperm will travel up through the vagina, through the uterus, and into the uterine tube. Of the millions of sperm that are ejaculated, only about 10,000 enter the correct uterine tube. Fertilization usually occurs near the junction of the ampulla and isthmus of the uterine tube. It may take anywhere from 30 min to 2 hours for the sperm to make this journey. Fewer than 100 sperm make it to this point. Dozens of sperm will begin to weaken the *corona radiata* (the protective outer covering of the oocyte). The tip of the head of the sperm (the *acrosomal cap*) contains enzymes called *hyaluronidase* and *acrosin*, used to weaken the corona. This team effort from dozens of sperm is required to weaken the corona enough to let one lucky sperm finally penetrate the corona and fertilize the oocyte. This one sperm entering the egg is called *monospermy*. If fertilization does not occur within 24 hours after ovulation, the oocyte will disintegrate.

The oocyte is not completely mature at ovulation. It will only fully mature when fertilization occurs. Upon penetration of the oocyte membrane by the sperm, the final steps of oocyte maturation (also called "oocyte activation") will occur. The egg will completely engulf the sperm. The genetic material in the female egg will organize and form the *female pronucleus*. The genetic material in the sperm will organize and form the *male pronucleus*. In *amphimixis*, the male and female pronucleus fuse- forming a zygote. The zygote immediately prepares to begin dividing (called cleavage) into two daughter cells. The division continues, forming a blastocyst by day 4-5.

Implantation and Placentation:

Implantation in the uterine wall begins 6-7 days after ovulation. The outer portion of the blastocyst is called a *trophoblast*. The trophoblast begins to secrete the enzyme hyaluronidase, which begins to erode the endometrium (the inner lining of the mother's uterus). The blastocyst is able to begin to burrow into the endometrium. By day 12 after ovulation, the blastocyst is completely inside the endometrium. The trophoblast will continue to expand in the endometrium. As it dissolves the endometrium, it releases nutrients stored in the endometrium for use by the blastocyst. Eventually, the trophoblast will encounter blood vessels in the endometrium, and siphon nutrients out of the capillaries to nourish itself as well. These nutrients will keep the blastocyst and embryo alive until the placenta is formed.

Placenta formation (called **placentation**) takes place in weeks 3-10. A fluid filled sac will form around the embryo called the *amniotic sac*. Gradually the embryo and fetus will move away from the uterine wall (weeks 5-10) in the amniotic sac. The fetus will be connected to the placenta by the *umbilical cord*. The placenta will take over the delivery of nutrients to the fetus and the removal of wastes from the fetus. The placenta receives blood from the umbilical arteries, and returns blood to the umbilical veins. The *chorionic villi* in the placenta allow for the exchange of wastes and nutrients between mother and baby. Mother's blood and fetal blood never directly touch one another. Nutrients and wastes are able to diffuse through the chorionic villi, while blood cells cannot. The placenta is fully formed and functional by the end of the third month.

In addition to supplying the embryo and fetus with nutrients, oxygen, and removing wastes- the placenta also produces a large amount of hormones: *Human chorionic gonadotropin (hCG)* prompts the corpus luteum to continue secretion of progesterone and estrogen. hCG levels rise until the end of the second month, and then decline as the placenta begins to secrete progesterone and estrogen. hCG is the hormone tested for in home pregnancy tests. *Placental prolactin* assists in stimulating the production of milk by mammary glands. *Relaxin* softens connective tissue to allow the pelvis and pelvic canal to widen during labor. *Placental progesterone* and *placental estrogen* are also produced. Large amounts of progesterone and estrogen are needed to sustain and maintain the fetus- much more than the ovaries can produce. So, the placenta makes large amounts of these hormones.

First Trimester:

The first trimester of pregnancy is the time from fertilization until the 12th developmental week. During this time, the embryo forms and the beginning structures of all major organ systems develop. Fertilization, implantation, and placentation all occur during the First Trimester. *Embryogenesis*, the development of the embryo, occurs during this time. Embryo development ends at the 8th week. Beginning in week 9, the embryo is now called the fetus. At this time, all organ systems are recognizable. During the first 12 weeks of development, *organogenesis* (development of organs) begins. The endoderm, ectoderm, and mesoderm (primitive tissues which form early in development) will mature and form our tissues and organs. Some things that begin to develop during the first trimester are:
- Neural tube, brain and spinal cord structure
- Eyes, ears, taste buds and olfactory epithelium
- Nail beds, sweat glands, hair follicles, epidermal layers
- Rudimentary muscular system
- Trachea, lungs, diaphragm
- Thymus, thyroid, pituitary, adrenal glands
- Tonsils, blood formation in bone marrow and spleen, lymphocyte migration to lymph organs
- Intestinal tract, liver, pancreas, gallbladder and pancreas formation
- Allantois (bladder predecessor) and embryonic kidneys
- Cartilage and basic skeletal formation
- Heartbeat, basic heart structures, major blood vessels, lymph nodes
- Gonad and external genitalia formation, oogonia formation in female

Second Trimester:

The second trimester is the fourth, fifth, and sixth month of development. The risk of miscarriage drops significantly now. All of the major organ systems have some form of development already accomplished. The fetus will grow to about one and a half pounds during this trimester. Some events during the second trimester include:
- Keratin and nail formation
- Facial bone structure, joint articulations
- Rapid expansion of cerebrum, CNS tract formation, myelination of spinal cord
- Nostrils open, alveoli form
- Eyes can blink, lips can do sucking motion, fetus will suck thumb
- Intestinal subdivisions
- Fetal movements can be felt by mother. Fetus was moving since late first trimester, but was not large enough to have movements sensed by mother.
- Gender can usually be detected by ultrasound

Third Trimester:

The third trimester is the seventh, eighth, and ninth months of development. Organ systems get ready to take over control of the needs of the fetus/infant. The fetus will gain about 5 and a half pounds on average- for a birth weight of around 7 pounds. Some events during the third trimester are:
- Eyes able to detect light
- Adrenal gland finishes development
- Hair formation
- Taste buds functional
- Testicular descent
- Nephron formation
- Lungs fully mature

Anatomical and Physiological Changes in a Pregnant Female:

Anatomically, many changes will occur in a pregnant female. Weight gain of ~13 kg (28lb), for a mother of normal weight prior to pregnancy is expected. Early in pregnancy, reproductive organs become engorged with blood. *Chadwick's sign* is when the vagina develops a purplish hue on gynecological examination. Breasts will enlarge and areolae darken. Pigmentation of facial skin many increase (*chloasma*). Her body may exhibit increased lumbar curvature (*hyperlordosis*) as the uterus grows and center of gravity shifts. This can lead to back pain, muscular soreness, and pubic pain. The hormone relaxin causes pelvic ligaments and the pubic symphysis to relax to ease birth passage. As relaxin levels increase towards the end of pregnancy, she may develop a "waddling" gait.

Physiologically, many organ systems in her body will alter their activity due to the stress of the pregnancy. In the digestive system, morning sickness (due to elevated levels of estrogen and progesterone) can occur usually in the first trimester. Heartburn and constipation are common, and hemorrhoids may develop. The maternal requirements for nutrients and vitamins increase by 10-30%. In the urinary system, urine production will increase due to increased metabolism and fetal wastes. The glomerular filtration rate (GFR) increases by 30%. Urination frequency increases as the fetus grows and reduces available bladder space. Stress incontinence may occur as the bladder is compressed. In the respiratory system, estrogens may cause nasal edema and congestion. Respiratory rate and tidal volume increases. Dyspnea (difficult breathing) may occur later in pregnancy, due to enlarging fetus interfering with diaphragm movement. For the cardiovascular system, the blood volume increases by 25-40%. Maternal blood pressure and pulse rate rise. Venous return from lower limbs may be impaired due to the growing fetus, resulting in varicose veins.

Parturition (Childbirth)-

Parturition is the term used to describe giving birth to the baby, "childbirth". This involves the labor events that expel the infant from the uterus. After labor is initiated, parturition is made up of three stages: Dilation, Expulsion, and the Placental stage. Oxytocin and prostaglandins are powerful uterine muscle stimulants, and help to initiate labor.

The **dilation stage** of parturition is the longest stage of labor: 6-12 hours or more. Initial weak contractions often begin this stage. They gradually become more vigorous and rapid. The cervix effaces and dilates fully to 10 cm. The amnion ruptures, releasing amniotic fluid. Engagement occurs, and the fetal head enters the mother's true pelvis.

Next, comes the **expulsion stage**. Here, strong contractions occur every 2-3 minutes, and are about 1 minute long. The urge to push increases (in absence of local anesthesia). Crowning occurs when the largest dimension of the head distends the vulva. The *vertex position* (head down) is the ideal position for vaginal delivery. *"Occiput facing anterior" (OA)* is the most common position of the infant during labor. Vertex, but *"occiput facing posterior" (OP)* increases chances for painful "back labor". The *breech position* is when the fetus is positioned in the uterus with the buttocks down. This presentation usually will be delivered via C-section. A *transverse lie position* is where the fetus is laying sideways. This will also usually be delivered via C- section. Delivery of the infant occurs finally at the end of the expulsion stage.

Lastly, is the **placental stage**. In this phase, strong contractions continue. These contractions cause detachment of the placenta and compression of uterine blood vessels. Delivery of the afterbirth (placenta and membranes) occurs approximately 30 minutes after birth. All placental fragments must be removed to prevent postpartum bleeding.

APGAR score and neonatal health care:

The neonatal period is the four-week period immediately after birth. Physical status of the newborn is assessed 1-5 minutes after birth using the **APGAR score**. The APGAR score is assessed by observing the following: ***heart rate, color, respiration, reflexes,*** and ***muscle tone***. For each of those criteria, 0-2 points are assessed for each category. A score of 8-10 is considered healthy. For the rest of the neonatal period, the newborn will be followed closely by their pediatrician. A hearing test will usually be conducted. Weekly checkups for the newborn will also be requested. Weight will be measured at every visit. It is normal for the weight of a neonate to drop initially after birth, but within two weeks after delivery, the weight should be back near the birth weight.

Multiple births

Multiple births include twins, triplets, quadruplets, etc. *Dizygotic "Fraternal" twins* result when two oocytes are ovulated by the ovary during one ovarian cycle and each oocyte is fertilized by a sperm. The twins will each have different genetic makeups. *Monozygotic "identical" twins* result when one egg is fertilized by one sperm, but the blastomeres separate into two embryos. These twins will have identical genetic makeups. Triplets, quadruplets, etc. can also arise in either one of the two methods of twin development listed above. Odds of naturally having multiples: Twins- 1:89 births; Triplets- 1:7921 births; Quadruplets- 1:704,969 births.

Physical Examination of the Genitourinary Systems (Urinary and Reproductive)

Inspection of the Female Genitourinary System

1. Inspect the area of the abdomen around the kidneys and bladder for lesions, discolorations, inflammation, swelling
2. Inspect for urinary incontinence as patient bears down
3. Inspect external genitalia, perineum, urethral and vaginal openings for: size, symmetry, caking or discharge, inflammation, irritation, swelling, or lesions
4. Utilizing speculum, inspect internal genitalia for: color, position of cervix and surface characteristics, discharge, and vaginal wall characteristics.
5. After inspection, collect Pap smear and other necessary specimens

Palpation of the Female Genitourinary System

1. Palpate kidney's bilaterally in abdomen
2. Palpate bladder in the lower abdomen
3. Palpate external genitalia structures for lumps, masses, tenderness, swelling or discharge
4. Palpate vaginal walls, cervix, uterus, and ovaries during bimanual examination for size, shape, location and tenderness

Percussion of the Kidney

1. With patient seated, percuss the kidney on the patient's back

Inspection of the Female Breast

1. Inspect breast (with woman seated with arms at side, and repeat with arms overhead) and compare them bilaterally for:
    *   Size and symmetry
    *   Contour
    *   Retractions or dimpling
    *   Skin color and texture
    *   Lesions
    *   Nipple size, shape, symmetry, inversion, eversion, retraction, discharge

Palpation of Female Breast

1. Systematically palpate all regions of breasts for lumps or nodules
2. Palpate for lymph nodes in axillae

Inspection of the Male Genitourinary System

1. Inspect the area of the abdomen around the kidneys and bladder for lesions, discolorations, inflammation, swelling
2. Inspect for urinary incontinence as patient bears down
3. Inspect male external genitalia (retracting foreskin, if present) for:
   - Penis color
   - Urethral opening
   - Presence of any discharge or lesions
   - Unusual thickening
   - Scrotum texture and asymmetry
   - Presence of inguinal hernia
4. Transilluminate any masses in the scrotum

Palpation of the Male Genitourinary System

1. Palpate kidney's bilaterally in abdomen
2. Palpate bladder in the lower abdomen
3. Palpate the external genitalia of the male, looking for any masses, nodules, swelling, tenderness, inflammation. Palpate the penis, testicles, epididymis, spermatic cords, and inguinal area
4. Palpate the prostate gland and assess for size, texture, tenderness, nodules, enlargement

Percussion of the Kidney

1. With patient seated, percuss the kidney on the patient's back

Inspection of the Male Breast

1. Inspect breast, areolae and nipples for:
   - Symmetry and surface characteristics
   - Enlargement
   - Nipple size, shape, symmetry, retraction, inversion, eversion, discharge

Palpation of Male Breast

1. Systematically palpate all regions of breasts for lumps or nodules
2. Palpate for lymph nodes in axillae

General Abnormal Findings of the Genitourinary System

Abnormal findings, if necessary, should be referred to patients PCP or the proper specialist: gynecologist, obstetrician, nephrologist, or urologist

Breast nodule- lump palpated in any region of breast, in either sex. Could be benign (fibrocystic or fibroadenoma), or malignant (breast cancer). May or may not be tender on palpation.

Dimpling- puckering or retraction of skin on the breast, suggests a malignancy

Peau d'orange- a late sign of breast cancer, thickening and pitting of breast skin (resembles an orange peel)

Nipple retraction- nipple inverting

Breast pain- most commonly is due to benign conditions like fibrocystic breast disease or mastitis

Polyuria- increased urination (more than 2500 ml of urine per day). One of the more common findings-usually results from Diabetes Mellitus, Diabetes Insipidus, or diuretic use.

Hematuria- blood in urine. Looks brown or bright red. Timing of the appearance of blood in the urine stream suggests the underlying problem: if blood is present at the beginning of urination this can indicate a urethral disorder; if it is present at the end of urinating or throughout urination it can indicate a bladder disorder.

Urinary frequency- increased frequency to urinate. This can be a result of decreased bladder capacity, pregnancy, uterine tumor, prostatic hypertrophy, or prostate cancer. It is also a very common symptom of a UTI.

Urinary hesitancy- difficulty with starting a stream of urine when attempting to urinate. In women, urinary hesitancy can occur with UTI, obstruction of lower urinary tract, neuromuscular disorders. In men, it could be the result of prostatic hypertrophy, prostate cancer, UTI, some medications.

Nocturia- excessive nighttime urination. Could be the result of kidney or urinary tract infections, overstimulation of nerve to bladder, or the use of diuretics

Urinary incontinence- unable to hold urine. Can be caused by stress incontinence, tumor of bladder or prostate, kidney stones, prostatic hypertrophy, neurologic disorders (Guillain Barre syndrome, multiple sclerosis, and spinal cord injury)

Dysuria- pain during urination- signals a lower UTI. If dysuria occurs just before urination it indicates a bladder infection. If it occurs at the start of urination it often indicates infection at bladder outlet. If the pain occurs at the end of urination it indicates bladder spasm and urethritis. If dysuria is present throughout the entire urination, it could indicate pyelonephrosis/pyelonephritis (especially if combined with flank pain, fever, chills, hematuria)

Dysmenorrhea- painful menses. Could be due to endometriosis, pelvic inflammatory disease, PMS

Amenorrhea- absence of menses

Vaginal discharge-
- Thick, white, lumpy and curd-like, with yeasty sweet odor= *Candidiasis*
- White or grayish discharge with a fishy odor (which can get worse after intercourse)= *Bacterial vaginosis*
- Yellow, odorless, or acrid= *Chlamydia*
- Yellow or cloudy foul smelling discharge= *Gonorrhea*

Penile discharge (urethritis)-
- White, yellow or green discharge= *Gonorrhea*
- Clear or cloudy discharge= *Chlamydia*

Genital lesions- visible on external genitalia (vaginal area, penile area). Could be indicative of:
- *Cancer-* painless, often ulcerative lesions
- *Genital warts-* painless, flesh colored, cauliflower like. Can be present for weeks, months, or longer. (Caused by human papilloma virus)
- *Genital herpes-* one or more painful, red, blistering lesions
- *Syphilis-* a painless, hard, round, firm nodule which eventually erodes to an ulcer

Chadwick's sign is a bluish discoloration of the cervix, vagina and vulva caused by venous congestion. It can be observed as early as 6-8 weeks after conception, and is often used as an early sign of pregnancy.

Goodell's sign- An indication of pregnancy in which the cervix and vagina soften.

Priapism- persistent painful erection, not caused by sexual excitation

Prostate enlargement: if prostate protrudes into rectal lumen on palpation, it is enlarged. Enlargement can be benign or cancerous and rated from Grade 1 (mildly enlarged) to Grade 4 (significantly enlarged)
- **Prostatic Hypertrophy-** enlargement of the prostate, which happens in nearly every elderly male. This enlargement will strangle the urethra, causing difficult urination. This impairment of urine flow can increase the risk of cystitis and kidney damage.
- **Prostate cancer-** Cancer of the prostate. Symptoms can mimic prostatic hypertrophy. It is the third most prevalent cancer in males. It is often a slow growing condition, which often times causes it to not be diagnosed. Can be deadly. Digital palpation of the prostate and PSA blood tests can be done for diagnosis.

Abdominal Pain: abdominal pain can indicate issues with the digestive, urinary and/or reproductive system.
- **Salpingitis-** is infection/inflammation of the uterine tubes. May have symptoms of lower quadrant pain- usually on left. Suprapubic tenderness may also be seen and pain on pelvic exam, with fever, nausea, and vomiting
- **Ectopic Pregnancy-** lower quadrant pain, referred to shoulder. With rupture of fallopian tubes- can be agonizing. May have symptoms of pregnancy, spotting, irregular menses, mass and tenderness on bimanual exam. Positive Kehr and Cullen signs. Blood lab tests may reveal lower than normal HCG levels.
- **Pelvic Inflammatory Disease-** lower quadrant pain, often increased with activity. Tender adenexa and cervix, discharge from vagina
- **Renal Calculi (Kidney Stone)-** intense flank pain, extending to groin and genitals. May be episodic. Fever, hematuria and positive Kehr's sign may be present

Advanced Imaging and Diagnostic Tests of the Genitourinary System

Amniocentesis- Analysis of amniotic fluid. The fluid is withdrawn by inserting a needle through the abdominal wall, and into the amniotic sac. Amnion is withdrawn and will be analyzed to determine abnormalities in the fetus.

Chorionic Villus Sampling- Removal of part of the chorionic villi of the placenta for examination. A catheter is inserted through the abdominal wall or through the cervix and a portion of the chorionic villi is removed. This procedure is done to detect some disorders of the fetus and is usually done between 10 and 12 weeks of pregnancy. Often the chorionic villus sampling can be done earlier in the pregnancy than amniocentesis.

Colposcopy- Direct examination of the cervix using a magnifying lens. Often done after an abnormal Pap smear result has been recorded.

Cone Biopsy- Removal of a cone shaped piece of tissue from the cervix. This is performed after abnormal Pap results, and is often done to assist in the detection of cervical cancer. (also can be called *Conization*)

Cystoscopy- insertion of a flexible viewing tube in the urethra and bladder. The tube often has a light to assist in viewing, and often also has a clipping device at the tip to remove bladder tissue for biopsy, if needed.

Cystography- A catheter is inserted into bladder which carries radioactive dye. X-rays are taken to assess for bladder tumors or reflux of urine from bladder into ureter.

Hysteroscopy- evaluation of the inside of the uterus with a fiber-optic tube

Intravenous pyelogram (urography)- Radioactive dye is injected into the bloodstream and is observed as it moves through the kidney and the urinary tract.

Mammography- The breast tissue is flattened between x-ray plates and x-rays are taken. All women over the age of 40 are recommended to have one done annually. (Please note, the age guidelines for mammography screenings may be changing). Women who have a family history of breast cancer may be asked to have mammograms performed earlier

Papanicolaou test (Pap test/ Pap smear)- After inserting a speculum, the doctor will scrape cells off of the outer surface of the cervix and the inner surface of the cervix. The cells are placed on a slide and then observed under a microscope.

Retrograde urography- A catheter is inserted through the urethra, into bladder and finally into the ureter. Radioopaque dye is injected, and an x-ray study of the bladder and ureters can be done.

Transvaginal Ultrasound- A small ultrasound transducer (probe) is inserted into the vagina. Is often done during the first few weeks of pregnancy (to determine presence of viable embryo or gestational sac). Can also be used to examine the ovaries.

Transrectal Ultrasound- A small ultrasound transducer (probe) is inserted into the rectum. Can be done in males to view the prostate.

Abdominal or pelvic ultrasound- Transducer wand is placed on the surface of the abdomen or pelvic cavity. Uses sound waves (ultrasound) to detect structural or functional abnormalities. This procedure can be done on many organs of the body including kidney, bladder, ovary, uterus, prostate and testes.

Urinalysis and **Blood Lab Panels** can also be done to assess health of the urinary and reproductive systems.

Pathologies of the Reproductive System

For additional infectious diseases that may affect this system, please refer to the Communicable/Infectious Disease Chart in Chapter 10.

Breast Cancer- One of the leading causes of death in American women (one in eight women will develop this pathology). Each year over 43,000 women will die from this disease. *Red Flag symptoms: Breast cancer is often detected by a change in skin texture, a palpable lump, puckering or leakage from the nipple.* Early detection by self-examination or mammography are the best ways to increase the chances of survival. Most common in females, but males CAN develop this pathology.

Cervical cancer- second most common cancer in women. Mostly caused by the *Human Papillomavirus (HPV),* which can be transmitted during sexual intercourse. There is a vaccine available now for this virus. PAP smear is commonly used to diagnose this condition. *Red Flag symptoms- there may not be any, but in later stages there may be bleeding after intercourse.*

Ectopic Pregnancy- This occurs when the fertilized egg does not implant in the uterus, instead, it implants in the uterine tube, ovary or in the abdominal/pelvic cavity and starts developing there. These pregnancies will not be able to survive to full term and substantial bleeding may be seen. *Red Flag symptoms include pain, cramping, and a bloody discharge in the first trimester of pregnancy. Pain may be in the lower abdominal area and refer into the shoulder.* Blood tests will show low HCG levels. Untreated, this could be fatal for the mother. Treatment could include surgery to remove the affected uterine tube or treatment with a chemotherapy drug called Methotrexate.

Endometrial/Uterine Cancer- Cancer of the uterus. Seen most often in postmenopausal women; high risk of spreading to other areas of the body. Risk factors increase with estrogen replacement therapy. Pap smears may be used for diagnosis, but they are not as effective as they are for cervical cancer. Endometrial biopsy is a better test. *Red Flag symptoms: abnormal bleeding may be seen, especially in postmenopausal women.*

Endometriosis- An inflammatory condition in which endometrial tissue grows outside of the uterus- often in the pelvic cavity. Characterized by abnormal uterine or rectal bleeding, dysmenorrhea and pelvic pain. May cause infertility. Diagnosis is done by endoscopy and biopsy.

Erectile Dysfunction (ED)- the inability to have or maintain an erection during intercourse. This could be an indication of an underlying health problem, such as hypertension, uncontrolled diabetes, atherosclerosis, heart disease, high cholesterol, Parkinson's, Multiple Sclerosis, depression, anxiety or a side effect of some medications.

Fibroadenoma- The most common benign (non-cancerous) tumors found in the breast. Usually appearing in young women and may be mistaken for cancer. Can be felt during palpation of breast tissue and seen on examination tests. Biopsies will be done to rule out cancer. These may be surgically removed.

Fibrocystic breast disease- formation of fluid filled cysts in the breast tissue. This is the most common disorder of the breast. Hormonal imbalances may be the cause. These may be removed surgically.

Gynecomastia- enlargement of breast tissue in males.

Hemolytic Disease of the Newborn (HDN) – aka **Erythroblastosis fetalis.** A disease process found in developing fetuses. It is found when a mother has a Rh- blood type and the fetus has a Rh+ blood type. Rh antibodies from the mom can pass through the placenta, and attack the fetuses RBC's- destroying them. Without treatment, the fetus will usually die in-utero or soon thereafter. Treatment- giving mother anti-Rh antibodies (called RhoGam), during the last 3 months of pregnancy and after delivery (for breast milk safety)

Hyperemesis gravidarum- Malignant nausea and excessive vomiting (beyond "normal" morning sickness), to the extent that the pregnant woman becomes dehydrated and her tissues and blood become acidic.

Mastitis- Infection of the breast tissue. Often seen in the first few weeks of breast-feeding. The nipples can become cracked and raw, allowing easy infection by the *Staphylococcus aureus* bacteria.

Menopause- not technically a "pathology". Seen in women as their estrogen levels naturally decline with age. Eventually, ovulation becomes irregular, menses become shorter in length, and will ultimately cease altogether. Menopause is officially diagnosed after a whole year has passed without menstruation.

Ovarian Cancer- Risk factor increases with age (most often 50-70). Irregular menstrual cycles, early menses, pain in abdomen, late menopause, and endometriosis may increase risk factors. Ultrasound or CT scan may be used to diagnose. Laparoscopy may be done to assess or perform a biopsy to rule out ovarian cysts (non-cancerous growths). *Red Flag symptoms: often there are none early on, but if there are symptoms they may include feeling bloated, frequent urination, appetite changes, pain in lower abdominal/pelvic region.*

Pelvic Inflammatory Disease- Because the uterine tubes do not attach onto the ovaries in a female, some sexually transmitted diseases (such as gonorrhea, chlamydia, and syphilis) can infect the peritoneal/abdominal cavity. These STD's are transmitted into the vagina, climb through the uterus, uterine tubes, and out into the peritoneal cavity. This infection can cause scarring and closure of the uterine tubes and is a leading cause of infertility.

Polycystic Ovary Syndrome (PCOS) – is a hormonal disorder in women where many cysts appear on the ovary. Often due to hormonal imbalances. Several symptoms may be seen: excessive hair growth (including on the face), acne, obesity, irregular menses, amenorrhea, infertility.

Prostatitis- swelling or inflammation of the prostate. Symptoms can include urination problems (pain, burning, difficulty urinating, nighttime urination, urgent need to urinate), painful ejaculation, or pain in groin or lower back. If it is caused by a bacterial infection, it can be treated with antibiotics.

Prostate cancer- Cancer of the prostate. Symptoms can mimic prostatic hypertrophy. It is the third most prevalent cancer in males. It is often a slow growing condition, which often times causes it to not be diagnosed. It can be deadly. *Red Flag symptoms: Urination troubles (difficulty urinating, weak flow of urine, blood in urine, nighttime urination), pain in abdomen or back, and erectile dysfunction.* Digital palpation of the prostate and PSA blood tests can be done for diagnosis.

Prostatic Hypertrophy (also known as ***Benign Prostatic Hypertrophy/Hyperplasia- BPH***) - enlargement of the prostate, which happens in nearly every elderly male. This enlargement will strangle the urethra, causing difficult urination. This can increase the risk of cystitis and kidney damage.

Testicular cancer- the most common cancer in men ages 18-34. Highly curable if caught and treated early. Leading risk factor is an undescended testicle, and family history increases risk. Self-examination of the testicles can often be the first detection of the tumor. The tumor on palpation is often painless; the area may eventually ache or have a sense of heaviness as the tumor grows. Diagnosis is often done by ultrasound, and blood tests looking for cancer markers.

Toxemia- also known as "***pre-eclampsia***". A pathological process in a pregnant mother. *Red Flag symptoms: hypertension, proteinuria, and excessive edema.* Without treatment and bed rest, pre-eclampsia can progress to eclampsia. If this occurs the mother could exhibit epilepsy, cerebral hemorrhage, liver failure or coma.

Uterine Fibroids- (also called *leiomyoma*, or *myoma*) - these are masses in the muscular tissue of the uterus. There may be a single fibroid growing, or multiple- and the size of fibroids can vary greatly. Women are most at risk if they are overweight, have a family history (especially mother) of fibroids, eat a lot of red meat, are African American and are in the age range of 30-menopause. Most uterine fibroids do not have any symptoms. If they grow large, they may enlarge the abdomen, cause heavy menstrual bleeding, cause pain during intercourse, and give the sensation of fullness in the pelvic area.

Practice Study and Test Questions:

1) Fertilization usually occurs in the:
    A) uterus
    B) vagina
    C) ovary
    D) uterine (fallopian) tubes

2) Peau d'orange and nipple retraction may be observed in the physical examination of a patient with
    A) mastitis
    B) prostatic hypertrophy
    C) breast cancer
    D) uterine cancer

3) Early symptoms of ovarian cancer are
    A) abnormal menstrual bleeding
    B) fever
    C) pain that radiates into the lumbar region
    D) often there are none

4) The inner mucosal layer of the uterus that is sloughed off approximately every 28 days is called the:
    A) endometrium
    B) myometrium
    C) epimetrium
    D) perimetrium

5) Surgery to remove a fallopian tube or methotrexate medication may be used to treat
    A) ectopic pregnancy
    B) fibroadenoma
    C) toxemia
    D) pelvic inflammatory disease

6) Risk factors for uterine fibroids are
    A) being African American
    B) being overweight
    C) family history of fibroids
    D) all of the above

7) Common diagnostic tests for prostate cancer are
    A) digital rectal examination
    B) PSA blood test
    C) cystography
    D) both A and B

8) Hypertension, proteinuria, and excessive edema may be signs of
    A) polycystic ovary syndrome
    B) uterine fibroids
    C) toxemia
    D) ectopic pregnancy

9) Each spermatid and ovum have:
    A) 46 pair of chromosomes
    B) 23 chromosomes
    C) 23 pair of chromosomes
    D) 46 chromosomes

10) An underlying health problem that may cause erectile dysfunction is
    A) hypertension
    B) celiac disease
    C) impetigo

11) The most common benign growth/tumor in breast tissue is called
    A) fibroadenoma
    B) fibrocystic breast disease
    C) endometriosis
    D) gynecomastia

12) Which test may be done to diagnose cervical cancer?
    A) cone biopsy
    B) conization
    C) papanicolaou test
    D) all of the above

13) The actual "sperm-forming factories" of the male reproductive system that empty sperm into the epididymis are called the:
    A) interstitial cells
    B) seminiferous tubules
    C) ductus deferens
    D) bulbourethral glands

14) An APGAR score of _____ is considered a healthy score
    A) 100
    B) 50-60
    C) 8-10
    D) 5

15) The path the sperm travels in the male duct system (from inside to outside) is:
    A) ejaculatory duct, ductus deferens, epididymis, urethra
    B) epididymis, ductus deferens, urethra, ejaculatory duct
    C) epididymis, ductus deferens, ejaculatory duct, urethra
    D) ductus deferens, epididymis, ejaculatory duct, urethra

16) The normal period of human gestation is calculated as _____ from the last menstrual period.
    A) exactly 9 lunar months
    B) 9 calendar months
    C) 280 days
    D) 265 days

Answers: 1) D 2) C 3) D 4) A 5) A 6) D 7) D 8) C 9) B 10) A 11) A 12) D 13) B 14) C 15) C 16) C

CHAPTER 15: LABORATORY TESTS AND SCREENING EXAMINATION GUIDELINES

The following laboratory tests are tests performed on blood, urine, or fecal materials of a patient. These tests are often done to help diagnose diseases and determine appropriate treatment.

Also included in this chapter are the screening examinations which are recommended for men and women.

There are some suffixes (word endings), word roots and prefixes (found at the beginning of the word) that are commonly used in the laboratory setting. Here is a partial list of some commonly used terms that you will find in the laboratory test results listed in this chapter.

Root, Prefix or Suffix	Meaning
Hemo-	Blood, usually red blood cells (RBC)
Hemato-	Blood, usually RBC
Leuko-	White blood cells
Hyper-	Increased levels
Hypo-	Decreased levels
-penia	Decreased levels
-philia	Increased levels
-cytosis	Abnormal levels (often increased)
-emia	Abnormal level in the blood
-uria	Related to urine

See the Medical Terminology chapter in this book for more roots, prefixes and suffixes.

For these lab tests, the patient will submit their specimen (blood, urine, feces) in the physician's office or at the hospital. Blood is usually collected via venipuncture. (**Venipuncture**- the process of withdrawing blood from the body by inserting a needle into a vein.) Urine and stool samples are usually collected by the patient in a provided sterile vessel. This collection can be done at the physician's office or hospital (usually) or at the patient's home. The physician then sends the specimen to a lab for processing.

****<u>Please Note</u>: for the test panels listed below, every laboratory that processes the sample (blood, urine, feces) has their own set of tests that they perform for the panel. Often, the different labs will process the specimen in the same way, BUT sometimes they choose to perform different tests on the specimen. So, there may be some differences in which tests are performed, depending on the lab used. For example, in the CBC (Complete Blood Count) - some labs do not perform the Reticulocyte Count in their CBC, but other labs will. This is usually why a physician has a certain lab that they like to work with- they will choose to send their specimens to a lab that performs the tests they like to see.**

On the following page is a sample blood lab result for a patient. (Patient's name has been removed). Note that the lab will send the standard reference range (normal range) for the items they test for. Each lab may have slightly different "normal" ranges for things (depending on their testing and processing techniques) - so, the physician must pay attention to the reference range provided by the laboratory in determining if the patient's values are normal or abnormal.

GENERAL HEALTH PANEL (CBC/Diff, CMP)   Patient: XXXXXXXXXXXXXXXXXXXX

Component	Your Value	Standard Range	Units
WBC	6.8	4.0 - 10.5	th/mm3
RBC	4.82	3.77 - 5.28	mil/mm3
HGB	13.5	11.1 - 15.9	g/dL
HCT	41.9	34.0 - 46.6	%
MCV	87	79 - 97	fL
MCH	28.0	26.6 - 33.0	pg
MCHC	32.2	31.5 - 35.7	g/dL
RDW	12.8	12.3 - 15.4	%
PLATELET CT	239	140 - 415	bil/L
POLYS-AUTO,%	54	40 - 75	%
LYMPHS,%	34	20 - 45	%
MONOS,%	5	0 - 14	%
EOSINOPHIL %	6	0 - 4	%
BASOPHILS,%	1	0 - 2	%
POTASSIUM	4.1	3.5 - 5.2	mEq/L
TOTAL CO2	25	19 - 28	mmol/L
New reference range effective 6/17/2013.			
CREATININE	0.77	0.57 - 1.00	mg/dL
CALCIUM	9.0	8.7 - 10.2	mg/dL
UREA NITROGEN	13	6 - 20	mg/dL
PROTEIN,TOTAL	7.3	6.0 - 8.5	g/dL
ALBUMIN, S	4.7	3.5 - 5.5	g/dL
BILIRUBIN,TOTAL	1.8	0.1 - 1.2	mg/dL
SODIUM	140	134 - 144	mEq/L
CHLORIDE	104	97 - 108	mEq/L
GLUCOSE	82	65 - 99	mg/dL
Normal printed is for fasting. No normals for random.			
ALT (GPT)	13	<33	U/L
AST(GOT)	19	0 - 50	U/L
ALK PTASE	40	25 - 150	U/L

The Complete Blood Count (CBC)

This is a commonly ordered laboratory test that examines the living components of the blood. The CBC is composed of the *White Blood Cell Count, White Blood Cell Differential, Red Blood Cell Count, Hematocrit, Hemoglobin, Mean Corpuscular Volume* and *Platelet Count*. For all of these criteria, normal amounts that should be found in the blood have been determined by the laboratory. Excessive (high) amounts or decreased (low) amounts could indicate pathology or abnormal functioning.

Test Name	Test use	Increased levels ↑	Decreased levels ↓
White Blood Cell Count (WBC count)	Counts the number of circulating White Blood Cells. Can be ordered if the physician is concerned with possible infection, inflammation, blood diseases.	**Leukocytosis-** ↑WBC count. Can be a sign of infection. WBC is also increased in certain types of leukemia	**Leukopenia-** ↓ WBC count. Can be a sign of bone marrow diseases, enlarged spleen, or sometimes seen in HIV infection.
WBC Differential (WBC Diff)	Counts the individual types of white blood cells: *(neutrophils, lymphocytes, monocytes, eosinophils, basophils)*. Each type of WBC responds to a different type of crisis in the body. For example, neutrophils respond to acute bacterial infections, monocytes respond to chronic/severe infections, eosinophils often respond in allergy situations. When crisis occurs in the body, the amount of the white blood cell that is best equipped to combat the situation will increase above the normal levels, and is assessed in this test.	**Neutrophilia-** ↑neutrophil count. Due to acute infections (especially bacterial), inflammation, smoking

Lymphocytosis- ↑ lymphocytes. Acute viral infection and some bacterial infections, lymphocytic leukemia

Monocytosis- ↑ monocytes. Chronic infections, some forms of leukemia

Eosinophilia- ↑ eosinophils. Seen in allergies, asthma, drug reactions, parasitic infections

Basophilia- ↑ basophils. Inflammation, hives, food allergies. | **Neutropenia-** ↓neutrophils. Due to bone marrow damage, nutritional deficiencies (B12, folate), autoimmune disorders, immunodeficiency diseases

Lymphopenia/ Lymphocytopenia- ↓ lymphocytes. Autoimmune disorders, immunodeficiency diseases, bone marrow damage

Monocytopenia- ↓ monocytes. Bone marrow damage.

Eosinopenia- ↓ eosinophils. Not usually indicative of a medical pathology.

Basopenia- ↓ basophils. Not usually indicative of a medical pathology. |
| **Red Blood Cell Count (RBC Count)** | Counts the total number of RBC's circulating. Performed if a physician is concerned about oxygenation of tissues or blood circulation. | **Polycythemia** or **Erythrocytosis-** ↑ RBC. Can be caused by lung diseases, polycythemia vera, kidney tumors, smoking | **Low red blood cell count** (sometimes called **anemia**)- can be caused by trauma, chronic bleeding, nutritional deficiency (B12, folate), bone marrow damage |
| **Hemoglobin (Hb or HGB)** | Measures the amount of Hemoglobin in the blood. Performed if a physician is concerned with anemia or polycythemia | **High Hemoglobin (Hb)-** can be due to polycythemia vera, lung disease, smoking, living at high altitudes, kidney tumor (producing too much EPO) | **Low Hemoglobin (Hb)-** due to thalassemia, excessive destruction of RBC's, acute or chronic bleeding, nutritional deficiency (iron, B12, folate), bone marrow damage |

Complete Blood Count (CBC) - continued

Test Name	Test use	Increased levels ↑	Decreased levels ↓
Hematocrit (HCT)	Tests the number of RBC's circulating and the volume of RBC's in the blood	**High Hematocrit (HCT)-** due to dehydration (most common), polycythemia vera, lung diseases, smoking	**Low Hematocrit (HCT)-** due to excessive destruction of RBC's or blood loss, thalassemia, nutritional deficiencies (iron, B12, folate)
RBC Indices: MCV, MCH, MCHC, RDW	**Mean corpuscular volume (MCV)** measures the average size of RBC's. **Mean corpuscular hemoglobin (MCH)** measures the amount of hemoglobin in an average red blood cell. **Mean corpuscular hemoglobin concentration (MCHC)** measures the concentration of hemoglobin in a red blood cell. These tests are all used in assisting the physician in diagnosing some different kinds of anemia. **Red Blood Cell Distribution Width (RDW)** measures size variations in red blood cells	**Macrocytic** RBC's- ↑MCV, RDW and MCH. Could indicate pernicious anemia (lack of B12), lack of folate **Hyperchromic** RBC's- ↑MCHC. Could indicate sickle cell anemia.	**Microcytic** RBC's- ↓ MCV and RDW. Could indicate iron deficiency anemia, thalassemia **Hypochromic** RBC's- ↓ MCH and MCHC. Could indicate iron deficiency anemia
Platelet Count	Counts the number of circulating platelets in the blood. Performed if a physician is concerned with clotting of the blood.	**Thrombocythemia and Thrombocytosis-** ↑ platelet count. Can occur with bleeding, cigarette smoking or excess production by the bone marrow.	**Thrombocytopenia-** ↓ platelet count. Due to Immune Thrombocytopenia (ITP), acute blood loss, drug effects (such as heparin) infections with sepsis, bone marrow failure
Reticulocyte count (*some labs do not include this test in their CBC)	Counts the number of immature Red Blood Cells (Reticulocytes) circulating. (often ordered if a patient has had a bone marrow transplant to see how transplant is functioning)	**High Reticulocyte Count-** can indicate bleeding, hemolytic anemia, Hemolytic Disease of the Newborn,	**Low Reticulocyte Count-** bone marrow transplant failure, iron deficiency anemia

Basic Metabolic Panel/Profile (BMP)

The Basic Metabolic Panel/Profile is a commonly ordered test. It gives information on: *glucose, calcium, sodium, potassium, carbon dioxide, chloride* and *kidney panel (functioning)*. This test can also be called the **CHEM 7 test** (not including calcium) or the **CHEM 8 test** (including calcium).

Test Name	Test use	Increased levels ↑	Decreased levels ↓
Glucose	Monitors glucose ("blood sugar"). Can be done either as a fasting test, post-prandial (anytime), or after consuming a prescribed glucose drink (OGTT- oral glucose tolerance test). Used to diagnose and monitor diabetes mellitus.	**Hyperglycemia-** ↑glucose levels. Can indicate diabetes, or poorly controlled diabetes, hyperthyroidism, pancreatitis, or pancreatic tumor.	**Hypoglycemia-** ↓ glucose levels. Can indicate too much insulin medication administered, not eating enough food, hypothyroidism, pituitary tumor.
Calcium (Ca^{+2})	Monitors calcium levels circulating in the blood (only 1% of the calcium in our body is found in the blood)	**Hypercalcemia-** ↑calcium levels. Can be caused by hyperparathyroidism, cancer in the bones, hyperthyroidism, side effects of medications (ex: thiazide diuretics)	**Hypocalcemia-** ↓ calcium levels. Can be a result of dietary deficiency (of calcium, Vitamin D, and/or magnesium), hypoparathyroidism, renal failure
Sodium (Na$^+$)	The main extracellular cation. Will be of particular interest in a patient with high blood pressure, dehydration or edema.	**Hypernatremia-** ↑sodium levels. Due to dehydration, Cushing's disease, Diabetes Insipidus, some medications, steroid usage.	**Hyponatremia-** ↓ sodium levels. Addison's disease, diarrhea, diuretic medications, *excessive* water consumption, kidney disease can all be causes.
Potassium (K$^+$)	The main cation in intracellular fluid. Often tested in patients with muscle weakness, cardiac arrhythmias.	**Hyperkalemia-** ↑potassium levels. Due to kidney disease/renal failure, some medications (NSAIDS, beta blockers, ACE inhibitors), dehydration, excessive potassium intake in foods.	**Hypokalemia-** ↓ potassium levels. Can be caused by excessive diarrhea and vomiting, hyperaldosteronism, some medications (corticosteroids, acetaminophen overdose)
Carbon Dioxide (CO$_2$)- Bicarbonate	Bicarbonate (HCO$_3^-$) is a common form of transporting carbon dioxide in the bloodstream. It can be used in regulating the acid/base (pH) balance in the blood.	**High Bicarbonate levels-** due to severe vomiting, COPD, and metabolic alkalosis.	**Low Bicarbonate levels-** due to chronic diarrhea, diabetic ketoacidosis, metabolic acidosis, kidney disease, aspirin overdose
Chloride (Cl$^-$)	Chloride is the most common negatively charged electrolyte in the extracellular fluid. It works closely with sodium in the body. It is used to maintain fluid balance in the body and maintain acid/base (pH) balance	**Hyperchloremia-** ↑chloride. Can be due to dehydration or starvation, Cushing's disease, metabolic acidosis, hyperventilation, increased sodium intake	**Hypochloremia-** ↓chloride. Due to prolonged vomiting, congestive heart failure, COPD, metabolic alkalosis, excessive antacid use.
Kidney Panel	Kidney Panel tests for ✓ **Blood Urea Nitrogen (BUN)** ✓ **Creatinine**	See Kidney Panel Chart	See Kidney Panel Chart

Comprehensive Metabolic Panel/Profile (CMP)

The Comprehensive Metabolic Panel/Profile (CMP) is the **Basic Metabolic Panel** plus **albumin, total protein**, and the **liver panel**.

Test Name	Test use	Increased levels ↑	Decreased levels ↓
Albumin	Albumin is a protein in the blood. Abnormal levels could indicate a liver problem, kidney problem or protein malabsorption issue.	**Increased blood albumin-** can be due to a high protein diet or dehydration.	**Decreased blood albumin-** can be due to kidney disease, hepatitis, cirrhosis, Crohn's disease, celiac disease, malnutrition
Total Protein	This test measures the levels of albumin and globulin proteins in the blood. Globulins are important proteins used in the immune system (antibodies, for example). Albumin helps to regulate fluid levels in the blood.	**Increased Total Protein levels-** due to chronic inflammation or infection (such as HIV, Hepatitis C), multiple myeloma (a bone marrow disorder)	**Decreased Total Protein levels-** can be a result of kidney disease, hepatitis, cirrhosis, Crohn's disease, celiac disease, malnutrition
Basic Metabolic Panel/Profile (BMP)	The Basic Metabolic Panel/Profile tests for: ✓ **Glucose** ✓ **Calcium** ✓ **Sodium** ✓ **Potassium** ✓ CO_2/HCO_3^- ✓ **Chloride** ✓ **Kidney Panel: Blood Urea Nitrogen (BUN)** and **Creatinine**	See Basic Metabolic Panel Chart	See Basic Metabolic Panel Chart
Liver Panel	The Liver Panel tests for: ✓ **ALP (Alkaline Phosphatase)** ✓ **ALT (Alanine aminotransferase)** ✓ **AST (Aspartate aminotransferase)** ✓ **Bilirubin**	See Liver Panel Chart	See Liver Panel Chart

Kidney Panel

This panel tests for proper functioning of the kidney. It can be ordered as a stand-alone panel, but most commonly is ordered as a part of the Basic Metabolic Panel (BMP) or Comprehensive Metabolic Panel (CMP) as a screening test to evaluate kidney health. The kidney panel is composed of *Blood Urea Nitrogen (BUN)* and *Creatinine*.

Test Name	Test use	Increased levels ↑	Decreased levels ↓
Blood Urea Nitrogen (BUN)	Often performed on a patient undergoing dialysis or suspected kidney disease. Or as a part of BMP or CMP (as a screening for kidney health)	↑ **BUN**- caused by kidney damage or failure, poor blood circulation to the kidney, dehydration, excessive protein in diet, medication side effect.	↓ **BUN**- caused by liver disease, malnutrition or very low protein diet, overhydration
Creatinine	Often performed on a patient undergoing dialysis or suspected kidney disease. Or as a part of BMP or CMP (as a screening for kidney health)	↑ **Creatinine**- can be due to glomerulonephritis, pyelonephritis, kidney damage or failure, urinary tract obstruction, poor blood supply to kidney.	↓ **Creatinine**- can be seen during pregnancy, but generally not a problem.

Liver (Hepatic) Panel

This panel tests for proper functioning of the liver. It can be ordered as a stand-alone panel, but most commonly is ordered as a part of Comprehensive Metabolic Panel (CMP) as a screening test to evaluate liver health. The liver panel is composed of *ALP, ALT, AST* and *Bilirubin*.

Test Name	Test use	Increased levels ↑	Decreased levels ↓
Alkaline Phosphatase (ALP)	To screen for a liver disease or monitor liver health when using certain medications. Can also be elevated in certain bone diseases	↑ ALP present with hepatitis, bile duct blockage, Paget's disease, bone cancer, liver cancer	↓ ALP may be due to malnutrition, diseases that affect nutrient absorption (celiac, Crohn's), protein deficiency
Alanine aminotransferase (ALT)	Usually used to screen for injury or damage to the liver. ALT and AST are the most important tests for liver damage.	↑ ALT (very high levels) indicate acute hepatitis. Moderate increases of ALT can indicate chronic hepatitis, bile duct blockage, or cirrhosis	↓ ALT does not usually indicate a health issue
Aspartate aminotransferase (AST)	Usually used to screen for injury or damage to the liver. Can also indicate cardiac muscle or muscle damage	↑ AST (very high levels) indicate acute hepatitis. Moderate increases of AST can indicate chronic hepatitis, bile duct blockage, or cirrhosis. Can also be increased after a heart attack	↓ AST does not usually indicate a health issue
Bilirubin	Usually used to screen for injury or damage to the liver. Can also indicate hemolytic anemia	↑ Bilirubin- patient may appear *jaundiced*. Indicates hepatitis, liver disease, bile duct blockage, hemolytic or pernicious anemia	↓ Bilirubin does not usually indicate a health issue

Cardiac Panel

This panel looks for markers in the blood that indicate that the cardiac tissue has been damaged or is under stress. For example: heart attack (myocardial infarction), angina, heart failure. Laboratories vary as far as what blood tests they include in their cardiac panel. Here are some of the main tests ordered to assess cardiac health: ***total Creatine Kinase, Creatine Kinase MB, Troponin, myoglobin,*** and (sometimes) ***C-reactive protein or high sensitivity C-reactive protein.***

Test Name	Test use	Increased levels ↑	Decreased levels ↓
Total Creatine Kinase (CK)	Used to detect cardiac muscle damage, and can also be used in skeletal muscle damage	↑ CK- seen in heart attack (peaks within 12-24 hours after heart attack and then declines), rhabdomyolysis	↓ CK can be seen in early pregnancy, alcoholic liver disease and rheumatoid arthritis.
Creatine Kinase MB (CK-MB)	Used to distinguish between cardiac muscle and skeletal muscle damage. CK-MB will be released into the blood during cardiac muscle damage	↑ CK-MB is seen in a heart attack or kidney failure (usually within 3-8 hours after onset of chest pain)	↓ CK-MB can be seen in alcoholic liver disease and rheumatoid arthritis.
Troponin	Used to detect cardiac muscle damage.	↑ Troponin is seen during a heart attack or other form of cardiac muscle damage (only 3-4 hours after chest pain onset).	↓ Troponin not usually indicative of a problem
Myoglobin	Used to detect cardiac muscle damage, and can also be used in skeletal muscle damage. Troponin is a more specific test for cardiac damage, but myoglobin appears quicker/earlier during testing for a patient with chest pain	↑ Myoglobin is seen during heart attack or other form of cardiac muscle damage (only 2-3 hours after chest pain onset).	↓ Myoglobin can indicate rheumatoid arthritis, myasthenia gravis
C-Reactive Protein (CRP) and the **high sensitivity CRP (hs-CRP)** (* some labs may not include this test in the cardiac panel)	A non-specific test- meaning it can be used in a variety of clinical situations. It tests for inflammation (which could be due to tissue trauma, injury, infection), but does not indicate specific location of the pathology. Often used with other tests to confirm injury or infection. A more specific type of CRP test called the **high sensitivity CRP (hs-CRP)** test can be ordered to determine risk of heart disease.	↑ CRP indicates cardiac damage, bacterial infections, lupus, rheumatoid arthritis. ↑ hs-CRP indicates increased risk of heart disease.	↓ CRP does not usually indicate problem. It is normally very low. ↓ hs-CRP does not usually indicate problem. It is normally very low.

Thyroid Panel

This panel tests the functioning of the thyroid gland. The thyroid gland produces hormones that are essential in regulating body metabolism. Lab tests included in the thyroid panel include: **TSH, T4 or Free T4,** and **T3 or Free T3.**

Test Name	Test use	Increased levels ↑	Decreased levels ↓
TSH- (Thyroid Stimulating Hormone/Thyrotropin)	TSH is the hormone released by the anterior pituitary. It travels to the thyroid and stimulates the thyroid to produce T3 and T4. If the thyroid is not producing enough T3 and T4 (hypothyroidism), the anterior pituitary will release higher and higher levels of TSH to try to stimulate the thyroid to increase its production.	↑ TSH- can indicate hypothyroidism	↓ TSH- can indicate hyperthyroidism
T4 or Free T4 (Thyroxine)	**T4** test is an older test; **Free T4** tends to give more specific results and is being more commonly ordered.	↑ T4 can indicate hyperthyroidism	↓ T4- can indicate hypothyroidism
T3 or Free T3 (Triiodothyronine)	This test can be very helpful in diagnosing a specific type of hyperthyroidism called Graves' Disease	↑ T3 can indicate hyperthyroidism	↓ T3 can indicate hypothyroidism

Lipid Profile

Tests the levels of lipid substances in the blood. Higher than normal levels can indicate cardiovascular risk. The lipid profile tests include: Total Cholesterol, HDL, LDL, Triglycerides. These tests are usually performed after a 9-12 hour fast (although some recent studies are indicating the fasting may not be necessary).

Test Name	Test use	Increased levels ↑	Decreased levels ↓
Total Cholesterol	Usually recommended as a screening (with the rest of the lipid profile) once every 5 years for an adult (more frequently for a patient with elevated levels or patients with high risk of heart disease) Desirable level= below 200 mg/dl	Borderline High= 200-239 mg/ml. Moderate risk of heart disease, depending on the rest of the lipid profile and other risk factors High risk- greater than 240 mg/dl. Treatment may be needed depending on cause.	Desirable level= below 200 mg/dl
HDL (High density lipoprotein)	The "good" cholesterol. Higher levels of this type of cholesterol are a good thing.	HDL above 60 mg/dl is associated with a *less* than average risk of heart disease	HDL below 40 mg/dl in men and 50 mg/dl for women increases risk of heart disease HDL 40-50 mg/dl in men and 50-59 mg/dl for women associated with average risk of heart disease
LDL (Low density lipoprotein)	The "bad" cholesterol. High levels of this type of cholesterol are associated with a higher risk of heart disease.	100-129 mg/dl is above optimal 130-159 mg/dl is borderline high 160-189 mg/dl is high Greater than 189 mg/dl is very high.	Optimal: Less than 100 mg/dl is optimal
Triglycerides	This test is ordered in conjunction with the other cholesterol tests and is usually not ordered alone.	Borderline high: 150-199 mg/dl High: 200-499 mg/dl Very high: Greater than 500 mg/dl If the patient is a diabetic and blood sugar levels are not being managed well, triglycerides may be high.	Desirable: less than 150 mg/dl

Reproductive Panel

These tests are ordered to assess the functioning of the reproductive system. They may be ordered individually, or a few may be chosen by the physician depending on patient symptoms or conditions. Some hormones used to assess reproductive functioning are: **Luteinizing Hormone (LH), Follicle Stimulating Hormone (FSH), Testosterone, Estrogen, Progesterone**

Test Name	Test use	Increased levels ↑	Decreased levels ↓
Luteinizing Hormone (LH)	Can be used to assess patients with irregular or heavy periods, low testosterone levels or fertility issues.	↑ LH in women can indicate primary ovarian failure (tumor, polycystic ovary syndrome, thyroid disease) ↑ LH in men can indicate primary testicular failure (trauma, tumor, infection- such as mumps)	↓ LH in women: indicates secondary ovarian failure (pituitary or hypothalamus problem) ↓ LH in men indicates secondary testicular failure (pituitary or hypothalamus)
Follicle Stimulating Hormone (FSH)	Can be tested in cases of infertility in men and women.	↑ FSH in women can indicate primary ovarian failure (tumor, polycystic ovary syndrome PCOS, thyroid disease) ↑ FSH in men can indicate primary testicular failure (trauma, tumor, infection- such as mumps)	↓ FSH in women can indicate secondary ovarian failure (pituitary or hypothalamus problem) ↓ FSH in men can indicate secondary testicular failure (pituitary or hypothalamus)
Testosterone	Can be tested in cases of ED, infertility, PCOS	↑ Testosterone in males- can indicate testicular or adrenal tumors, use of anabolic steroids, hyperthyroidism ↑ Testosterone in females- can indicate polycystic ovary disease (PCOS), ovarian tumor, adrenal tumor, anabolic steroid use, medications (clomiphene and ERT)	**Hypogonadism -** ↓ Testosterone in males, due to hypothalamus or pituitary disease, testicular failure, testicle damage (alcohol, mumps, physical injury)
Estrogen (E1, E2, E3)	Estrogen tests can measure **Estrone (E1), Estradiol (E2),** and/or **Estrone (E3).** Estradiol is the most common form in the body and is needed for proper ovulation, fertilization of the egg, and healthy bone structure.	↑ Estrogens in females can indicate: early puberty, hyperthyroidism, ovary or adrenal glands tumors, (can be normal depending on where the female is in her menstrual cycle or if she is pregnant). ↑ Estrogens in males can indicate: tumors adrenal glands and gynecomastia	↓ Estrogens in females are seen in menopause, pituitary issues, failing pregnancy, anorexia nervosa, medications (clomiphene and oral contraceptives) ↓ Estrogens in males can be a result of pituitary issues
Progesterone	Used in determining cause of infertility, diagnosing an ectopic or failing pregnancy, abnormal bleeding in non-pregnant female	↑ Progesterone- can be present with some ovarian cysts, molar pregnancies (non-viable pregnancies), adrenal gland tumor or overproduction, healthy pregnancy	↓ progesterone can be present in toxemia, decreased ovarian function, amenorrhea

Pregnancy Tests:

The following list details some laboratory tests that may be performed during pregnancy. Not every pregnant woman will have all of these tests administered to them during their pregnancy. Some tests are used more commonly than others. A CBC is also commonly ordered, in addition to the tests listed below.

Pregnancy Test	Test Use
hCG- Human Chorionic Gonadotropin	This test looks for the presence of hCG- a hormone produced by the placenta. This is the test that is usually done to initially confirm a pregnancy. This test can be performed at home using a home pregnancy test (testing the urine) or in a physician's office using blood. The blood hCG test may be repeatedly performed early in pregnancy if the woman has a history of ectopic pregnancy or failed pregnancies.
Progesterone	This test looks at the level of progesterone in the blood. Early in pregnancy, the progesterone levels should increase. In a woman with a history of failed pregnancies, progesterone levels may be monitored in the first trimester.
IgG Rubella Test	This test is performed on the blood and looks for antibodies to Rubella (German Measles). A positive Rubella Test indicates that the patient has been exposed to the Rubella virus before (either through illness or vaccination)
HIV Antibody Test	This test is performed on the blood and looks for antibodies to HIV (Human Immunodeficiency Virus). A positive HIV Test indicates that the patient has been exposed to the HIV virus.
Hepatitis B Screening	This test is performed on the blood and looks for antibodies to hepatitis B. A positive Hepatitis B Test indicates that the patient has been exposed to the Hepatitis B virus (HBV) before (either through illness or vaccination)
First Trimester Downs Syndrome Screen	Usually performed between 10.5 weeks and 13 weeks of pregnancy. This screening test involves blood analysis- looking at pregnancy associated plasma protein A (PAPP-A) and hCG levels. And, a nuchal translucency ultrasound will be performed. This test looks for *risk factors* that could indicate Down's Syndrome or other chromosomal abnormalities. It does not diagnose the fetus as having the chromosomal abnormalities. Other tests would need to be done to offer more of an actual diagnosis.
Triple Marker or Quad Marker Screen	Usually performed between 15-20 weeks gestation (2nd trimester of pregnancy). This is a blood screening panel that assesses levels of: alpha-fetoprotein (AFP), hCG, unconjugated estriol (for triple marker screen). To perform a Quad Marker, the previous levels will be measured in addition to inhibin A. These tests look for markers for Down's Syndrome and neural tube defects. Further testing would need to be done to confirm diagnosis.
Group B strep	This test looks to see if the mother is infected with Group B Streptococcus (GBS) bacteria. GBS can be passed from mother to baby. If positive, antibiotics will be administered. This test is performed by obtaining a vaginal swab- usually between weeks 35-37 of pregnancy.
Urine screen for glucose and protein	Urinalysis of a pregnant mother measuring glucose and protein levels. This is done to monitor the mother for gestational diabetes or toxemia (pre-eclampsia). This urinalysis will be done periodically throughout the pregnancy.
Blood ABO and Rh type	Blood analysis to determine mother's blood type (Type A, B, AB, O, Rh+, Rh-)
Cell Free Fetal DNA	A sample of the mother's blood is taken after the 10th week of pregnancy. Fetal DNA is detected in the mother's blood and is analyzed for Down's Syndrome (Trisomy 21), Trisomy 18, and Trisomy 13. Gender can be identified also.

Urinalysis

Urine tests are typically evaluated with a reagent strip that is briefly dipped into a urine sample. The technician reads the colors of each test and compares them with a reference chart. The items in a urinalysis that can be tested using a reagent strip are: *specific gravity, pH, protein, glucose, ketones, leukocyte esterase, nitrite, bilirubin* and *urobilinogen*. A few items in the urinalysis may need to be performed using a microscope to examine the urine. They are: *red blood cells RBC, white blood cells WBC, epithelial cells,* and *microorganisms*. These tests are semi-quantitative; there can be some variation from one sample to another on how the tests are scored.

Urinalysis Test	Test use
Specific Gravity (SG)	This test measures how dilute or concentrated the urine is. Water would have a SG of 1.000. Most urine is around 1.010, but it can vary greatly depending on when the patient drank fluids last, or if the patient is dehydrated.
pH	This is a measure of acidity of the urine. Diet can influence the acidity/alkalinity of the body- and in turn the urine. Other pathologies can also create alkalosis or acidosis in the body. This shift in pH of the blood can also be seen in the urine.
Protein	Normally there is no protein detectable on a urinalysis strip. Protein can indicate kidney damage, blood in the urine, or an infection. Up to 10% of children can have protein in their urine. Certain diseases require the use of a special, more sensitive (and more expensive) test for protein called a microalbumin test. A microalbumin test is very useful in screening for early damage to the kidneys from diabetes, for instance.
Glucose	Normally negative (meaning not usually found in the urine). A positive glucose result occurs in diabetes. There are a small number of people that have glucose in their urine with normal blood glucose levels; however any glucose in the urine would raise the possibility of diabetes, glucose intolerance, liver disease, or pregnancy.
Ketones	Normally negative. Ketones are present in the urine of a patient who is undergoing fat metabolism in their body (starvation, high protein diets, diabetes and severe exercise)
Leukocyte Esterase	Normally negative. A positive leukocyte esterase test suggests a urinary tract infection.
Nitrite	Normally negative, this usually indicates a urinary tract infection.
Bilirubin	Normally negative. This pigment is normally cleared from the blood by the liver. In liver or gallbladder disease bilirubin may appear in the urine.
Urobilinogen	Normally there is no urobilinogen in the urine. This pigment is normally cleared from the blood by the liver. In liver or gallbladder disease urobilinogen may appear in the urine.
Red Blood Cell (RBC)	Normally a low amount in the urine. If amount is elevated, it could indicate kidney, bladder or urethra damage.
White Blood Cell (WBC)	Normally a low amount in the urine. If amount is elevated, it indicates infection or inflammation in the urinary tract.
Epithelial cells	Normally a low amount in the urine. If amount is elevated, it indicates infection or inflammation in the urinary tract. Specific epithelial cells will be identified, and that can show where in the urinary tract the problem is (for example: bladder or nephron)
Microorganisms	Normally, urine is *sterile* (meaning no microorganisms are present). Microorganisms can be bacteria, viruses, fungi, parasites. Presence of microorganisms can indicate a urinary tract infection.

Stool Tests

Stool tests are performed on fecal material obtained from the patient.

Stool test	Test Use
Fecal Fat Stool Test	Stool fats, also known as fecal fats, or fecal lipids, are fats that are excreted in the feces. When secretions from the pancreas, gall bladder and liver are adequate, emulsified dietary fats are almost completely absorbed in the small intestine. When a malabsorption disorder or other disease disrupts this process, excretion of fat in the stool increases. This test evaluates digestion of fats by determining if there is an excessive excretion of lipids in the fecal material. This may occur in patients exhibiting signs of malabsorption, such as: weight loss, abdominal distention, and scaly skin. Drugs that may increase fecal fat levels include enemas and laxatives, especially mineral oil. Drugs that may decrease fecal fat include Metamucil and barium. Other substances that can affect test results include alcohol, potassium chloride, calcium carbonate, neomycin, and other broad-spectrum antibiotics. Excessive excretion of fecal fat is called *steatorrhea*, a condition that is suspected when the patient has large, "greasy," and foul-smelling stools. Both digestive and absorptive disorders can cause steatorrhea- such as, cystic fibrosis, celiac disease, bile duct blockage, gall stones.
Ova and Parasite Test	Stool analysis has the advantage of looking for parasites and/or their eggs (ova), including *Giardia lamblia* and *E. histolytica*. This test can be helpful when the diagnosis of a specific type of parasitic infection is unclear. For example, if a patient presents with symptoms of prolonged diarrhea, abdominal pain, and/or blood and mucous in the stool, there can be many pathogens that could cause these symptoms. This test may be ordered when the patient is exhibiting symptoms- especially if the patient has recently traveled outside the U.S., drunk stream or lake water while camping, or been exposed to someone who has a parasitic infection (like a family member).
Stool Culture	This test assesses the possibility of a bacterial infection in the gastrointestinal tract. Often done in conjunction with the Ova and Parasite test to ensure proper diagnosis of the pathogen.
Fecal Occult Blood Test (aka Guaiac Test)	This test looks for blood in the stool. Indicates bleeding in the gastrointestinal tract.

LABORATORY TEST SUMMARY CHART

Complete Blood Count (CBC)
White Blood Cell Count
White Blood Cell
   Differential
Red Blood Cell
Red Blood Cell Indices
   (MCV. MCH, MCHC)
Hemoglobin
Hematocrit
Platelet Count
*Reticulocyte Count

Basic Metabolic Profile/Panel (BMP)
Glucose
Calcium
Sodium
Potassium
CO2/Bicarbonate
Chloride
Kidney Panel Tests

Comprehensive Metabolic Profile/Panel (CMP)
Glucose
Calcium
Sodium
Potassium
CO2/Bicarbonate
Chloride
Albumin
Total Protein
Kidney Panel Tests
Liver Panel Tests

Kidney Panel
Blood Urea Nitrogen
Creatinine

Liver (Hepatic) Panel
ALP
ALT
AST
Bilirubin

Cardiac Panel
Total Creatine Kinase (CK)
Creatine Kinase MB
Troponin
Myoglobin
*C-reactive Protein and
   hc-CRP

Thyroid Panel
TSH
T4 or Free T4
T3 or Free T3

Reproductive Panel
LH
FSH
Testosterone
Estrogens
Progesterone

Lipid Profile
Total Cholesterol
HDL
LDL
Triglycerides

Pregnancy Tests
HCG
Progesterone
IgG Rubella Test
HIV antibody test
Hepatitis B screening
First trimester Downs
   Syndrome Screen
Triple Marker or Quad
   Marker Screen
Group B Strep
Urine Screen for glucose
   and protein
Blood ABO and Rh type
Cell Free Fetal DNA Test

Urinalysis
Specific Gravity
pH
Protein
Glucose
Ketones
Leukocyte Esterase
Nitrite
Bilirubin
Urobilinogen
RBC's
WBC's
Epithelial Cells
Microorganisms

Stool Tests
Fecal Fat Stool Test
Ova and Parasite test
Stool Culture
Fecal Occult Blood Test
(aka Guaiac Test)

Screening Examination Schedule Guidelines:

These recommendations are from the **United States Department of Health and Human Services (HHS) Recommendations and the U.S. Preventive Services Task Force (USPSTF). Guidelines can be viewed at** *uspreventiveservicestaskforce.org*

The following recommendations are for a woman or man with no prior history of the following health conditions and no strong family history of these conditions. Should a patient have past history or strong family history or the following conditions, these guidelines may be altered by their PCP or specialist.

Screening Examination Recommendations for Women and Men	
Screening Exam	**Recommendation**
Obesity	Have BMI evaluated to screen for obesity.
Blood Pressure	Have BP screening at least every 2 years if BP <120/80. High blood pressure is 140/90 or higher. Patients with high blood pressure should be screened yearly.
Colorectal Cancer	Have a test for colorectal cancer starting at age 50. Prior family history may require earlier testing.
Diabetes	Test for diabetes if you have high blood pressure or high cholesterol
Depression	If patient has felt "down", sad, or hopeless for more than two weeks, have doctor screen for depression
HIV	Have an HIV screening if: the patient has had unprotected sex with multiple partners; if pregnant (woman); have used or currently use injection drugs; exchange sex for money or drugs- or have sex partners that do; have past or present sex partners who are HIV+, are bisexual or use injection drugs; are being treated for other STD's, or have had a blood transfusion between 1978-1985.
Hepatitis B	Recommended for men and women at risk of infection and in all pregnant women
Lung Cancer	Annual screening (low dose CT scan) for adults age 55- 80 years old who have a 30 pack smoking history and currently smoke or have quit within the last 15 years
Additional Screening Examinations For Women	
Breast Cancer	Have a mammogram every 1-2 years starting at age 40 (please note- a current research report has stated that women in their 40's should not get mammograms, and should wait until they are 50 to begin. So, guidelines could be changing over the next few years). Many health care providers also encourage a monthly self-breast exam done by the patient. BRCA1 or BRCA2 screening should be done for women with family history of breast, ovarian or peritoneal cancer.
Cervical Cancer	Have a pap smear every 1-3 years if the woman has ever been sexually active, and is the ages of 21-65.
Cholesterol	Have it checked regularly (once every 5 years if levels are normal) starting at age 45. If younger than 45, talk to doctor about earlier screenings if the woman has diabetes, high blood pressure, a history of heart disease in family, or smokes.
Osteoporosis	Have bone density test beginning at age 65. If ages 61-64 and less than 154 pounds, talk to doctor about getting screened earlier
Chlamydia and other STD/STI	Have a test for Chlamydia if woman is 25 or younger and sexually active. If older, talk to doctor about being screened. Pregnant women should also be screened.
Additional Screening Examinations For Men	
Cholesterol	Have it checked regularly starting at age 35. If younger than 35, talk to doctor about earlier screenings if the man has diabetes, high blood pressure, a history of heart disease in family, or smokes.
Osteoporosis	Have bone density test beginning at age 70. Screening can begin for men ages 50-69 if there is concern for osteoporosis based on their risk profile.
STD/STI	Speak with doctor about being screened, based on sexual history
Abdominal Aortic Aneurysm	If between ages 60-75 and have ever smoked, should be screened.

Practice Study and Test Questions:

1) Which of the following tests is not a part of the hepatic panel?
   A) alkaline phosphatase (ALP)
   B) creatinine
   C) aspartate aminotransferase (ALT)
   D) bilirubin

2) Acute bacterial infections would cause which abnormal CBC finding?
   A) neutrophilia
   B) lymphopenia
   C) eosinophilia
   D) polycythemia

3) Excessive potassium in the blood is called
   A) hyperkalemia
   B) hypernatremia
   C) hypokalemia
   D) hyponatremia

4) Increased levels of _____ in the blood could indicate that a heart attack or cardiac muscle damage has occurred within the past few hours.
   A) albumin
   B) alanine aminotransferase
   C) hemoglobin
   D) troponin

5) A patient with gall stones or any other form of bile duct blockage could have which abnormal blood test findings?
   A) increased bilirubin
   B) increased ALT
   C) increased AST
   D) all of the above

6) According to the United States Department of Health and Human Services, a woman should be screened for cervical cancer via a pap smear
   A) yearly from age 5-65
   B) every 1-3 years between the ages of 21-65
   C) every year from the onset of menses until the woman dies
   D) once every 5 years while the woman is sexually active

7) Which laboratory findings might be present in a patient with uncontrolled diabetes?
   A) decreased blood glucose levels, no glucose in the urine, decreased bicarbonate blood levels
   B) increased blood glucose levels, glucose in the urine, increased bicarbonate blood levels
   C) increased blood glucose levels, glucose in the urine, decreased bicarbonate blood levels
   D) increased blood glucose levels, no glucose in the urine, low bicarbonate blood levels

8) Polycystic ovary disease could cause which abnormal finding in a blood test?
   A) Increased testosterone levels
   B) Decreased testosterone levels
   C) Decreased follicle stimulating hormone levels
   D) Decreased luteinizing hormone levels

9) Which pregnancy test may be done early in the first trimester?
   A) Group B strep
   B) triple marker test
   C) hCG test
   D) all of the above

10) Which type of cholesterol is the "good" type; and, which type of cholesterol is the "bad" type?
   A) LDL; VDL
   B) GDL; LDL
   C) HDL; LDL
   D) LDL; HDL

11) According to the United States Department of Health and Human Services, a man should be screened for cholesterol
   A) regularly once he is sexually active
   B) regularly starting at age 55
   C) regularly starting at age 35; possibly earlier if the male has certain health conditions or risk factors
   D) regularly starting at age 65, but only if he smokes

12) A patient is diagnosed with sickle cell anemia. What abnormal blood findings may be present?
   A) thrombocythemia
   B) decreased mean corpuscular hemoglobin concentration
   C) increased mean corpuscular hemoglobin concentration
   D) leukocytosis

13) This stool test is used to diagnose a bacterial infection
   A) ova and parasite test
   B) occult blood test
   C) fecal fat stool test
   D) stool culture

14) Which substances might be detected in a urinalysis in a patient with a urinary tract infection?
   A) epithelial cells
   B) nitrite
   C) white blood cells
   D) all of the above

15) Which blood findings can indicate hypothyroidism?
   A) Increased TSH, decreased T4, decreased T3
   B) Decreased TSH, decreased T4, decreased T3
   C) Increased TSH, increased T4, increased T3
   D) Decreased TSH, increased T4, decreased T3

16) Decreased white blood cell count is called
   A) leukocytosis
   B) neutrophilia
   C) erythrocytosis
   D) leukopenia

Answers: 1) B 2) A 3) A 4) D 5) D 6) B 7) C 8) A 9) C 10) C 11) C 12) C 13) D 14) D 15) A 16) D

CHAPTER 16: PHARMACEUTICALS

Pharmacology Terminology:

Drug: any chemical that can affect living processes (a very wide range definition!). For therapeutic use, the three most important characteristics of a drug are: effectiveness, safety, and selectivity (no side effects)

Drug prototypes: Considered to be the first pure compound to have been discovered in any series of chemically or developmentally related therapeutic agents.

Pharmacology: study of drugs and their interactions with living systems

OTC: Over the counter (able to be bought without a prescription)

Side effect: a nearly unavoidable secondary drug effect produced at therapeutic doses

Adverse drug reaction (ADR): any noxious, unintended, and undesired effect that occurs at normal drug doses. People at most risk for adverse drug reactions are the very young, the elderly, the very ill, and those taking multiple medications.

Iatrogenic disease: a drug or physician induced disease

Hepatotoxic: drugs that may cause liver failure

QT interval drugs: drugs that can cause dangerous cardiac dysrhythmias

Physical dependence: develops during long term use of certain drugs, such as opioids, alcohol, barbiturates, and amphetamines (some people refer to this as an "addiction")

Allergic reaction: an immune response. For an immune response to occur there must be prior sensitization (exposure) of the drug to the immune system. First exposure does not produce the allergic response, but re-exposure to the drug can. **Anaphylaxis** is a potentially life threatening allergic reaction.

Idiosyncratic effect: an adverse drug reaction based on a genetic predisposition

Carcinogenic effect: drug induced cancer

Teratogenic effect: drug induced birth defect

Drug Names:

Drugs have three types of names
1. **Chemical name-** name uses the nomenclature of chemistry. Due to complexity, not usually used. Example: N-acetyl-para-aminophenol

2. **Generic name-** each drug is assigned a generic name by the United States Adopted Names Council. The generic name is also known as the non-proprietary name. Generic names are less complicated than chemical names, but typically more complex than trade names. Example: acetaminophen

3. **Trade name-** also known as proprietary or brand names. These are the names under which a drug is marketed. Must be approved by the FDA, to ensure that two names for different drugs are not too similar. In addition trade names cannot imply efficacy. So, the name may not sound anything like its intended effect. Example: Tylenol

Things to note about names:
- A single drug can have multiple trade names. A drug can have only one generic name, but can have multiple trade names.
  - Ibuprofen (generic name) has multiple trade names (Advil, Motrin, Nuprin)
- Products with the same trade name may have different active ingredients
  - Monistat has the active ingredient Miconazole
  - Monistat 1 has the active ingredient Tioconazole
- Products with the same trade name in the United States and abroad may contain different active ingredients (and totally different therapeutic uses!)
  - Allegra in US contains the active drug Fexofenadine and is used for allergies
  - Allegra in Germany contains the active drug Frovatriptin and is used for migraines

Administration Routes of Drugs:

Two major methods:
1. <u>Enteral</u>: via the gastrointestinal tract
   - **Oral (PO)-** swallowed by mouth

2. <u>Parenteral</u>: Outside the GI tract
   - **Intravenous (IV)** - medication administered directly into the bloodstream via a vein.
   - **Intramuscular (IM)-** medication injected into a muscle (often deltoid, vastus lateralis, or the gluteal muscles)
   - **Subcutaneous (subQ)** - medication injected into the hypodermis (adipose) layer under the skin.
   - **Intrathecal-** medication injected into the subarachnoid space of the spine

Additional methods of administration:
- Topically and Transdermal
- Inhaled
- Rectal suppositories and Vaginal suppositories
- Direct injection into a specific site (joints, nerves, etc.)
- Sublingual (under the tongue)

Drug Interactions:

Drug-Drug interaction: when 2 drugs interact, there are three possible outcomes.
1. One drug may intensify the effects of another.
   - May increase therapeutic effects- this is ideal
   - May increase adverse effects
2. One drug may reduce the effects of another.
   - May reduce therapeutic effects- a detrimental inhibitory effect
   - May reduce adverse effects- a beneficial inhibitory effect
3. The combination may produce a new response not seen with either drug alone

Drug-Food interaction: important possible interaction, but still not very well understood
1. Food may decrease the rate of absorption of certain medications. This delays onset of the effects of the medication. Some examples:
   - Eating calcium containing foods while taking tetracycline antibiotics. Tetracycline's bind with calcium to make an insoluble and non-absorbable complex.
   - High fiber foods can reduce absorption of some drugs
2. Foods may increase the absorption of medications.
3. Foods may alter the metabolism (break down) of medications in the body
   - Grapefruit juice can inhibit metabolism of certain drugs, thereby raising blood levels (possibly to dangerous levels)
4. Foods may increase toxicity of drugs
   - Monoamine oxidase (MAO) inhibitors (an antidepressant) combined with foods high in tyramine (found in aged cheeses, yeast extracts, Chianti wine) can cause blood pressure to rise to a dangerous level.
5. Foods may directly impact drug action
   - Foods rich in vitamin K (broccoli, Brussels sprouts, cabbage) can reduce the effect of anticoagulants- such as warfarin (Coumadin)
6. Timing of drug administration with meals:
   - "with food" means administer it with or shortly after a meal. Some medications may upset the stomach if taken on an empty stomach. If food does not decrease the rate of absorption of the drug, then the drug should be taken with a meal.
   - "empty stomach" means to administer it one hour before a meal or 2 hours after.

Drug- supplement interactions: are unfortunately not well researched or understood. Interactions can lead to possible reduction of therapeutic effects of the drug or increased toxicity of the drug. Some common interactions include:
1. *American Ginseng*: may interact with NSAIDs, anticoagulants, antiplatelet medications, digoxin, diuretics, antiretroviral medications, and some chemotherapy medications.
2. *St John's Wort*: may decrease levels of antihyperlipidemic medications (statins) and some calcium channel blockers (antihypertensives). Should not be taken by a patient who takes SSRI's, anticoagulant, antiretroviral, antiseizure, oral contraceptive, and some chemotherapy medications.
3. *Psyllium or other bulk forming laxatives*- should not be taken at the same time as oral medications as it may decrease absorption (should wait about 4 hours between taking meds and psyllium).
4. *Iron* can decrease availability of some medications (tetracycline, ciprofloxacin, Synthroid)
5. *Garlic* may increase risk of bleeding in patients taking NSAIDs, anticoagulant or antiplatelet medications. May also decrease effectiveness of antiretrovirals and hypoglycemic medications.
6. *Ginkgo*- may increase risk of bleeding in patients taking NSAIDs, anticoagulant or antiplatelet medications. It may also interact with antiseizure, hypoglycemic and diuretic medications.
7. *Saw palmetto*- may increase bleeding in patients taking NSAIDs, anticoagulants or antiplatelet meds.
8. *Ginger*- may increase risk of bleeding in patients taking NSAIDs, anticoagulants or antiplatelet meds.
9. *Kava*- may cause liver damage. Should not be taken with meds that affect the liver or are hepatotoxic.

Identifying Adverse Drug Reactions (ADR):

To identify an ADR, the following questions should be asked:
1. Did symptoms appear shortly after the drug was first used?
2. Did symptoms abate when the drug was discontinued?
3. Did symptoms reappear when the drug was reinstated?
4. Are the symptoms of the illness able to explain the event?
5. Could other drugs the patient is taking explain the event?

If a possible ADR is occurring, instruct the patient to contact the prescribing physician immediately if reaction is not causing life threatening reaction (for example: a skin rash, redness at injection site, etc.), If a life threatening reaction is occurring involving respiratory, cardiac, or neurologic (consciousness), call 911.

Pregnancy and medications:

The risks for most drugs used in pregnancy have not been determined. (The benefits of treatment must balance the risks.)
- Category A: Remote risk of fetal harm
- Category B: Slightly more risk than A
- Category C: Greater risk than B
- Category D: Proven risk of fetal harm
- Category X: Proven risk of fetal harm

Drugs that should be avoided in pregnancy due to teratogenicity:
- Anticancer/Immunosuppressant drugs (methotrexate)
- Antiseizure drugs (carbamazepine, valproic acid, phenytoin, and others)
- Androgens (danazol, finasteride, dutasteride)
- ACE inhibitors (lisinopril and others)
- Angiotensin-receptor blockers (losartan and others)
- Anti-thyroid drugs (propylthiouracil, methimazole)
- Fluoroquinolone antibiotics (ciprofloxacin, levofloxacin)
- HMG-CoA reductase inhibitors [i.e., statins] (atorvastatin and others)
- Isotretinoin (Accutane) used for acne
- Lithium used for bipolar disorder
- Non-steroidal anti-inflammatory drugs (ibuprofen and others)
- Megadoses of vitamin A
- Tetracycline antibiotics (minocycline, doxycycline)
- Warfarin (Coumadin)

Commonly used suffixes (endings) in drug names

Suffix	Drug type which uses the name	Drug Example
-tidine:	Histamine2 blocker- acid reducer	Cimetidine
-prazole	Protein pump inhibitor- acid reducer	Omeprazole
-cillin	In the penicillin antibiotic family	Amoxicillin
-cycline	In the tetracycline antibiotic family	Tetracycline
-floxacin	In the fluoroquinolone antibiotic family	Levofloxacin
-thromycin	In the macrolide antibiotic family	Azithromycin
-micin, -mycin	In the aminoglycoside antibiotic family	Gentamicin
-azole	Antifungal	Itraconazole
-triptan	Serotonin-receptor agonists used for migraines	Sumatriptan
-denafil, -dalafil	Phosphodiesterase type 5 inhibitors for erectile dysfunction	Sildenafil
-curium, -curonium	Neuromuscular blockers used for muscle relaxation during surgery	Pancuronium
-zosin	Alpha-adrenergic blocker used for hypertension and benign prostatic hypertrophy	Prazosin
-olol, -lol	Beta- adrenergic blocker (BB)	Metoprolol
-zepam, -zolam	Benzodiazepine (BDZ)- antianxiety med.	Diazepam
-pril	Angiotensin-converting enzyme (ACE) inhibitor	Lisinopril
-artan	Angiotensin-receptor blocker (ARB)	Candesartan
-dipine	Calcium channel blocker (CCB)	Amlodipine
-statin	Lipid (cholesterol) lowering drug	Atorvastatin
-ase, -plase	Thrombolytic used to dissolve clots	Alteplase
-parin	Anticoagulant	Enoxaparin
-sone, -olone	Corticosteroid	Prednisone
-dronate	Bisphosphonate for osteoporosis	Alendronate
-terol	Bronchodilator used for asthma and COPD	Albuterol
-thiazide	Diuretic	Hydrochlorothiazide
-vir	Antiviral	Acyclovir

Prescription and OTC Medications: Classifications, Mechanism of Action, Actions (uses) and Side Effects

**Please note: when medication names are listed you will see: Generic Name (Trade Name, if applicable). For example: Atorvastatin (Lipitor)*

This list is NOT meant to be an all-inclusive list of ALL prescription and OTC medications- but will hopefully be a starting place for a review of pharmaceuticals utilized by a physician. Please refer to a pharmacology text to view more medications (or further detail of the medications listed here) - if you need more information.

Nervous System

Classification: Antiseizure Medications /Antiepileptic Drugs (AED's)

> **Prototypes**: Phenytoin (Dilantin) and Valproic Acid (Depakote)
>   - **Mechanism of Action**: Stabilizes neuron cell membranes by inhibiting entry of sodium into neuron. This decreases action potentials and limits spread of seizure activity
>   - **Action (Uses)**: Epilepsy (grand mal, psychomotor, and status epilepticus), can also be used for cardiac dysrhythmias, and some may be used for migraines and bipolar disorder
>   - **Adverse Effects/ Side effects**: Do not use in pregnancy. May cause constipation, nausea, diarrhea, headache, nystagmus, ataxia, gingival hyperplasia, sedation, insomnia, hepatotoxicity, may increase suicidal thoughts and behaviors
>   - **Other examples of this class of medication**: Carbamazepine (Tegretol), Ethosuxamide (Zarontin), Phenobarbital, Fosphenytion (Cerebyx), Topiramate (Topamax), Gabapentin (Neurontin), Oxcarbazepine (Trileptal), Pregabalin (Lyrica)

Classification: Anti-Parkinson's Medications

> **Prototype**: Levodopa
>   - **Mechanism of Action**: Increased dopamine concentration in the brain. Usually Levodopa is combined with Carbidopa to increase effectiveness
>   - **Action (Uses)**: Treatment of Parkinson's disease
>   - **Adverse Effects/ Side effects**: dyskinesia's, nausea
>   - **Other examples of Levodopa-Carbidopa combinations**: Parcopa, Sinemet, Stalevo (contains levodopa, carbidopa and entacapone)

Classification: CNS Stimulants

- ➤ **Category: Amphetamines**
  - **Mechanism of Action**: Promotes release of NE (norepinephrine) and dopamine, and inhibits reuptake in CNS and peripheral nerves. Causes increased wakefulness, alertness, decreased fatigue, increased mood, augmented self-confidence and initiative. Can suppress appetite and perception of pain
  - **Action (Uses)**: ADHD, narcolepsy, obesity
  - **Adverse Effects/ Side effects**: tolerance and physical dependence, CNS stimulation (insomnia), cardiovascular effects, weight loss
  - **Other examples of this class of medication**: Dextroamphetamine Sulfate, Lisdexamfetamine, Methamphetamine

- ➤ **Category: Attention Deficit Medications**
  - **Prototype**: Methylphenidate (Ritalin, Metadate, Concerta, Daytrana)
  - **Mechanism of Action**: Promotes release of NE and dopamine and prevents re-uptake
  - **Action (Uses)**: ADHD, narcolepsy
  - **Adverse Effects/ Side effects**: Insomnia, reduced appetite, weight loss, palpitations, hypertension, angina dysrhythmias, psychosis

- ➤ **Category: Methylxanthines**
  - **Prototype**: Caffeine
  - **Mechanism of Action**: enhancement of calcium permeability, blockade of adenosine receptors
  - **Action (Uses)**: Promoting wakefulness
  - **Adverse Effects/ Side effects**: dysrhythmias with high levels, nervousness, insomnia, tremors, diuretic

Classification: Alzheimers Medications

- ➤ **Category: NMDA receptor antagonist**
  - **Prototype**: Memantine (Namenda)
  - **Mechanism of Action**: Blocks the receptors on brain cells of glutamate (an excitatory neurotransmitter). Overstimulation of neurons by glutamate may damage the neurons. This medication blocks glutamate receptors in the brain (the receptors are called NMDA receptors).
  - **Action (Uses)**: Alzheimers disease, dementia
  - **Adverse Effects/ Side effects**: fatigue, pain, increased blood pressure, dizziness, headache, constipation, vomiting, and confusion.

Psychiatric

Classification: Antidepressants

➤ **Category: Tricyclic Antidepressants (TCA's)**
  - **Prototype:** Imipramine (Tofranil)
  - **Mechanism of Action:** Blocks re-uptake of norepinephrine (NE) and serotonin. This allows more serotonin and NE to be available at the synapses (and increases mood)
  - **Action (Uses):** Depression, bipolar disorder, ADHD, obsessive compulsive disorder (OCD)
  - **Adverse Effects/ Side effects:** orthostatic hypotension, sedation, cardiotoxicity, increased risk of suicide, anticholinergic effects- BUDCAT *(B= Blurry vision, photophobia, increased ocular pressure. U= Urinary retention. D= dry mouth. C= Constipation. A= Anhidrosis (absence of sweat). T= tachycardia*
  - **Other examples of this class of medication:** Amitriptyline, Clomipramine (Anafranil), Doxepin (Sinequan)

➤ **Category: Selective Serotonin Reuptake Inhibitors (SSRI)**
  - **Prototype:** Fluoxetine (Prozac, Sarafem)
  - **Mechanism of Action:** Inhibits serotonin reuptake (therefore, more serotonin is available at the synapse). This increases mood and decreases anxiety.
  - **Action (Uses):** Most widely prescribed antidepressant. Also used for bipolar disorder, OCD
  - **Adverse Effects/ Side effects:** sexual dysfunction, nausea, headache, insomnia, weight gain, increased risk of suicide, serotonin syndrome (agitation, confusion, disorientation, hallucinations)
  - **Other examples of this class of medication:** Paroxetine (Paxil, Paxil CR, Pexeva), Sertraline (Zoloft), Citalopram (Celexa), Fluvoxamine (Luvox), Escitalopram (Lexapro)

➤ **Category: Monoamine Oxidase Inhibitors (MAOI's)**
  - **Prototype:** Isocarboxazid (Marplan)
  - **Mechanism of Action:** Monoamine Oxidase (MAO) is an enzyme which breaks down NE and serotonin. MAOI's block this enzyme- allowing NE and serotonin to have longer lasting effects.
  - **Action (Uses):** Used in patients with depression who have not responded to SSRI's or Tricyclic's. For Atypical Depression, MAOI's are drug of first choice. Also can be used in OCD.
  - **Adverse Effects/ Side effects:** CNS stimulation (anxiety, insomnia, agitation, mania), orthostatic hypotension, hypertensive crisis if individual consumes high levels of tyramine in their diet)
  - **Other examples of this class of medication:** Phenelzine (Nardil), Tranylcypromine (Parnate), Transdermal selegiline (Emsam)

➤ **Category: Serotonin- Norepinephrine Re-uptake Inhibitor (SNRI)**
  - **Prototype:** Venlafaxine (Effexor)
  - **Mechanism of Action:** inhibits serotonin and norepinephrine re-uptake. Increases mood and decreases anxiety
  - **Action (Uses):** Antidepressant, decreases anxiety, reduces neuropathic pain, fibromyalgia
  - **Adverse Effects/ Side effects:** sexual dysfunction, nausea, headache, insomnia, weight gain, increased risk of suicide, serotonin syndrome (agitation, confusion, disorientation, hallucinations)
  - **Other examples of this class of medication:** Duloxetine (Cymbalta), Minacipran (Dalcipran)

Classification: Antipsychotics

- ➤ **Category: Conventional Antipsychotics (First generation)**
  - **Prototypes:** Haloperidol (Haldol)- high potency; Chlorpromazine (Thorazine)- low potency
  - **Mechanism of Action:** Blocks receptors for dopamine, acetylcholine, histamine, and NE
  - **Action (Uses):** Schizophrenia
  - **Adverse Effects/ Side effects:** Extrapyramidal syndrome (acute dystonia, parkinsonism, tardive dyskinesia), neuroleptic malignant syndrome (lead pipe rigidity, high fever, autonomic instability), anticholinergic effects (BUDCAT)
  - **Other examples of this class of medication:** Low potency: Thioridazine (Mellaril). High potency: Trifluoperazine, Thiothixene (Navane), Pimozide (Orap)

- ➤ **Category: Atypical Antipsychotics (Second generation)**
  - **Prototype:** Clozapine (Clozaril)
  - **Mechanism of Action:** Blocks receptors for serotonin, acetylcholine, histamine, and NE
  - **Action (Uses):** Schizophrenia. Atypical outsells conventional antipsychotics by 10 to 1 (but costs 10 times as much). Also used for bipolar disorder
  - **Adverse Effects/ Side effects:** Metabolic effects (weight gain, diabetes, dyslipidemia), seizures, orthostatic hypotension, weight gain, anticholinergic effects (BUDCAT)
  - **Other examples of this class of medication:** Aripiprazole (Abilify), Risperdine (Risperdal), Olanzapine (Zyprexa), Quetiapine (Seroquel), Ziprasidone (Geodon)

Classification: Mood Stabilizing Medications

- ➤ **Prototype:** Lithium (Lithobid, Lithonte, Lithotabs)
  - **Mechanism of Action:** mechanism not fully understood, may alter ions and neurotransmitters to stabilize mood
  - **Action (Uses):** Bipolar disorder, preferred for patients with classic (euphoric) mania
  - **Adverse Effects/ Side effects:** Accumulates to toxic levels in presence of low sodium levels, lithium blood levels must be monitored (mandatory)- with blood levels being drawn 12 hours after evening dose.

- ➤ **Other Categories used as Mood stabilizing drugs: Antiepileptic drugs** (see previous discussion in other section), **Antipsychotic drugs** (see previous discussion in other section)

Classification: Antianxiety medications

- ➤ **Other Categories Used As Antianxiety medications: Benzodiazepines** (see previous discussion in Sedative Drugs), **SSRI's** (see previous discussion in Antidepressants)

Classification: Sedative Drugs (CNS Depressants) and Sleep Medications

- ➢ **Category: Benzodiazepines (BZDs)**
  - **Prototype**: Alprazolam (Xanax)
  - **Mechanism of Action**: Increases actions of GABA (an inhibitory CNS neurotransmitter). Depresses CNS functions, reduces anxiety, promotes sleep
  - **Action (Uses)**: Anxiety, insomnia, seizure disorder
  - **Adverse Effects/ Side effects**: CNS depression, anterograde amnesia, sleep driving and other complex sleep related behaviors, respiratory depression
  - **Other examples of this class of medication**: Diazepam (Valium), Triazolam (Halcion), Lorazepam (Ativan), Clonazepam (Klonopin), Midazolam (Versed), Temazepam (Restoril)

- ➢ **Category: Benzodiazepine-like drugs**
  - **Prototype**: Zolpidem (Ambien)
  - **Mechanism of Action**: Increases actions of GABA (an inhibitory CNS neurotransmitter). Depresses CNS functions, reduces anxiety, promotes sleep
  - **Action (Uses)**: Insomnia
  - **Adverse Effects/ Side effects**: daytime drowsiness, dizziness, sleep driving and other complex sleep related behaviors
  - **Other examples of this class of medication**: Zaleplon (Sonata), Eszopiclone (Lunesta)

- ➢ **Category: Barbiturates**
  - **Prototype**: Phenobarbital
  - **Mechanism of Action**: Increases actions of GABA (an inhibitory CNS neurotransmitter). Depresses CNS functions, reduces anxiety, promotes sleep
  - **Action (Uses)**: Insomnia, treatment of manic states
  - **Adverse Effects/ Side effects**: respiratory depression (can be fatal in overdose), many drug interactions, may lead to tolerance and dependence
  - **Other examples of this class of medication**: Secobarbital, thiopental

Musculoskeletal

Classification: Bisphosphonates (Osteoporosis Medications)

> **Prototype**: Alendronate (Fosamax)
>   - **Mechanism of Action**: Suppresses reabsorption of bone. Reduces number and activity of osteoclasts
>   - **Action (Uses)**: Osteoporosis, Paget's disease
>   - **Adverse Effects/ Side effects**: Esophagitis, musculoskeletal pain, osteonecrosis of the jaw
>   - **Other examples of this class of medication**: Risedronate (Actonel), Ibandronate (Boniva), Zoledronate (Reclast, Zometa)

Classification: Muscle Relaxants

> **Prototype**: Metaxalone (Skelaxin)
>   - **Mechanism of Action**: Unclear, sedative properties may cause relaxation
>   - **Action (Uses)**: Relief of muscle spasms
>   - **Adverse Effects/ Side effects**: CNS depression, hepatotoxicity. physical dependence
>   - **Other examples of this class of medication**: Baclofen (Lioresal), Diazepam (Valium), Cyclobenzaprine (Flexaril, Fexmid), Chlorzoxazone (Paraflex, Parafon Forte, Remular-S), Methocarbamol (Robaxin)

Diuretics

Classification: Diuretics

- ➢ **Category: Loop Diuretics (High Ceiling)**
  - **Prototype**: Furosemide (Lasix)
  - **Mechanism of Action**: Inhibit sodium and chloride reabsorption in the ascending portion of the Loop of Henle in the kidney nephron. This causes increased urination. This is a better diuretic in patients with kidney conditions
  - **Action (Uses)**: Edema, hypertension
  - **Adverse Effects/ Side effects**: hyponatremia, hypochloremia, dehydration, hypokalemia, hypotension
  - **Other examples of this class of medication**: Ethacrynic acid (Edecrin), Bumetanide (Bumex), Torsemide (Demadex)

- ➢ **Category: Thiazide diuretics**
  - **Prototype**: Hydrochlorothiazide (HCTZ)
  - **Mechanism of Action**: Inhibit sodium and chloride reabsorption in the distal convoluted tubule of the kidney nephron. This causes increased urination. This is a better diuretic in patients with normal kidney function
  - **Action (Uses)**: Hypertension, edema
  - **Adverse Effects/ Side effects**: hyponatremia, hypochloremia, dehydration, hypokalemia, hypotension
  - **Other examples of this class of medication**: Chlorothiazide (Diuril), Methyclothiazide (Enduron), Chlorthalidone (Hygroton, Thalitone), Metolazone (Zaroxylin)

Cardiovascular

Classification: Antihypertension Medications

> **Category: Beta-Adrenergic Antagonists (Beta Blockers)**
> - **Prototypes**: Non-selective: Propranolol (Inderal, Innopran)
>   - Cardioselective: Metoprolol (Lopressor, Toprol XL); Nebivolol (Bystolic)
>   - Alpha/Beta Blocker: Labetalol (Normodyne, Trandate)
> - **Mechanism of Action**: Beta$_1$ (B$_1$) blockers affect the heart; Beta$_2$ (B$_2$) blockers affect the lungs. These drugs block sympathetic nervous system catecholamines from stimulating tissues in the body. Non selective (1st generation) beta blockers will have an effect on both the heart ($\downarrow$ HR, $\downarrow$force of contraction, $\downarrow$ conduction at AV node, $\downarrow$cardiac output) and lungs (bronchoconstriction). Non-selective beta blockers should not be used with patients with asthma or COPD because of these lung effects. Cardioselective (2nd generation) beta blockers only create the heart effects. Alpha/Beta Blockers are 3rd generation beta blockers.
> - **Action (Uses)**: Hypertension, angina, cardiac dysrhythmias, myocardial infarction
> - **Adverse Effects/ Side effects**: More adverse events present with nonselective beta blockers- do not use them with patients with asthma, diabetes, COPD. Side effects: bradycardia, AV heart block, heart failure, inhibition of glycogenolysis, drowsiness, depression, bronchospasm
> - **Other examples of this class of medication**:
>   - Nonselective: Nadolol (Corgard), Sotalol (Betapace)
>   - Cardioselective: Acebutolol (secretal), Atenolol (Tenormin)

> **Category: Calcium Channel Blockers (CCB's)**
> - **Prototypes**: Non- dihydropyridines: Verapamil (Calan) and Diltiazem (Cardizem)
>   - Dihydropyradines: Amlodipine (Norvasc) and Nifedipine (Adalat)
> - **Mechanism of Action**: Blocks calcium channels in blood vessels, which decreases calcium access to cells. This decreases contractility and conductivity of heart; and causes vasodilation of peripheral blood vessels. Dihydropyradines do not have much effect on the heart, only blood vessels (useful for treating hypertension, not useful for dysrhythmias)
> - **Action (Uses)**: Hypertension (Non- dihydropyridines and Dihydropyradines), Cardiac dysrhythmias (Non- dihydropyridines), Angina
> - **Adverse Effects/ Side effects**: Edema in extremities, hypotension, dizziness, headache, bradycardia (Non- dihydropyridines)
> - **Other examples of this class of medication**: Nicarpidine (Cardene), Isradipine (DynaCirc), Felodipine (Plendinl), Nimodipine (Nimotop)

> **Category: Angiotensin Converting Enzyme (ACE) Inhibitor**
> - **Prototype**: Ramipril (Altace)
> - **Mechanism of Action**: Blocks ACE (which prevents conversion of angiotensin I to angiotensin II in the kidney). Angiotensin II is a vasoconstrictor, so by preventing the formation of angiotensin II this leads to vasodilation of blood vessels- reducing blood pressure.
> - **Action (Uses)**: Hypertension, heart failure, myocardial infarction
> - **Adverse Effects/ Side effects**: Hypotension, cough, angioedema
> - **Other examples of this class of medication**: Benazepril (Lotensin), Captopril (Capoten), Enalapril (Vasotec), Lisinopril (Prinivil and Zestril), Fosinopril (Monopril)

> ### Category: Alpha-Adrenergic Antagonists (Alpha Blockers)
> - **Prototype**: Prazosin (Minipress)
> - **Mechanism of Action**: blocks alpha$_1$ receptors- this decreases sympathetic nervous system effects and leads to dilation of arteries and veins (decreases peripheral resistance). Can also decrease smooth muscle activity on bladder and prostate
> - **Action (Uses)**: Essential hypertension (mild to moderate). Also can be used in benign prostatic hyperplasia (BPH) and Raynaud's Disease
> - **Adverse Effects/ Side effects**: Orthostatic hypotension, tachycardia, vertigo, nasal congestion, sexual dysfunction
> - **Other examples of this class of medication**: Doxazosin (Cardura), Terazosin (Hytrin), Tamsulosin (Flomax) for BPH only, Alfuzosin (Uroxatral) for BPH only

> ### Category: Angiotensin Receptor Blocker (ARB)/ Angiotensin II Inhibitor
> - **Prototype**: Valsartan (Diovan)
> - **Mechanism of Action**: blocks receptors for Angiotensin II. This encourages vasodilation (which decreases blood pressure)
> - **Action (Uses)**: Hypertension, heart failure
> - **Adverse Effects/ Side effects**: Headache, dizziness, fatigue, diarrhea, nausea, kidney problems, skin rash
> - **Other examples of this class of medication**: Amiodipine (Norvasc), Irbesartan (Avapro), Iosartan (Cozaar)

Classification: Cardiac Antidysrhythmic Medications

> ### Category: Sodium Channel Blockers
> - **Prototypes**: Procainamide (Procanbid) and Lidocaine (Xylocaine)
> - **Mechanism of Action**: Block sodium, which slows transmission of impulses in the atria, ventricles, bundles of His, and Purkinje fibers
> - **Action (Uses)**: Atrial and ventricular dysrhythmias
> - **Adverse Effects/ Side effects**: dizziness, tinnitus, drowsiness, fatigue
> - **Other examples of this class of medication**: Quinidine, Disopyramide (Norpace), Mexiletine (Mexitil), Phenytoin (Dilantin)

> ### Category: Potassium Channel Blockers
> - **Prototype**: Amiodarone (Cordarone, Pacerone)
> - **Mechanism of Action**: Blocks transmission of potassium in the repolarization period. This delays repolarization, and reduces conduction through the AV node, bundles of His and Purkinje fibers
> - **Action (Uses)**: Ventricular fibrillation, ventricular tachycardia
> - **Adverse Effects/ Side effects**: pulmonary toxicities, disruption of heart rhythm (QRS complex, PR and QT intervals), AV block, hypotension, visual impairment
> - **Other examples of this class of medication**: Bretylium, Sotalol (Betapace), Dofetilide (Tikosyn)

> ### Other Categories that act as Antidysrhythmics: Beta Blockers (see Antihypertensives) and Calcium Channel Blockers (see Antihypertensives)

Classification: Antihyperlipidemic (Antilipidemic) Medications

- ➢ **Category**: HMG-CoA Reductase Inhibitors (Statins)
  - **Prototype**: Atorvastatin (Lipitor)
  - **Mechanism of Action**: HMG-CoA reductase is an enzyme produced in the liver which helps the liver produce 80% of the cholesterol in our body. Statin drugs inhibit HMG-CoA reductase. It also increases the number of LDL receptors on liver cells to remove more LDL (the "bad" cholesterol)
  - **Action (Uses)**: Hypercholesterolemia, prevention of cardiovascular events, post MI therapy
  - **Adverse Effects/ Side effects**: headache, myopathy, hepatotoxicity, rash, GI complaints
  - **Other examples of this class of medication**: Fluvastatin (Lescol), Lovastatin (Mevacor, Altoprev), Provastatin (Pravachol), Rosuvastatin (Crestor), Simvastatin (Zocor), Ezetmibe (Zetia)

Classification: Angina Medications

- ➢ **Category: Organic Nitrates**
  - **Prototype**: Nitroglycerine
  - **Mechanism of Action**: Dilates veins, decreases venous return to the heart. This reduces ventricular filling and wall tension. Also reduces cardiac oxygen demand.
  - **Action (Uses)**: Angina, myocardial infarction
  - **Adverse Effects/ Side effects**: headache, orthostatic hypotension, reflex tachycardia, tolerance to drug effect
  - **Similar agents of this class of medication**: Isosorbide mononitrate, isosorbide dinitrate, amyl nitrate

- ➢ **Other Categories used for Angina: Beta blockers** (See earlier discussion), **Calcium Channel Blockers** (See earlier discussion)

Classification: Anticoagulant Medications

- ➢ **Prototype**: Heparin
  - **Mechanism of Action**: Suppresses formation of fibrin in veins, inactivates clotting factors thrombin and Xa. Anticoagulant effect develops quickly
  - **Action (Uses)**: Pulmonary embolism (PE), stroke, DVT, prevention of postoperative thrombosis, acute myocardial infarction (MI)
  - **Adverse Effects/ Side effects**: Bleeding, heparin induced thrombocytopenia (HIT), hypersensitivity reaction (fever, chills, urticaria)
  - **Other examples of this class of medication**: Enoxaparin (Lovenox), Dalteparin (Fragmin), Tinzaparin (Innohep)

- ➢ **Prototype**: Warfarin (Coumadin, Jantoven)
  - **Mechanism of Action**: Reduces production of clotting factors, antagonizes Vitamin K, blocks synthesis of clotting factors and prothrombin. It takes a few days for effects to occur.
  - **Action (Uses)**: Long term prophylaxis of venous thrombosis and PE, prevention of thromboembolism in patients with mechanical heart valves and atrial fibrillation
  - **Adverse Effects/ Side effects**: Hemorrhage, skin disorders, GI disturbances, increased risk of fractures with long term use, many drug interactions, must keep intake of vitamin K foods constant

Classification: Antiplatelet Medications

➢ **Category: Cyclooxygenase (COX) Inhibitors**
- **Prototype**: Aspirin
- **Mechanism of Action**: Irreversible inhibition of COX-1 and COX-2. Suppresses platelet aggregation, decreases prostaglandin synthesis, reduces inflammation, pain and fever
- **Action (Uses)**: Ischemic stroke, myocardial infarction (previous MI or prevention), reduction of pain, inflammation, fever
- **Adverse Effects/ Side effects**: Gastric distress, GI bleeding, gastric ulceration and bleeding, not used in children because of risk of Reye's syndrome, renal impairment

➢ **Category: Adenosine diphosphate (ADP) receptor antagonists**
- **Prototype**: Clopidogrel (Plavix)
- **Mechanism of Action**: Blocks ADP receptors so that platelets are unable to aggregate (stick together)
- **Action (Uses)**: Prevents blockage of coronary artery stents, reduces thrombotic events (MI, ischemic stroke)
- **Adverse Effects/ Side effects**: Dyspepsia, diarrhea, rash, GI bleeding, intracranial hemorrhage

➢ **Category: Glycoprotein IIb/IIIa- Receptor antagonists**
- **Prototype**: Abciximab (RePro)
- **Mechanism of Action**: Causes reversible blockade of platelet GP IIb/IIIa receptors which interferes with the final step of platelet aggregation
- **Action (Uses)**: Prevents ischemic events in patients with acute coronary syndrome
- **Adverse Effects/ Side effects**: Hemorrhage

Classification: Thrombolytic Drugs

➢ **Prototype**: Alteplase (tPA)
- **Mechanism of Action**: Converts plasminogen to plasmin. (Plasmin is an enzyme that digests the fibrin matrix of clots.) Dissolves existing clots
- **Action (Uses)**: Acute myocardial infarction (MI), pulmonary embolism, ischemic stroke
- **Adverse Effects/ Side Effects**: Bleeding, intracranial hemorrhage

Antibiotics, Antivirals, Antiretrovirals, Antifungals

Classification: Antibiotics (following are a few examples of categories)

> **Category: Aminoglycosides**
> - **Prototype**: Gentamicin
> - **Mechanism of Action**: Disrupts bacterial protein synthesis
> - **Action (Uses)**: Effective against aerobic gram negative bacteria
> - **Adverse Effects/ Side effects**: Nephrotoxicity, ototoxicity, respiratory arrest
> - **Other examples of this class of medication**: Tobramycin, Amikacin (Amikin)

> **Category: Fluoroquinolones**
> - **Prototype**: Ciprofloxacin (Cipro)
> - **Mechanism of Action**: Inhibits bacterial DNA and cell division
> - **Action (Uses)**: infections of urinary, respiratory, and GI tracts, bones, joints, skin, soft tissues, anthrax
> - **Adverse Effects/ Side effects**: Achilles tendon rupture and tendinitis, GI upset, CNS effects (dizziness, headache, restlessness). Do not take with dairy or iron
> - **Other examples of this class of medication**: Moxifloxacin (Avelox), Levofloxacin (Levaquin), Gemifloxacin (Factive)

> **Category: Penicillin**
> - **Prototypes**: Amoxicillin (Novamox, Amoxil), Benzylpenicillin (Penicillin G), Nafcillin (Unipen), Ticarcillin (Ticar), Piperacillin (Pipracil)- many other types and examples of penicillin's are also available.
> - **Mechanism of Action**: Inhibits bacterial cell wall synthesis
> - **Action (Uses)**: used for wide range of bacterial infections (most gram positive and some gram negative) including streptococcal, syphilis, Lyme disease,
> - **Adverse Effects/ Side effects**: GI effects, diarrhea, nausea, rash & allergic reactions

> **Category: Cephalosporins**
> - **Prototype**: 1st generation: Cephalexin (Keflex)
>   - 2nd generation: Cefprozil (Cefzil)
>   - 3rd generation: Ceftriaxone (Rocephin)
>   - 4th generation: Cefepime (Maxipime)
>   - 5th generation: Ceftobiprole (Zeftera)
> - **Mechanism of Action**: Inhibits bacterial cell wall synthesis
> - **Action (Uses)**: 1st gen: Gram + infections, 2nd gen: increased ability to fight Gram – infections, 3rd gen: better against Gram – infections and able to penetrate cerebrospinal fluid (useful with bacterial meningitis), 4th gen: pseudomonal infections, 5th gen: MRSA
> - **Adverse Effects/ Side effects**: Allergic reaction, thrombophlebitis, GI upset, diarrhea, nausea (especially with alcohol use)

➢ **Category: Macrolides**
  - **Prototype**: Azithromycin (Erythocin)
  - **Mechanism of Action**: Inhibits bacterial cell wall synthesis
  - **Action (Uses)**: broad spectrum- active against most Gram + and Gram- bacteria. Can be used as an alternative to penicillin in PCN allergic individuals
  - **Adverse Effects/ Side effects**: GI effects, liver injury
  - **Other examples of this class of medication**: Azithromycin (Zithromax), Clarithromycin (Biaxin), Dirithromycin (Dynabac)

➢ **Category: Tetracyclines**
  - **Prototype**: Doxycycline (Vibramycin)
  - **Mechanism of Action**: Inhibits bacterial cell wall synthesis
  - **Action (Uses)**: Broad spectrum antibiotics, Rocky mountain spotted fever, typhus fever, brucella, cholera, pneumonia, Lyme disease, anthrax, peptic ulcer disease (H. pylori), CA-MRSA
  - **Adverse Effects/ Side effects**: GI irritation, candida albicans infections, discoloration of teeth, sensitivity to sunlight
  - **Other examples of this class of medication**: Tetracycline (Sumycin), Minocycline (Minocin), Demeclocycline (Declomycin)

➢ **Category: Vancomycin (Vancocin)**
  - **Mechanism of Action**: Inhibits bacterial cell wall synthesis
  - **Action (Uses)**: Gram + bacteria, MRSA, patients allergic to penicillin
  - **Adverse Effects/ Side effects**: Ototoxicity, thrombophlebitis, flushing, tachycardia

Classification: Antiprotozoal Medications

➢ **Prototype**: Metronidazole (Flagyl)
  - **Mechanism of Action**: Blocks internal functions of protozoa and some anaerobic bacteria
  - **Action (Uses)**: Protozoal infections (Entamoeba histolytica, Giardia lamblia, Trichomonas vaginalis) and anaerobic bacterial infections
  - **Adverse Effects/ Side effects**: Nausea, diarrhea, metallic taste in mouth

Classification: Antiviral Medications

➢ **Prototype**: Acyclovir (Zovirax)
  - **Mechanism of Action**: Suppresses synthesis of viral DNA
  - **Action (Uses)**: Genital herpes, mucocutaneous herpes simplex infections (cold sores), varicella zoster infections
  - **Adverse Effects/ Side effects**: Nausea, headache, vomiting, diarrhea
  - **Other examples of this class of medication**: Valacyclovir (Valtrex), Famciclovir (Famvir), Docosanol (Abbreva)

Classification: Antiretroviral Medications

➤ **Category:** Nucleoside/Nucleotide Reverse Transcriptase Inhibitors (NRTI's)
  - **Prototype:** Zidovudine (Retrovir)
  - **Mechanism of Action:** inhibit viral replication by blocking DNA synthesis
  - **Action (Uses):** HIV
  - **Adverse Effects/ Side effects:** anemia, neutropenia, GI upset
  - **Other examples of this class of medication:** Didanosine (Videx), Stavudine (Zerit), Lamivudine (Epivir)

➤ **Category: Non-Nucleoside Reverse Transcriptase Inhibitors (NNRTI's)**
  - **Prototype:** Efavirenz (Sustiva)
  - **Mechanism of Action:** Binds directly to HIV reverse transcriptase and inhibits reverse transcriptase
  - **Action (Uses):** HIV
  - **Adverse Effects/ Side effects:** CNS symptoms, rash, liver damage
  - **Other examples of this class of medication:** Etravirine (Intelence), Nevirapine (Viramune)

➤ **Category: Protease Inhibitors**
  - **Prototype:** Ritonavir (Norvir)
  - **Mechanism of Action:** inhibits the enzyme protease, which the virus needs to mature
  - **Action (Uses):** HIV
  - **Adverse Effects/ Side effects:** hyperglycemia, fat maldistribution, hyperlipidemia, bone loss
  - **Other examples of this class of medication:** Nelfinavir (Viracept), Saquinavir (Invirase), Indinavir (Crixivan)

Classification: Antifungal Medications

➤ **Prototype:** Itraconazole (Sporanox)
  - **Mechanism of Action:** Causes cell wall of mycoses to leak
  - **Action (Uses):** Systemic and superficial mycoses (fungi)
  - **Adverse Effects/ Side effects:** GI effects, headache, abdominal pain, edema
  - **Other examples of this class of medication:** Fluconazole (Diflucan), Clotrimazole (Lotrimin), Miconazole (Monistat, Desenex), Ketoconazole (Nizoral), Terbinafine (Lamisil)

Digestive (Gastrointestinal)

Classification: Antinausea / Antiemetic Medications

- **Prototypes**: Hydroxyzine (Vistaril, Atarax), Ondansetron (Zofran), Prochlorperazine (Compazine)
  - **Mechanism of Action**: The different prototypes will block some of the following receptors: serotonin, 5-HT$_3$, dopamine, histaminergic, cholinergic
  - **Action (Uses)**: Nausea, nausea after chemotherapy
  - **Adverse Effects/ Side effects**: headache, diarrhea, dizziness, hypotension, sedation, blurry vision, anticholinergic effects (BUDCAT)

Classification: Gastric Acid Inhibitors

- **Category: Histamine$_2$ Receptor Antagonist**
  - **Prototype**: Cimetidine (Tagamet)
  - **Mechanism of Action**: Blocks H$_2$ receptors on parietal cells of stomach, therefore decreasing gastric acid production
  - **Action (Uses)**: Gastric and duodenal ulcers, heartburn, GERD, acid indigestion
  - **Adverse Effects/ Side effects**: Rare- confusion, hallucinations, CNS depression or excitation
  - **Other examples of this class of medication**: Ranitidine (Zantac), Famotidine (Pepcid), Nizatidine (Axid)

- **Category: Proton Pump Inhibitors**
  - **Prototype**: Omeprazole (Prilosec)
  - **Mechanism of Action**: Inhibits enzyme that generates acid production
  - **Action (Uses)**: Gastric and duodenal ulcers, heartburn, GERD, acid indigestion
  - **Adverse Effects/ Side effects**: Headache, diarrhea, nausea, vomiting, gastric cancer, hip fracture
  - **Other examples of this class of medication**: Esomeprazole (Nexium), Lansoprazole (Prevacid)

Classification: Antidiarrheal medications

- **Prototype: Loperamide (Imodium)**
  - **Mechanism of Action**: Decreases muscular activity in the intestines, slowing down the number of times the person needs to go to the bathroom
  - **Action (Uses)**: Diarrhea, traveler's diarrhea, diarrhea in people with inflammatory bowel disease
  - **Adverse Effects/ Side effects**: dizziness, drowsiness, constipation
  - **Other examples of this class of medication**: Kaopectate 1-D

Classification: Weight Management Medications

- ➤ **Category: Appetite Suppressant Medications**
  - **Prototype**: Phentermine (Lonamin)
  - **Mechanism of Action**: Acts as a sympathomimetic agent (mimics sympathetic nervous system responses, including appetite suppression)
  - **Action (Uses)**: Appetite suppression in obese individuals (BMI of 30 or over)
  - **Adverse Effects/ Side effects**: Only for use in short term (a few weeks), high risk of addiction (very similar chemically to amphetamines), dizziness, dry mouth, difficulty sleeping, irritability, nausea, vomiting, diarrhea
  - **Other examples of this class of medication**: Adipex-P, Profast

- ➤ **Category: Fat Absorption Inhibitor**
  - **Prototype**: Orlistat (Prescription name= Xenical; Over the counter name= Alli)
  - **Mechanism of Action**: Blocks the digestive enzymes which break fats down into their smaller building blocks- fatty acids. The undigested fats are unable to be absorbed and are then excreted from the body via the feces.
  - **Action (Uses)**: Weight loss for significantly overweight individuals
  - **Adverse Effects/ Side effects**: Fatty oily stools, increased gas and bloating, poor bowel control, increased urge to defecate

Classification: Stool Softeners/Laxatives

- ➤ **Category: Bulk Producing Agent**
  - **Prototype**: Psyllium Husk (Metamucil), methylcellulose (Citrucel)
  - **Mechanism of Action**: The fiber in these agents acts to absorb water, which adds moisture to the fecal material. This makes it easier for the large intestine to expel the feces.
  - **Action (Uses)**: Constipation; Soften the fecal material and make it easier to expel feces
  - **Adverse Effects/ Side effects**: Should be taken with a lot of water. Can impair absorption of other medications,
  - **Other examples of this class of medication**: Dietary fiber in foods (apples, bran, broccoli, prunes)

- ➤ **Category: Stool Softeners**
  - **Prototype**: Docuset (Colase, Correctol)
  - **Mechanism of Action**: Acts as a surfactant, allows water and fat to be incorporated into the fecal material- softening it. This makes it easier for the body to expel the fecal material.
  - **Action (Uses)**: Constipation, used after surgery to prevent straining while defecating
  - **Adverse Effects/ Side effects**: Diarrhea, stomach pain, cramping
  - **Other examples of this class of medication**: Ex-lax, Senocot

Respiratory

Classification: Anti-Asthmatic Medications

> **Category: Beta₂-Adrenergic Agonists Bronchodilators**
>   - **Prototype**: Short acting: Albuterol (Proventil, Ventolin, Accuneb); Long lasting: Salmeterol (Serevent)
>   - **Mechanism of Action**: Activates Beta₂-Adrenergic receptors in the lungs, promoting bronchodilation
>   - **Action (Uses)**: Asthma. Short acting can be used as rescue inhaler
>   - **Adverse Effects/ Side effects**: Tachycardia, angina, tremor, leg cramps

> **Category: Anti-inflammatory Drugs for Asthma**
>   - **Prototype**: Cromolyn (Intal)
>   - **Mechanism of Action**: Suppresses inflammation, prevents release of histamine. Not a bronchodilator. Not used for rescue, must be taken on a fixed schedule
>   - **Action (Uses)**: Asthma
>   - **Adverse Effects/ Side effects**: Rare- cough or bronchospasm. Safest of all anti-asthma meds

> **Category: Inhaled Corticosteroids**
>   - **Prototype**: Fluticasone Propionate (Flovent, Advair Diskus)
>   - **Mechanism of Action**: Suppresses inflammation of asthma, decreases leukotrienes, histamine, prostaglandin, eosinophils, and leukocytes. Reduces edema of airway and mucus production.
>   - **Action (Uses)**: Asthma- given on fixed schedule. Takes 2-8 days to see effects. Maximum benefit in 4-6 weeks; COPD
>   - **Adverse Effects/ Side effects**: oropharyngeal candidiasis, adrenal suppression, bone loss, cataracts, glaucoma
>   - **Other examples of this class of medication**: Beclomethasone dipropionate (QVAR), Budesonide (Pulmicort Turbohaler, Pulmocort Respules), Budesonide/Formoterol (Symbicort)

> **Category: Leukotriene Modifiers**
>   - **Prototype**: Montelukast (Singulair)
>   - **Mechanism of Action**: Blocks leukotriene receptors- reduces inflammation, bronchoconstriction, and edema
>   - **Action (Uses)**: Asthma (not used for rescue), prevention of exercise induced asthma, allergic rhinitis
>   - **Adverse Effects/ Side effects**: GI upset, delayed effect, possible rare neuropsychiatric effects

Classification: Cough Medications

> **Category: Cough Suppressors (Antitussive medications)**
> - **Prototype**: Dextromethorphan (DM) (Robitussin)
> - **Mechanism of Action**: Elevates the threshold for coughing
> - **Action (Uses)**: For non-productive coughs, chronic coughing, acute illness
> - **Adverse Effects/ Side effects**: Nausea, drowsiness, gastrointestinal disturbances. At higher doses can be a drug of abuse due to sensations such as euphoria, elevated mood, creative dreaming – called "robbo-tripping".
> - **Other examples of this class of medication**: Codeine (has high addiction possibility), Pertussin, Sucrets, Vicks Formula 44, can also be combined with an expectorant such as guaifenesin.

> **Category: Expectorants**
> - **Prototype**: Guaifenesin (Mucinex)
> - **Mechanism of Action**: Thins mucus, making it easier to expel when coughing
> - **Action (Uses)**: Productive coughing
> - **Adverse Effects/ Side effects**: Should not be used on children under age of 4. Children ages 4-11 must use children's formula and should be supervised closely for any adverse side effects. Nausea, vomiting, diarrhea, kidney stones. Severe allergic reactions may be seen.
> - **Other examples of this class of medication**: Tussin, KidsEEZE, Vicks Day-Quil

Classification: Bronchodilator Anticholinergic/Antimuscarinic

- **Prototype**: Ipratropium bromide (Atrovent)
- **Mechanism of Action**: Inhibits muscarinic receptors, leading to bronchodilation. This opens airways and makes breathing easier
- **Action (Uses)**: Bronchodilation in patients with COPD (emphysema and chronic bronchitis)
- **Adverse Effects/ Side effects**: Dry mouth, arthritis, coughing, influenza-like symptoms
- **Other examples of this class of medication**: Tiotropium bromide (Spiriva Handihaler)

Allergy Medications

Classification: Allergy medications

➢ **Category: Intranasal Glucocorticoids**
- **Prototype:** Fluticasone (Flonase)
- **Mechanism of Action:** Acts as an anti-inflammatory medication
- **Action (Uses):** seasonal and perennial rhinitis, sneezing, nasal itching
- **Adverse Effects/ Side effects:** Drying of nasal mucosa, burning or itching, sore throat, headache, nose bleeds
- **Other examples of this class of medication:** Flunisolide (Nasarel), Mometasone (Nasonex), Budesonide (Rhinocort Aqua)

➢ **Category: H_1 antagonist antihistamines**
- **Prototype:** 1st Generation: Diphenhydramine (Benadryl); 2nd Generation (Non-sedating): Loratadine (Claritin)
- **Mechanism of Action:** Blocks H1 receptors, reducing actions of histamine.
- **Action (Uses):** allergic rhinitis, urticaria. 1st generation can be used for insomnia and as an antitussive
- **Adverse Effects/ Side effects:** 1st generation: sedation, confusion, fatigue, GI disturbances. 2nd generation: hepatic or renal impairment
- **Other examples of this class of medication:** 1st gen: Chlorpheniramine (Chlor-trimeton), Clemastine (Tavist), Dexchlorpheniramine

Smoking Cessation Medications

Classification: Smoking Cessation Medications

> **Category: Nicotine Replacement Therapy**
> - **Prototype**: Nicoderm
> - **Mechanism of Action**: Replaces the nicotine from cigarettes
> - **Action (Uses)**: Smoking cessation
> - **Adverse Effects/ Side effects**: Can be taken in as patch placed on the skin, or chewed as gum. If using the patch, side effects can include itching and redness at the site of the patch application. Headache, dizziness, nausea, flushing can occur
> - **Other examples of this class of medication**: Habitrol, Nicotrol

> **Category: Sustained Release Bupropion**
> - **Prototype**: Wellbutrin, Zyban
> - **Mechanism of Action**: Is a nicotinic acetylcholine receptor antagonist. Reduces nicotine craving and withdrawal symptoms.
> - **Action (Uses)**: Smoking cessation, antidepressant
> - **Adverse Effects/ Side effects**: Dry mouth, nausea, epileptic seizures, hypertension, insomnia, tremor
> - **Other examples of this class of medication**: Voxra

> **Category: Nicotine Receptor Partial Agonist**
> - **Prototype**: Varenicline (Chantix)
> - **Mechanism of Action**: Stimulates nicotine receptors in the body less strongly than nicotine does.
> - **Action (Uses)**: Smoking cessation
> - **Adverse Effects/ Side effects**: Headache, nausea, constipation, difficulty sleeping, depressed mood, suicidal thoughts, possible cardiovascular side effects

Pain Relief

Classification: Non-Steroidal Anti-Inflammatory Drug (NSAIDS)

> **Category: Cyclooxygenase Inhibitors (Aspirin)-** see earlier discussion

> **Category: Non Aspirin Cyclooxygenase Inhibitors**
> - **Prototype:** Ibuprofen (Advil, Motrin)
> - **Mechanism of Action:** Inhibits COX-1 and COX-2, inhibits prostaglandin synthesis.
> - **Action (Uses):** Has anti-inflammatory and anti-pyretic actions. Fever, pain, arthritis, inflammation
> - **Adverse Effects/ Side effects:** Bleeding, renal impairment, gastric ulceration, Reye's syndrome, risk of MI and stroke
> - **Other examples of this class of medication:** Naproxen (Aleve, Naprelan, Naprosyn). 2nd generation: Celecoxib (Celebrex)

Classification: Aniline analgesic and antipyretic

> **Prototype:** Acetaminophen (Tylenol)
> - **Mechanism of Action:** Reduces prostaglandin synthesis
> - **Action (Uses):** No anti-inflammatory properties (therefore not technically an NSAID), fever, headache, pain reliever, preferred in children
> - **Adverse Effects/ Side effects:** Hepatic necrosis

Classification: Local Anesthetics

> **Prototype:** Lidocaine
> - **Mechanism of Action:** Blocks sodium channels in neuron membrane, therefore stopping nerve conduction
> - **Action (Uses):** Surgical local anesthesia
> - **Adverse Effects/ Side effects:** CNS excitation followed by depression, confusion, convulsions, respiratory depression, bradycardia, heart block, cardiac arrest, drowsiness, loss of sensation
> - **Other examples of this class of medication:** Procaine (Novocain), Bupivacaine (Marcaine)

Classification: General Anesthetics

➢ **Prototype:** See below for examples
- **Mechanism of Action:** Enhances transmission at inhibitory neuron synapses, Depresses transmission at excitatory neuron synapses
- **Action (Uses):** General anesthesia for surgery
- **Adverse Effects/ Side effects:** respiratory and cardiac depression, cardiac dysrhythmias, malignant hyperthermia, aspiration of gastric contents, hepatotoxicity
- **Other examples of this class of medication:**
  - <u>Inhaled Anesthetics:</u> Halothane (Fluothane), Isoflurane (Forane), Enflurane (Ethrane), Desflurane (Suprane), Sevoflurane (Ultane), Nitrous Oxide
  - <u>Intravenous Anesthetics:</u> Thiopental sodium (Pentothal), Methohexital sodium (Brevital), Diazepam (Valium), Midazolam (Versed), Propofol (Diprivan), Ketaminhe (Ketalar)

Classification: Opioids

➢ **Prototype:** Morphine
- **Mechanism of Action:** Activates mu opioid receptors. When mu receptors are activated it causes analgesia, euphoria, and sedation
- **Action (Uses):** Relief of pain
- **Adverse Effects/ Side effects:** respiratory depression, constipation, orthostatic hypotension, urinary retention, cough suppression, euphoria, sedation, tolerance and physical dependence
- **Other examples of opioid agonists:** Meperidine (Demerol), Methadone (Diskets, Dolophine, Methadose), Heroin, Codeine, Oxycodone (OxyContin, Percodan, Percoset), Hydrocodone (Vicodin, Loriah), Propoxyphene (Darvon), Buprenorphine (Suboxone)

Endocrine

Classification: Glucocorticoids (Steroids)

➤ **Prototype: Prednisone**
- **Mechanism of Action**: Suppresses immune response and inflammation, inhibits prostaglandins, leukotrienes, and histamine
- **Action (Uses)**: anaphylaxis, rheumatoid arthritis, arthritis, SLE, bursitis, skin disorder, replacement therapy for people with Addison's Disease
- **Adverse Effects/ Side effects**: adrenal insufficiency, osteoporosis, myopathy, sodium and water retention, potassium loss
- **Other examples of this class of medication**: Cortisone, Hydrocortisone, Prednisolone, Pethylprednisone

Classification: Antidiabetic Medications

➤ **Category: Oral agents for Type 2 diabetes-Biguanides**
- **Prototype**: Metformin (Glucophage, Fortamet, Glumetza, Riomet)
- **Mechanism of Action**: Inhibits glucose production in liver, reduces glucose absorption in gut, increases insulin sensitivity in tissue cells
- **Action (Uses)**: Preferred drug of choice for Type 2 diabetes
- **Adverse Effects/ Side effects**: GI disturbances, decreased appetite, nausea, diarrhea
- **Other examples of this class of medication**: Sitagliptin (Januvia)

➤ **Category: Insulin**
- **Prototypes**:
  o Short duration, rapid acting: Insulin Lispro (Humalog), Insulin aspart (Novolog)
  o Short duration, slow acting: Regular insulin (Humilin R)
  o Intermediate duration: NPH insulin (Humilin N), Insulin detemir (levemir)
  o Long duration: Insulin glargine (Lantus)
- **Mechanism of Action**: does the actions of insulin (hormone produced by pancreas)
- **Action (Uses)**: All Type 1 diabetics, some type 2 and some gestational diabetics
- **Adverse Effects/ Side effects**: Hypoglycemia

Classification: Thyroid Medications

➤ **Category: Thyroid Hormones**
- **Prototype**: Levothyroxine (Synthroid, Levoxyl)
- **Mechanism of Action**: Converted to T3 in the body, thyroid hormone replacement
- **Action (Uses)**: Hypothyroidism
- **Adverse Effects/ Side effects**: Irritability, insomnia, weight loss, tachycardia

Reproductive

Classification: Erectile Dysfunction Drugs (Sexual Dysfunction Drugs)

- ➢ **Category: PDE-5 Inhibitors**
  - **Prototype**: Sildenafil (Viagra)
  - **Mechanism of Action**: Inhibits PDE-5, enhances normal erectile response to sexual stimuli
  - **Action (Uses)**: Erectile dysfunction (ED)
  - **Adverse Effects/ Side effects**: Hypotension, priapism, optic neuropathy, dyspepsia, headache, nasal congestion, rhinitis, severe hypotension if used within 24 hours of nitrates
  - **Other examples of this class of medication**: Tadalafil (Cialis), Vardenafil (Levitra)

Classification: Birth Control

- ➢ **Category: Oral Contraceptives (Combination)**
  - **Mechanism of Action**: Inhibition of ovulation
  - **Action (Uses)**: Prevention of pregnancy
  - **Adverse Effects/ Side effects**: breast tenderness, nausea, bloating, edema, weight gain, thromboembolic disorders,
  - **Other examples of this class of medication**: Many examples of oral contraceptive brands, here are a few: Ortho-Novum, Ortho-Cyclen, Loestrin, YAZ, Junel, Microgestin

- ➢ **Category: Long Acting Contraceptives/ Subdermal Implants and Injections**
  - **Prototype**: Depot Medrooxyprogesterone Acetate (Depo-Provera)-
    - ▪ Implanon
  - **Mechanism of Action**: delays ovulation. Depo-Provera is injected every three months, Implanon is a rod implant that lasts for 3 years
  - **Action (Uses)**: Prevent pregnancy
  - **Adverse Effects/ Side effects**: Implanon: irregular bleeding. Depo-Provera: bone loss, irregular menses, weight gain, bloating, headache, depression

Classification: Hormone Replacement Therapy (HRT)

- ➢ **Categories: Estrogen Replacement Therapy; Progestin Replacement Therapy and Estrogen/Progestin Combination Replacement Therapy**
  - **Prototypes**: **Estrogen only-** Estrace, Dienestrol, Estraderm; **Progestin only-** Medroxyprogesterone (Cycrin, Prometrium); **Estrogen/Progestin Combination Therapy-** Prempro, Premphase
  - **Mechanism of Action**: Estrogen, progestin, and/or estrogen+progesterone combination replacement
  - **Action (Uses)**: Treatment of menopause, osteoporosis, hysterectomy patients
  - **Adverse Effects/ Side effects**: Comes in the form of oral pill, skin patch, gel, cream, or vaginal suppository. Side effects: monthly bleeding, irregular spotting, breast tenderness. May increase risk of heart attack, stroke, blood clots in legs and lungs, breast cancer
  - **Other examples of this class of medication**: Climara-Pro, FemHRT, Ortho-Prefest, Aygestin, Climara, Menset, Premarin,

Topical Skin Medications

Classification: Acne Medications (Anti-Acne)

- **Prototype: Benzoyl Peroxide**
  - **Mechanism of Action**: Slowly releases oxygen, acts as an antibacterial, can help with drying of acne lesions (comedo)
  - **Action (Uses)**: Acne, can also be used to treat decubitus ulcers
  - **Adverse Effects/ Side effects**: Burning sensation, redness of skin, stinging of skin

- **Prototype: Salicylic Acid**
  - **Mechanism of Action**: Weakens the keratin in the stratum corneum of the skin, allowing outer layers of the stratum corneum to slough off. This is useful in treating warts. Can also act as an antiseptic.
  - **Action (Uses)**: Acne, wart removal, psoriasis
  - **Adverse Effects/ Side effects**: Burning sensation, redness of skin, stinging of skin

- **Prototype: Tretinoin (Retin A)**
  - **Mechanism of Action**: Not totally understood. Researchers think that it increases activity and cell turn over in follicles of the skin- helping to release contents of the comedo
  - **Action (Uses)**: Acne, wrinkles on the skin, hyperpigmentation of the skin, acute promyelocytic leukemia
  - **Adverse Effects/ Side effects**: Skin will be very sensitive to sunlight- so avoid sun exposure on treated areas. Burning, redness, peeling, inflammation of the skin. Allergic reactions such as hives, swelling of tongue or lips may also occur.

Classification: Antifungal Medications

- Please see this discussion earlier in this chapter

Classification: Glucocorticoids (Steroids)

- Please see this discussion earlier in this chapter

Anticancer Medications (Antineoplastic Medications)

Also known as "Chemotherapy"

Classification: Antimetabolite Medications

> **Prototypes: Methotrexate, Pemetrexed (Alimta)**
> - **Mechanism of Action**: Block DNA replication in cancerous cells, by mimicking components of nucleotides needed in replication. Unable to complete replication and mitosis, the cell dies.
> - **Action (Uses)**: Cancer treatment, autoimmune diseases, ectopic pregnancy (methotrexate)
> - **Adverse Effects/ Side effects**: Increased risk of bleeding, nausea, vomiting, hair loss, immunosuppression, fatigue
> - **Other examples of this class of medication**: Gemcitabine, Capecitabine

Classification: Alkylating Agents

> **Prototypes: Cyclophosphamide (Neosar, Cytoxan);**
> - **Mechanism of Action**: These drugs bind onto DNA of the cancerous cells, triggering the cells to die when they try to attempt mitosis.
> - **Action (Uses)**: Cancer treatment, autoimmune diseases
> - **Adverse Effects/ Side effects**: Increases risk of developing leukemia,   Increased risk of bleeding, nausea, vomiting, hair loss, immunosuppression, fatigue

Classification: Anti-tumor Antibiotics

> **Prototypes: Anthracyclines (Doxorubicin, Daunorubicin, Epirubicin, Idarubicin)**
> - **Mechanism of Action**: Can lodge themselves in-between the strands of DNA in the cancer cell or can generate free radicals which damage the cancer cells
> - **Action (Uses)**: Cancer treatment
> - **Adverse Effects/ Side effects**: Heart damage if used in high doses. Increased risk of bleeding, nausea, vomiting, hair loss, immunosuppression, fatigue
> - **Other examples of this class of medication**: Mitomycin-C, Actinomycin-D, Bleomycin

Classification: Mitotic Inhibitors

> **Prototypes: Vinca alkaloids: vincristine (Oncovin), vinblastine (Velban)**
> - **Mechanism of Action**: Interfere in the mitosis of cancer cells, by preventing proper functioning of the microtubules.
> - **Action (Uses)**: Cancer treatment
> - **Adverse Effects/ Side effects**: May cause peripheral nerve damage. Increased risk of bleeding, nausea, vomiting, hair loss, immunosuppression, fatigue
> - **Other examples of this class of medication**: Taxanes: paclitaxel (Taxol), docetaxel (Taxotere)

Immune Modulators

Classification: Antirheumatic medications

> **Prototypes: Adalimumab (Humira)**
> - **Mechanism of Action**: Adalimumab stops Tissue Necrosis Factor activity (TNF). Abatacept blocks cytotoxic T-cell activity.
> - **Action (Uses)**: Rheumatoid Arthritis, Plaque Psoriasis, Crohn's disease, Ulcerative Colitis, Ankylosing Spondylitis
> - **Adverse Effects/ Side effects**: Increased risk of bleeding, increased risk of infections, headache, body aches, gas with abdominal pain, light headedness, insomnia, hives
> - **Other examples of this class of medication**: Abatacept (Orencia)

Classification: Immunologic Agents

> **Prototypes: Infliximab (Remicade)**
> - **Mechanism of Action**: Stops Tissue Necrosis Factor activity (TNF).
> - **Action (Uses)**: Rheumatoid Arthritis, Crohn's disease, Ulcerative Colitis, Ankylosing Spondylitis, Plaque Psoriasis
> - **Adverse Effects/ Side effects**: Increased risk of bleeding, increased risk of infections, headache, body aches, abdominal pain, chest pain, chill, cough, hives, itching
> - **Other examples of this class of medication**: Ustekinumab (Stelara)

Classification: Immune Suppressant Medications

> **Prototypes: Etanercept (Enbrel), Cyclosporin**
> - **Mechanism of Action**: Stops Tissue Necrosis Factor activity (TNF) or blocks Cytotoxic T-cell activity
> - **Action (Uses)**: Rheumatoid Arthritis, Ankylosing Spondylitis, Plaque Psoriasis, after tissue transplant to prevent rejection (Cyclosporin)
> - **Adverse Effects/ Side effects**: Increased risk of bleeding, increased risk of infections, skin reaction at site of injection, rhinitis, upper respiratory tract infection,
> - **Other examples of this class of medication**: Alefacept (Amevive)

Classification: Granulocyte Colony Stimulating Factor

> **Prototypes: Pegfilgrastim (Neulasta)**
> - **Mechanism of Action**: Stimulates production of neutrophils (a type of WBC) to decrease risk of infection in chemotherapy patients
> - **Action (Uses)**: Prevents neutropenia in chemotherapy patients
> - **Adverse Effects/ Side effects**: bone pain, tenderness at injection site, dizziness, rash, shortness of breath. Do not use in patients with sickle cell anemia, latex allergy, or myeloid leukemia. Administer at least 24 hours *after* a chemotherapy session

Drugs of Abuse

Classification: Drugs of Abuse (including alcohol and tobacco)

➤ **Alcohol:** Effects- depression of CNS, activation of the dopamine reward circuit in the brain, leading to adaptive changes in the circuit which can make it more difficult to control use. Other effects are: nutritional deficiencies, sleep disruption, dilation of cutaneous blood vessels, elevation of blood pressure, hepatitis, cirrhosis, diuresis

➤ **Nicotine:** Cigarette smoking is the greatest single cause of preventable illness and premature death. Nicotine acts on nicotinic receptors. Low doses activate nicotinic receptors, where high doses block them. Effects are: elevated blood pressure and increased strain on the heart, increased secretion of gastric secretions, may induce vomiting, increases alertness, decreases aggression, suppresses appetite, and may increase stimulation of the dopamine pleasure centers in the brain. Can cause cardiovascular disease, many cancers (lung, larynx, mouth, pharynx, bladder, cervix, kidney, pancreas, and stomach), leukemia, type 2 diabetes. Can be harmful to fetal development. For information on Smoking Cessation medications, see the discussion on them earlier in this chapter.

➤ **Cocaine/Crack:** is a psychostimulant and a sympathomimetic. Similar CNS effects as amphetamines. It increases activation of dopamine receptors in the brain, causing euphoria. It also can produce local anesthesia, vasoconstriction and cardiac stimulation. Can be inhaled (cocaine) or rarely through an IV. Crack is more heat stabile and is usually smoked (freebasing). At usual doses, cocaine produces euphoria- often followed by dysphoria. Users will re-ingest more cocaine or crack after the euphoria stage to try to avoid the dysphoria. Overdose is frequent and may be fatal. Overdose can cause cardiac and neurological complications. Chronic cocaine use can cause atrophy of nasal mucosa and loss of sense of smell. Chronic crack use can damage lung tissue.

➤ **Marijuana:** Most commonly used illicit drug (according to Federal laws) in the US. The major psychoactive component in marijuana is delta-9-tetrahydrocannabinol (THC). Promotes release of dopamine in brain's reward circuit. Also increases production of prostaglandin E2 and changes neuronal membrane fluidity. Can be administered by smoking or oral ingestion. Marijuana produces three main effects: euphoria, sedation, and hallucination. In low to moderate doses the person may experience euphoria and relaxation, increased appetite, distortion of time perception, increased senses (smell, taste, touch), impairment of driving skills, impairment of short term memory, and temporal disintegration. High doses can lead to hallucinations, delusions, intense anxiety and paranoia. Other physiological effects are; increased heart rate, bronchitis, sinusitis, asthma, decreased spermatogenesis, decreased testosterone, and decreased reproductive hormones in the female.

➤ **D-Lysergic Acid Diethylamide (LSD):** Has effects at cerebral cortex by activating serotonin receptors. Usually is taken orally. LSD alters perception, thinking, feeling, sense of self, emotions, and sense of relationship with the environment. Exactly what will be experienced with each usage varies widely –some perceptions and hallucinations may be positive, some terrifying- and there is no control over what the user will experience. LSD has few physiologic effects- it may stimulate sympathetic nervous system responses.

➤ **Phencyclidine ("PCP", "angel dust")-** Acts in the cerebral cortex and limbic system where it blocks glutamate receptors. Low doses can cause euphoria, release of inhibitions, slurred speech, and motor incoordination. High doses can cause hallucinations, combativeness, and psychosis (which can last for weeks). Suicide may be attempted. Hypertension, coma, seizures, and muscular rigidity may also result.

➤ **3,4-Methylenedioxymethamphetamine (MDMA, Ecstasy):** Has stimulant and psychedelic properties. It promotes the release of serotonin, dopamine, and norepinephrine. It can cause elevated mood, elevated sensory awareness, increased sensitivity to music, increased sociability. It can also cause neurotoxicity, seizures, hyperthermia, and excessive cardiovascular stimulation. It can damage serotonergic neurons, perhaps irreversibly.

➤ **Opioids (Heroin, Oxycodone, Morphine):** See earlier discussion

➤ **Barbiturates (Amobarbital, Secobarbital, pentobarbital):** See earlier discussion

➤ **Amphetamines (Methamphetamine):** See earlier discussion

SUMMARY CHARTS

TOP 10 DRUGS IN SALES (REVENUE) FOR 2013

Rank	Trade Name	Generic Name	Drug Usage	Sales Revenue
1	Abilify	Aripiprazole	Depression, bipolar, schitzophrenia	6.5 billion
2	Nexium	Esomeprazole	Acid reflux (proton pump inhibitor)	6.1 billion
3	Humira	Adalimumab	Rheumatoid Arthritis, Crohn's Disease, Ankylosing Spondylitis	5.5 billion
4	Crestor	Rosuvastatin	Lowering Cholesterol (Antihyperlipidemic)	5.3 billion
5	Cymbalta	Duloxetine	Antidepressant, Anti-anxiety, Fibromyalgia, Neuropathic Pain	5.2 billion
6	Advar Diskus	Fluticasone	Asthma, COPD	5.1 billion
7	Enbrel	Etanercept	Rheumatoid Arthritis, Plaque Psoriasis, Ankylosing Spondylitis	4.7 billion
8	Remicade	Infliximab	Rheumatoid Arthritis, Crohn's Disease, Ankylosing Spondylitis	4.1 billion
9	Copaxone	Glatiramir Acetate	Multiple Sclerosis	3.7 billion
10	Neulasta	Pegfilgrastim	Stimulate WBC production in chemotherapy patients	3.6 billion

TOP 25 PRESCRIBED DRUGS IN 2013

Rank	Trade Name	Generic Name	Drug Usage
1	Synthroid	Levothyroxine	Thyroid medication
2	Crestor	Rosuvastatin	Lowering Cholesterol (Antihyperlipidemic)
3	Nexium	Esomeprazole	Acid reflux (proton pump inhibitor)
4	Cymbalta	Duloxetine	Antidepressant, Anti-anxiety, Fibromyalgia, Neuropathic Pain
5	Ventolin Hfa	Albuterol	Asthma
6	Advair Diskus	Fluticasone	Asthma, COPD
7	Diovan	Valsartan	High Blood Pressure, Heart Failure
8	Vyvanse	Lisdexamfetamine	ADHD (a CNS stimulant)
9	Lyrica	Pregabalin	Seizures, Neuropathic Pain, Fibromyalgia
10	Spiriva Handihaler	Tiotropium Bromide	COPD, Emphysema, Chronic Bronchitis
11	Lantus Solostar	Insulin Glargine	Type I and II Diabetes
12	Lantus	Insulin Glargine	Type I and II Diabetes
13	Celebrex	Celecoxib	Arthritis Pain (a NSAID)
14	Abilify	Aripiprazole	Depression, bipolar, schitzophrenia
15	Januvia	Sitagliptin	Type II Diabetes
16	Namenda	Memantine	Alzheimer's Disease, Dementia
17	Nasonex	Mometasone	Allergy Medication
18	Viagra	Sildenafil	Erectile Dysfunction
19	Zetia	Ezetimibe	Lowering Cholesterol (Antihyperlipidemic)
20	Cialis	Tadalafil	Erectile Dysfunction
21	Suboxone	Buprenorphine	Pain Relief
22	Bystolic	Nebivolol	High Blood Pressure (Beta Blocker)
23	Symbicort	Budesonide/Formoterol	Asthma, COPD
24	Flovent Hfa	Fluticasone Propionate	Asthma
25	Oxycontin	Oxycodone	Pain Relief

The Top 10 Drugs in Sales/Revenue and the Top 25 Prescribed Drugs information is from the IMS Institute for Healthcare Informatics. They produce a report each year on the top drugs in sales and prescriptions (the report tends to be released in late spring for the prior year). I will try to update this manual each year to show the current trends in sales and prescriptions (along with other information in this book). If you would like to view the IMS report on these statistics, the report is titled: "Medicine Use and Shifting Costs of Healthcare: A Review of the Use of Medicines in the U.S. in 2013." The report was released on April 9, 2014. The website to view the report is:

http://www.imshealth.com/portal/site/imshealth/menuitem.762a961826aad98f53c753c71ad8c22a/?vgnextoid=2684d47626745410VgnVCM10000076192ca2RCRD

The goal of giving you the top prescribed drugs and drugs sold is NOT to have you memorize rankings or dollar values. But, being aware of the drugs most commonly prescribed will most likely translate into the prescribed drugs you will most commonly see your patients taking.

Also, some students ask why the top prescribed drugs are not necessarily the same ones in the top revenue sales list. The reason comes down to the cost per dose (which is set by the manufacturer). For example, 30 tablets of Synthroid (the top prescribed drug) costs on average $31. The top drug in revenue (sales) is Abilify. The average cost of 30 tablets of Abilify is $830. This is what allows a drug which might not be as frequently prescribed, to generate more revenue in sales.

Practice Study and Test Questions:

1) Which of the following medication is a benzodiazepine?
      A) Alprazolam (Xanax)
      B) Fluoxetine (Prozac)
      C) Paroxetene (Paxil)
      D) Aripiprazole (Abilify)

2) What are some common general side effects of Anticancer (Antineoplastic) Medications?
      A) hypertension, excessive blood clotting and headaches
      B) increased risk of bleeding, nausea, vomiting, hair loss, immunosuppression, fatigue
      C) tremors, fluid retention, bloating, weight gain
      D) tachycardia, fever, chills, urticaria

3) Which medications might be prescribed for a patient who has rheumatoid arthritis?
      A) Remicade
      B) Humira
      C) Enbrel
      D) all of the above

4) Which medication prototype may be used to treat ADHD?
      A) Phenytoin
      B) Methylphenidate
      C) Levodopa
      D) Ciprofloxacin

5) If a patient has their medication injected into the hypodermis, which route of administration is this?
      A) Oral (PO)
      B) Intravenous (IV)
      C) Intramuscular (IM)
      D) Subcutaneous (subQ)

6) Which of the following medications is not a Non-Steroidal Anti-Inflammatory Medication (NSAIDS)?
      A) Naproxen (Aleve)
      B) Ibuprofen (Advil, Motrin)
      C) Aspirin
      D) Acetaminophen (Tylenol)

7) Which class of medication blocks HMG-CoA reductase as its mechanism of action?
      A) Antiviral medications
      B) Anticoagulant medications
      C) Antihyperlipidemic medications
      D) Smoking cessation medications

8) Which of the following categories is the most commonly prescribed antidepressant?
      A) CCB's
      B) MAOI's
      C) SSRI's
      D) TCA's

9) Which drug of abuse is a sympathomimetic and a psychostimulant?
  A) cocaine
  B) alcohol
  C) marijuana
  D) phencyclidine "PCP"

10) Which category of asthma medications can be used as a "rescue" inhaler (for use during an asthma attack)?
  A) Short Acting Beta2-Adrenergic Agonist Bronchodilator
  B) Inhaled Corticosteroids
  C) Leukotriene Modifiers
  D) Anti-inflammatory Asthma Medications

11) What are possible side effects of Sildenafil (Viagra)?
  A) osteoporosis, water retention, and headache
  B) hypotension, priapism, and headache
  C) bloating, edema and weight gain
  D) hypoglycemia and arrhythmia

12) Which allergy medication blocks H1 receptors?
  A) Mometasone
  B) Diphenhydramine
  C) Fluticasone
  D) Flunisolide

13) Which medication may be utilized for smoking cessation?
  A) Wellbutrin
  B) Zyban
  C) Chantix
  D) All of the above

14) Acyclovir, Valacyclovir (Valtrex), and Famciclovir (Famvir) are examples of
  A) Diuretics
  B) Muscle relaxants
  C) Antiviral medications
  D) Antiplatelet medications

15) Foods rich in Vitamin K, may reduce the effect of
  A) antihyperlipidemics
  B) anticoagulants
  C) antiseizure medications
  D) erectile dysfunction drugs

16) The mechanism of action of Bisphosphonates is
  A) reduces number and activity of osteoclasts
  B) increases activity and number of osteoblasts
  C) increases activity and number of osteoclasts
  D) reduces number and activity of osteoblasts

17) Which of the following is not a category of antihypertension medication?
  A) beta adrenergic blocker
  B) monoamine oxidase inhibitors
  C) calcium channel blocker
  D) angiotensin converting enzyme inhibitor

18) St. John's Wort may interact with the effects of
    A) statin medications
    B) SSRI's
    C) anticoagulants
    D) all of the above

19) Which drug of abuse is the single greatest cause of preventable illness and premature death?
    A) Nicotine
    B) Cocaine/Crack
    C) Heroin
    D) Amphetamines

20) Which of the following medications is a steroid?
    A) Benadryl
    B) Levoxyl
    C) Prednisone
    D) Wellbutrin

21) Which of the following drugs is used to treat thyroid issues?
    A) Esomeprazole (Nexium)
    B) Fluticasone (Advair Diskus)
    C) Levothyroxine (Synthroid)
    D) Aripiprazole (Abilify)

22) Which drug treats COPD?
    A) Symbicort
    B) Advair Diskus
    C) Spiriva Handihaler
    D) All of the above

23) Which of the following medications treats Type I and Type II Diabetes?
    A) Lantus
    B) Cymbalta
    C) Diovan
    D) Humira

24) Which drug is used in patients with Alzheimer's disease?
    A) Pregabalin
    B) Memantine
    C) Nebivolol
    D) Celexicob

25) Which of the following is NOT used in the treatment of a patient with high cholesterol??
    A) Crestor
    B) Zetia
    C) Celebrex
    D) Lipitor

Answers: 1) A 2) B 3) D 4) B 5) D 6) D 7) C 8) C 9) A 10) A 11) B 12) B 13) D 14) C 15) B 16) A 17) B 18) D 19) A 20) C 21) C 22) D 23) A 24) B 25) C

CHAPTER 17: NUTRITION AND SUPPLEMENTS

When discussing nutrition, a few terms and concepts should be defined.

Kilocalories (kcal) also called a "**Calorie**"- this is the energy value found in foods. Carbohydrates, fats and proteins all contain kilocalories. Vitamins and minerals do not contain kilocalories. When a person is looking at the number of "calories" in a food, this is what they are looking at.
- Carbohydrates contain 4 kilocalories/gram
- Proteins contain 4 kilocalories/gram
- Fats contain 9 kilocalories/gram

ATP- Adenosine triphosphate: this is the energy molecule used by body cells to power and fuel their activities. Carbohydrates, fats and proteins can be converted into ATP.

Nutrient: a food substance that is needed for normal physiological processes in the body (such as growth, repair, and normal maintenance).

Recommended Dietary Allowances (RDA) and Adequate Intake (AI)- these are the calculated values of nutrients which should be consumed daily for proper health. These values will change with age, gender, pregnancy or lactation.

Tolerable Upper Intake Level (UL)- highest level of daily intake that should not create any harmful effects. These values will change with age, gender, pregnancy or lactation.

Dietary Reference Intake (DRI) tables- these tables contain the RDA's, AI's, and UL's. The DRI tables are developed by the Food and Nutrition Board of the Institute of Medicine- a division of the National Academy of Sciences.

Nutrient Categories

- **Carbohydrates-** are obtained mostly when consuming plant products. Starches and sugars in fruits, vegetables, and grains are wonderful sources of carbohydrates. Carbohydrates are composed of long chains of sugars- and these long chains of sugars are digested and broken down into simple sugars (like glucose, for example). Carbohydrates are the body's preferred source of energy to make ATP.
- **Proteins-** Are often consumed in the form of meat or dairy- but plant products can also contain proteins (soy, legumes, cereals). Proteins are composed of long chains of amino acids. These long chains are digested in the stomach and small intestine.
- **Lipids (Fats)-** Can be found in animal products (meat and dairy) and plant products (nuts, seeds, vegetable oils). Most animal products (and coconut) contain saturated fats. Most plant products contain unsaturated fats. Lipids are digested in the small intestine and are broken down into fatty acids for use in the body.
- **Vitamins-** absorbed into the bloodstream in the small and large intestine. Vitamins are found in all food groups- so eat a good variety of foods to ensure proper intake. They usually function as coenzymes (they help facilitate chemical reactions in the body). Vitamins usually do not need to be digested in the digestive system- they are simply absorbed in the intestines.
- **Minerals-** Vegetables, legumes, dairy and meat are good sources. Minerals usually do not need to be digested in the digestive system- they are simply absorbed in the small and large intestine.
- **Water-** Water may or may not be considered a nutrient (depends on the text being referenced). But, regardless, water is essential for life.

Determining Normal and Abnormal Weight

Determining a healthy weight value for patients is important. Risk factors for many diseases are weight dependent. Abnormal weight can mean overweight, obese, or underweight. Poor dietary choices, inactivity, medical conditions (for example: anorexia nervosa, hypothyroidism, hyperthyroidism, Crohn's disease, bulimia nervosa) can all cause body weight to move into an abnormal range.

There are many methods for determining the amount of body fat in a patient: skinfold thickness measured with a caliper, underwater weighing, and bioelectric impedance are a few examples. But, these methods are not easily performed by many health care providers (they may need special equipment to perform it). So, two more commonly used methods for assessing abnormal weight are the Body Mass Index (BMI) and the Ideal Body Weight (IBW).

Body Mass Index (BMI)

The Body Mass Index (BMI) is a commonly used and recommended method of determining if someone is underweight or overweight. The BMI is a measure of weight relative to height. BMI values correlate fairly well with chronic disease risk factors. Approximately ½ of the US adults are overweight or obese (BMI ≥25). Mortality significantly increases at a BMI ≥27.

The mathematical formula for determining BMI (using pounds for weight) is:
$$[\text{Weight} \div \text{Height (in)}^2] \times 703 = BMI$$

For example- Height: 5'6" (66") and Weight: 160 lbs. $\Rightarrow$ $[160 \div (66)^2] \times 703 = 25.8$ BMI

BMI (kg/m²)	Weight Status Classification
<18.5	Underweight
18.5 - 24.9	Normal
25.0 - 29.9	Overweight
30.0 - 39.0	Obese
≥40	Severely Obese

** Please note that there are many BMI charts available for use which simplify the process of determining BMI. The health care provider simply needs the patient's height and weight information and they can refer to the chart for the corresponding BMI value (no math!)

Ideal Body Weight (IBW)

The Hamwi formula is another way to determine Ideal Body Weight (IBW) for a patient. IBW can be computed as follows. (Please also remember to allow an additional range of ±10% to allow for frame size and variations in body composition):
- **Females**: 100 pounds for the first 60 inches of height. Add 5 pounds for each additional inch.
  - *Example: For a female who is 5'5" tall (65 inches tall), her ideal body weight is 100 + 25 = 125 pounds.* This value can increase or decrease up to 10% for frame size and composition

- **Males**: 106 pounds for the first 60 inches of height. Add 6 pounds for each additional inch
  - *Example: For a male who is 6'0" tall (72 inches tall), his ideal body weight is 106 + 72 = 178 pounds.* This value can increase or decrease up to 10% for frame size and composition

Abnormal Weight

When dealing with a patient who is underweight or overweight, referral may be needed to another healthcare provider for both medical care and psychological support, if needed.

Overweight and Obesity

The American Heart Association states that obesity rates are climbing in the United States. 29.3 million (33% of boys and 30.4% of girls) children ages 2-9 are overweight or obese. For adults age 20 and older, 157.7 million are overweight or obese (79.9 million men and 74.8 million women). Currently, it is estimated that medical related costs for obesity might cost as much as $147 billion annually. The excess medical costs related to obesity are projected to reach $861-957 billion by 2030.

Where (the location of) the fat is distributed may be more important than quantity. An **android "apple" shape** of the body has fat distribution located around the stomach. A **gynoid "pear" shape** has more weight below the waist. The android "apple" shape has more health risks associated with it. This shape is more common in males than in females. The android "apple" shape could be a sign of *metabolic syndrome*-especially if it is combined with hypertension, high blood sugar (insulin resistance), high triglycerides and low HDL. If a patient has three of those factors, that qualifies as having metabolic syndrome. Metabolic syndrome increases the patient's risk of developing *diabetes or cardiovascular issues (atherosclerosis, heart attack, and stroke).* **Visceral fat**, often seen in the android "apple" shape, is fat which wraps around the internal abdominal organs (the viscera). Visceral fat increases the risk of *insulin resistance (leading to diabetes), heart disease, stroke, and dementia.* A patient can have a healthy BMI, but still have increased visceral fat- which will still raise their risk levels for those conditions.

Obesity raises the risk factors for these conditions: *Stroke, gallbladder disease, hypertension, low HDL, high LDL, high triglycerides, coronary artery disease, cerebral artery disease, type II diabetes and infertility. Other conditions will also be worsened by obesity.*

Underweight

Being underweight also causes health issues. An "underweight person" is usually 15-20% below accepted weight standards. A person may be underweight due to poor nutrition, starvation, or medical conditions such as: anorexia nervosa, bulimia, malabsorption diseases (celiac, Crohn's).

An underweight person increases the risk factors for these conditions: *poor function of the pituitary, thyroid, gonads, and adrenals (leading to many different endocrine disorders), loss of energy, increased susceptibility to infection and injury; osteoporosis, cardiac arrhythmias, distorted body image and other psychological problems.*

Nutritional Supplements:

Definition and Regulation of Dietary Supplements

As defined by Congress in the Dietary Supplement Health and Education Act (DSHEA), which became law in 1994, a dietary supplement is a product that
- is intended to supplement the diet
- contains one or more dietary ingredients (including vitamins; minerals; herbs or other botanicals; amino acids; and other substances) or their constituents;
- is intended to be taken by mouth as a pill, capsule, tablet, or liquid; and
- is labeled on the front panel as being a dietary supplement.

Dietary supplements are regulated by FDA. The types of claims that can be made on the labels of dietary supplements and pharmaceutical drugs differ. Drug manufacturers may claim that their product will diagnose, cure, treat, or prevent a disease (as long as those claims have been approved by the FDA). Dietary supplements may NOT make those same types of claims (although some products will try to do that- until the FDA steps in and tells them to quit). It is difficult to determine the quality of a dietary supplement product from its label. The degree of quality control depends on the manufacturer, the supplier, and others in the production process. There are some third party companies which will test the content of supplements, but no supplement manufacturer is required to have additional testing for quality. So, buyer beware!

Major Classifications of Supplements

The following classes of supplements will be discussed in more detail in this chapter. Here is an overview of the major classifications. The PDR (Physician's Desk Reference) and the Dietary Reference Intake Tables (DRI) are two good references for information on supplements.

Here is a brief overview of a few of the classes of supplements that will be covered in this chapter.

Vitamins: Vitamins are found in foods (and a few are manufactured in our large intestine), they do not need to be chemically digested by our body, and are essential for normal physiologic function. Having too much or too little of certain vitamins can lead to some negative symptoms. There are two main categories of vitamins:
- *Fat soluble vitamins*: A, D, E and K. Fat soluble vitamins are stored in body lipids and pose greater risk of deficiency or toxicity.
- *Water soluble vitamins*: B1, B2, B3, B5, B6, B7, B9, B12, and C. Water soluble vitamins cannot be stored for long periods by the body. Excess levels are usually excreted from the body in the urine.

Minerals: Also are consumed in our diet and do not need to be chemically digested by our body.
- *Macrominerals* are required in larger amounts. We need to consume over 100 mg of these minerals per day (ex. calcium, phosphorus).
- *Microminerals* are required in smaller amounts, usually less than 15 milligrams or in micrograms. Examples of microminerals are the trace elements (ex: iron, selenium)

Amino acids: Are the building blocks of proteins. We consume amino acids when we eat protein. Our digestive system breaks down proteins into these amino acids. The amino acids can then be absorbed into the bloodstream and transported to our body cells for use. *Essential amino acids* must be obtained from the food we eat (we cannot make them in our body). A *"complete" protein* food source contains all of the essential amino acids. *Non-Essential amino acids* can be made in our body (usually by the liver).

Antioxidants: Function to neutralize free radicals, which can be harmful and damage our body cells. Antioxidant vitamins are Vitamin C, E, carotenoids (Vitamin A precursors). Some minerals can have antioxidant properties (selenium, for example). Other materials can be taken as a supplement for antioxidant properties (CoQ10, lycopene, resveratrol, lutein).

FAT SOLUBLE VITAMINS

Vitamin Name	Mechanism/actions in the body	Symptoms of excessive intake	Symptoms of deficiency
Vitamin A (retinol):	Antioxidant; Used in the synthesis of light receptor pigments (retinol) in the retina of the eye; hormone synthesis; growth and development of epithelial, nervous, bone tissue; and immune function	*Hypervitaminosis A-* most commonly due to taking too many supplements (not usually due to natural intake). Vitamin A accumulates in liver and can cause liver damage. Anorexia; nausea and vomiting; dry, itchy, and flaking skin; alopecia; headache	Dry, scaling skin; anorexia; increased susceptibility to infections; night blindness (called xeropthalmia) and conjunctival and cornea abnormalities.
Vitamin D:	Promotes proper absorption and use of calcium and phosphorous, immune regulation, cell growth and proliferation	Hypercalcemia and calcification of soft tissues and blood vessels, kidney stones, fatigue	Deficiency can cause soft, poorly mineralized bones. This is called **rickets** (in children and infants) or **osteomalacia** (in adults).
Vitamin E	Antioxidant- prevents cell membrane damage; dilates blood vessels	Increased risk of bleeding in patients on anticoagulant meds and in patients who are Vitamin K deficient. May increase risk of stroke. Dizziness, weakness.	Rare, mostly seen with low birth weight infants and fat malabsorption conditions (Crohn's, cystic fibrosis). Hemolytic anemia; muscle weakness; degenerative neurological problems
Vitamin K	Obtained from foods in our diet and synthesized in large intestine by our intestinal flora bacteria. Stimulates blood clotting factors and facilitates binding of calcium ions. May help bone density in elderly. People who are taking anticoagulant medications should not take Vitamin K supplements.	Natural forms do not usually cause symptoms of toxicity; synthetic can decrease glutathione, cause liver damage, anemia	May occur with chronic antibiotic use. Newborns also at higher risk of deficiency (due to gut not yet populated with bacterial flora). Recommendations are to supplement all infants with Vitamin K. Defective blood coagulation (severe bleeding on injury) can occur. Symptoms can also include bruising, mineral loss from bone, osteoporosis

WATER SOLUBLE VITAMINS

Vitamin Name	Mechanism/actions in the body	Symptoms of excessive intake	Symptoms of deficiency
Vitamin B1, Thiamin	Co-enzyme for energy metabolism, used in Krebs cycle, nerve function	Rapid pulse, weakness, headache, stomach upset, insomnia	*Beriberi*- muscle weakness; anorexia; enlarged heart; edema, tingling and burning in hands and feet. **Wernike-Korsakoff syndrome**- a disorder of the brain caused by B1 deficiency. Memory problems and nerve damage can be seen.
Vitamin B2, Riboflavin	Used in processing amino acids and fats. Needed to help activate Folate and Vitamin B6 metabolism.	None reported	Cheilosis of lips, glossitis of tongue, oral and pharyngeal edema, peripheral neuropathy, skin rash
Vitamin B3, Niacin	Used in energy metabolism. Used to make adrenal gland hormones. It also lowers LDL and raises HDL.	Liver injury can occur. *Niacin flush*- vasodilation of blood vessels, leading to redness in skin, itching sensation, and increased warmth of skin	*Rare in the developed world. May occur in alcoholics.* **Pellagra**- diarrhea, dermatitis, dementia. Can also cause swelling and redness in the mouth, weakness, dizziness, loss of appetite.
Vitamin B5, Pantothenic Acid	Used in fatty acid synthesis, and Krebs cycle	Generally non-toxic, may cause abdominal discomfort or diarrhea.	Very rare, extreme malnutrition can cause neuropathy, "burning feet", fatigue, vomiting
Vitamin B6, Pyridoxine	Needed to make serotonin, norepinephrine, and myelin. Can lower homocysteine levels	1-6 g/day chronic doses have exhibited peripheral neuropathy, weakness, bloating.	Can occur in alcoholics, patients with hyperthyroidism. Symptoms: dermatitis, glossitis, depression, anemia
Vitamin B7, Biotin	Formed by intestinal bacteria. Coenzyme in energy metabolism (Krebs cycle)	None reported	very rare (can be seen in people who eat more than 2 raw egg whites per day); hallucinations, depression, nausea, scaly dermatitis, alopecia
Vitamin B9, Folic Acid	Needed in amino acid and nucleic acid (DNA/RNA) metabolism, works with Vitamin B12 to make RBC's	Stomach problems, seizures, insomnia. Can mask B12 deficiency	Megaloblastic, macrocytic anemia; diarrhea; fatigue; depression; abnormal cell division and birth defects
Vitamin B12, Cobalamin	Helps form nucleic acids in DNA. Needed for healthy RBC's.	None reported	Mostly due to inadequate absorption. Can cause *pernicious anemia* and/or nerve problems, depression, dementia
Vitamin C, Ascorbic Acid	Antioxidant; needed for collagen formation; used by immune system, assists in iron absorption.	Diarrhea, kidney stones, fatigue	<10mg/day may result in *scurvy*- bleeding gums, petichiae, easy bruising, decaying and loose teeth, delayed wound healing, impaired immune response

MACROMINERALS

Vitamin Name	Mechanism/actions in the body	Symptoms of excessive intake	Symptoms of deficiency
Calcium	Nerve transmissions, muscle contraction, blood clotting. Primary mineral in bone and tooth structure and health	**Hypercalcemia:** >3g/day may result in hypercalcemia, may lead to soft tissue calcification.	**Hypocalcemia:** Rickets, osteomalacia, osteoporosis, tetany
Chloride	Primary anion in body fluids. Maintains pH (acid-base) balance, formation of gastric juice (hydrochloric acid). Commonly consumed as NaCl (table salt).	**Hyperchloremia:** Not seen with normal circulation and renal function. If it occurs, can lead to vomiting, increased blood pressure and/or edema	**Hypochloremia:** Does not occur under normal conditions. Can be seen in a person with severe diarrhea or vomiting. In infants- deficiency can cause anorexia, failure to thrive, weakness, poor growth
Magnesium	Bone strength, nerve impulse transmission, protein synthesis. Magnesium supplementation used for constipation, muscle cramps, restless legs, arrhythmias	Not seen with normal circulation and renal function; 3-5g of Magnesium sulfate can cause diarrhea and possible dehydration.	Depression, weakness, convulsions, growth failure in children, confusion
Phosphorous	Cell membrane structure (phospholipids), bone and tooth formation, energy metabolism and pH regulation	Rare. Can combine with calcium to form mineral deposits in soft tissue. Usually only seen in patients with kidney disease.	Rare, only with malabsorption disorders and malnutrition- rickets, osteomalacia, anorexia, muscle weakness, decreased oxygen utilization
Potassium	Main cation in intracellular fluid. Fluid balance, electrolyte, pH regulation, nerve and muscle function.	**Hyperkalemia-** cardiac arrhythmias and cardiac arrest	**Hypokalemia-** muscle weakness, arrhythmias, fatigue, confusion. Subclinical deficiency can result in muscle cramps
Sodium	Main cation in extracellular fluid. Fluid balance, pH, and electrolyte regulation; nerve transmission; muscle contraction	**Hypernatremia-** High blood pressure; edema in patients with CHF, cirrhosis, or kidney disease	**Hyponatremia-** Not usually seen; excess water intake can lead to *dilutional hyponatremia-* muscle atrophy, weight loss, cramps, disorientation, severe- brain damage
Sulfur	The 3rd most abundant mineral in body tissues. Found in MSM which assists in joint health and connective tissue such as cartilage, tendons and ligaments	Poor growth and possible liver damage.	Deficiencies not conclusively identified, but may be a factor in obesity, joint pain and osteoarthritis, muscle weakness

MICROMINERALS

Vitamin Name	Mechanisms/actions in the body	Symptoms of excessive intake	Symptoms of deficiency
Chromium	Needed for normal use of blood glucose and function of insulin. Important in the metabolism of carbohydrates and fats. Can be supplemented via brewer's yeast.	Lung and kidney damage (though excessive occupational exposure only), otherwise, generally non-toxic	Widespread due to low intake (poor soil), age, and impaired glucose tolerance- insulin resistance, hyperinsulinemia. , Mild deficiency manifests as Syndrome X/Metabolic syndrome (minus the hypertension) and can cause impaired glucose metabolism
Copper	Used in iron utilization, hemoglobin formation, lipid metabolism, neurotransmitters	Rare, seen in *Wilson's disease.* Kayser- Fleischer rings in the eye, muscle weakness, poor coordination, speech difficulties, depression, vomiting, diarrhea	Seen in malabsorption syndromes or excessive antacid ingestion: anemia, neutropenia, bone abnormalities, decreased glutathione
Fluorine	Formation of teeth and bone	**Fluorosis**- mottling of teeth, skeletal deformation, nausea/vomiting	Increased tooth decay, bone development problems
Iodine	Thyroid hormone synthesis. Commonly found added to table salt "iodized salt". Naturally found in seafood.	Intakes up to 2mg/day are safe. Rare to reach toxic levels, but very high intake can damage the thyroid.	Goiter, hypothyroidism, cretinism in infants
Iron	Enzyme Cofactor- iron is needed for oxygen transport to cells. It helps form myoglobin and hemoglobin. Iron supplements should be kept out of reach of children to avoid iron poisoning. Iron supplements need to be taken with vitamin C or other acid	Iron overload can be from excess supplementation or hemochromatosis. Ferritin >200mcg/dL linked to heart disease. Iron poisoning can lead to fatigue, nausea, vomiting, weight loss, shortness of breath, liver damage, cardiac failure, death.	Iron deficiency anemia, fatigue, heart palpitations, headache, irritability, dysphagia, and decreased immune resistance. Iron supplements will increase Hgb and RBCs often within 2 weeks, replenishing body stores can take 6mo-1yr
Manganese	Enzyme Cofactor- brain function, collagen and bone, glucose and lipid metabolism	Can be found in air near industries such as mining, metal processing plants, pesticide producers. Toxic levels can damage brain. Lack of muscle coordination, mental changes, difficulty breathing or swallowing, possible infertility and birth defects may occur.	Skeletal deformation and inhibits collagen production in wound healing.

MICROMINERALS (CONTINUED)

Vitamin Name	Mechanisms/actions in the body	Symptoms of excessive intake	Symptoms of deficiency
Molybdenum	Enzyme Cofactor- acts as a catalyst to break down some amino acids, metabolism of fats and carbohydrates. Also found in tooth enamel.	Up to 1500mcg/day safe. Excess intake can cause uric acid accumulation and gout in areas with high soil molybdenum concentrations	Rare, but can cause defects in uric acid production and decreased metabolism of sulfur containing amino acids
Selenium	Antioxidant- offers cell protection from peroxides and free radicals. Used in reproduction, thyroid hormone metabolism, DNA synthesis. Brazil nuts contain a very high level of selenium (one serving contains 777% of the recommended daily value)	**Selenosis**: most common symptoms are fatigue, hair and nail loss. Patient may have a garlic odor to the breath and metallic taste in the mouth. May also show nausea, skin rashes, diarrhea, and mottled teeth.	Myalgia, Keshan's Disease (a type of heart disease), pancreatic degeneration, male infertility, Kashin-Beck disease (a type of osteoarthritis). *Keshan's and Kashin-Beck disease seen in China, Tibet and Siberia- where low levels of selenium are found.*
Zinc	Used in energy metabolism, protein and collagen synthesis, taste and smell, wound healing, immune system, DNA formation	Chronic doses of ~25mg/day lead to copper deficiency. Can also cause nausea, vomiting, diarrhea, abdominal cramps, headache, and low HDL levels.	Poor wound healing, stunted growth, anorexia, taste and smell changes, hair, skin, and nails, delayed sexual maturation, impotence, mental lethargy

FATS

Type of Fat	Mechanisms/actions in the body	Symptoms of excessive intake	Symptoms of deficiency
Omega 3 Fatty Acids: Eicosapentaenoic acid (EPA) and Docosahexaenioc acid (DHA)	Are anti-atherogenic, anti-inflammatory, decreases triglyceride levels and are used in cell membrane formation. EPA may decrease depression symptoms. Found in fish, plant and nut oils. Should not be used in patients who bruise easily, have a clotting disorder, or people who are taking blood thinning medications	>3000-4000mg/d may result in blood thinning (hemorrhage, bruising, bleeding)	Dermatitis, dry hair, dandruff, brittle nails, polydipsia, polyuria, fatty liver, neuropathy, vision and memory problems, cardiac arrhythmias, inflammatory conditions
Medium Chain Triglycerides (MCT)	To improve the health status of individuals with fat malabsorption problems (celiac disease, Crohn's, liver disease). Made by processing coconut and palm kernel oils. Should not be taken by diabetic patients.	Side effects with supplementation can be: diarrhea, vomiting, irritability, intestinal gas, ketosis (in diabetic patients).	Muscle breakdown in critically ill patients.

PHYTOESTROGENS:

Phytoestrogens are a supplement which has mixed or conflicting opinions on health benefits or risks, depending on the studies that are referenced. Here are some of the reported health benefits and health risks that various studies have described. These risks and benefits will most likely continue to change and be updated as more research is done. And, these risks and benefits may vary depending on the age, gender, ethnicity, and other health conditions of each patient.

Sources of Phytoestrogens	Proposed Health Benefits	Proposed Health Risks
• Soy (Isoflavonoids) • Flax (lignans) • Grape skin and wine (polyphenols-resveratrol) • Kale, Broccoli, Citrus, Green Tea, Chocolate (Flavonoids)	Lowered risk of • osteoporosis • heart disease • coronary artery disease (CAD) • breast cancer • menopausal symptoms	Act as an *Endocrine Disruptor*. This may increase risk of • recurrence of breast cancer in breast cancer patient • dysmenorrhea • abnormal uterine bleeding • abnormal ovulatory cycle • may be involved in low sperm count • may lead to developmental issues in a child such as earlier menarche, sexual precocity, hypospadias in male infants • babies fed a soy base formula may have a higher risk for developing uterine fibroids, longer menstrual bleeding, increased menstrual discomfort.

PLANT STEROL/STANOLS: PHYTOSTEROLS

More studies are currently being done on the *phytosterols (plant sterols and stanols)*. These substances are being added to many food products (margarine, yogurt, mayonnaise, orange juice, milk, snack bars) due to the premise of their LDL lowering ability.

Sources of Phytosterols	Proposed Health Benefits	Proposed Health Risks
• Unrefined vegetable oils • Whole grains • Nuts • Legumes	• Inhibit intestinal absorption of cholesterol • Lowers serum LDL levels (2-3 gm/day can lower LDL 9-14%) • May cause improvement of urinary tract functioning in men with benign prostatic hypertrophy (BPH) • May decrease some types of cancer, may have an anti-inflammatory effect	• Nausea, indigestion, diarrhea, and constipation have occasionally been reported • May interfere with absorption of dietary carotenoids (alpha carotene, beta carotene, lycopene)

AMINO ACIDS

Amino acids are the building blocks of proteins. There are around 20 amino acids used by the human body. The **essential amino acids** are the amino acids which can only be obtained through the diet (they are unable to be manufactured within our bodies). The 9 essential amino acids for adults are: *histidine, isoleucine, leucine, lysine, methionine, phenylalanine, threonine, tryptophan,* and *valine.* Eggs and soy protein are two examples of natural dietary sources of the essential amino acids. The **non-essential amino acids** are amino acids which can be manufactured in our bodies (often by the liver). Some examples of non-essential amino acids are: glutamine, tyrosine, cysteine, and alanine. *Listed below are a few of the amino acids that can be taken as a supplement. The "health benefits" and "health risks" listed below may not be backed by a lot of strong scientific evidence at this time- hence using the word "proposed" with those categories.*

Amino Acid	Proposed Health Benefits	Proposed Health Risks
L-glutamine	May be used by patients undergoing chemotherapy to help lessen side effects. Can be used by HIV/AIDS, Crohn's or Ulcerative Colitis patients to assist in absorbing nutrients when eating. Some say it may improve athletic performance.	Should not be used by people with severe liver disease, those diagnosed with mania or manic mental health conditions, epilepsy, or people with MSG sensitivity.
Lysine	Used to treat cold sores or to improve athletic performance	Can cause stomach pain or diarrhea
Choline	Very similar to B vitamins (more than an amino acid). Can be used in liver diseases (hepatitis, cirrhosis) and asthma. Some people take it to treat or slow neurological conditions (Alzheimer's, depression, dementia, Tourette's, schizophrenia and seizures). Can be taken by pregnant women to prevent neural tube defects.	High levels of intake may cause sweating, diarrhea, vomiting, low blood pressure and a fishy body odor.
Methionine	May be used to treat acetaminophen (Tylenol) overdose to prevent liver damage. May be taken to prevent colon cancer, treat depression, maintain normal liver function, and treat arthritis. A form of methionine called SAMe is used as a supplement for mood support.	High levels of methionine intake may worsen atherosclerosis, promote growth of tumors, or cause brain damage. It may worsen symptoms in patients with schizophrenia.
Tyrosine	Is used in patients with phenylketonuria (PKU). PKU patients cannot make tyrosine in their bodies naturally, so must get their tyrosine through supplement form. It may also increase alertness and wakefulness in a person who did not get much sleep the prior night.	Nausea, headache, fatigue, joint pain.
L-carnitine	The FDA has approved L-carnitine for people with genetic diseases that have caused L-carnitine deficiency. The FDA has also approved L-carnitine for people with severe kidney disease to help increase RBC numbers. Non approved uses include taking it to promote fatty acid breakdown and conversion into energy.	Nausea, vomiting, heartburn, diarrhea. May also cause a fishy odor in the breath, sweat and urine.

ANTIOXIDANTS

Antioxidants are substances that may be able to fight and neutralize free radicals. Free radicals are molecules made in our body that can damage healthy cells and tissues. *Listed below are a few of the antioxidants that can be taken as a supplement. The "health benefits" and "health risks" listed below may not be backed by a lot of strong scientific evidence at this time- hence using the word "proposed" with those categories.*

Antioxidant	Proposed Health Benefits	Proposed Health Risks
Vitamin A, C, E	See discussion earlier in this chapter	
Selenium	See discussion earlier in this chapter. Often taken as a treatment for Hashimoto's thyroiditis and to lower LDL cholesterol.	
Coenzyme Q10 (CoQ10)	Is naturally produced in the body. Levels can drop as we age, as a result of disease, or as a side effect of some medications. It is used in the biological processes which produce energy for the functioning of body cells. It may be taken as a supplement to replace low natural Coenzyme Q10 levels in a deficient person. It may also be taken to reduce blood pressure, slow down age related macular degeneration (AMD), and slow down the progression of Alzheimer's and to prevent or treat migraines. Many other health conditions are being researched to determine any effects that Coenzyme Q10 supplementation might have.	Insomnia, rashes, abdominal pain, nausea, heartburn, fatigue. Coenzyme Q10 may interfere with the effects of warfarin (Coumadin) - an anticoagulant medication.
Beta-carotene	Colored pigments which can form Vitamin A. May be useful when consumed (in foods- not in supplement form) for prevention of breast cancer and in treating age related macular degeneration (AMD). FDA approval for use in treating erythropoietic protoprophyria (an inherited disease that can cause photosensitivity).	High doses may increase lung cancer risk in smokers and increase the risk of prostate cancer in men. High doses can turn the skin yellow or orange.
Lycopene	Found naturally in tomatoes, watermelons, and pink grapefruit. It is often taken to reduce risk of atherosclerosis, heart disease, cancer (lung, prostate, ovarian, etc.).	Studies are being done to see if lycopene reduces the risk of developing prostate cancer; BUT if the cancer is already established, high doses of lycopene may worsen the cancer.
Lutein	Many take this supplement to help with eye health. It has been taken to try to prevent AMD and cataracts. Some people take it to reduce risk of breast or colon cancer.	Not many risks have been reported.
Resveratrol	Found in the skin of red grapes. It is often taken to lower cholesterol, as an anti-inflammatory, to prevent heart disease, to prevent insulin resistance, and to prevent cancer.	May negatively interact with warfarin (Coumadin) and NSAIDs
Acai	Used to treat osteoarthritis, erectile dysfunction, high cholesterol, obesity, detoxification	More studies are needed

BONE AND JOINT SUPPLEMENTS

The following supplements are a few examples of supplements often taken to improve bone and joint health. Some are more studied and verified (Calcium, Vitamin D, etc.) and some have not been studied as much (MSM).

Bone and/or Joint Health Supplement	Proposed Health Benefits	Proposed Health Risks
Calcium	See discussion earlier in this chapter	
Vitamin D	See discussion earlier in this chapter	
Glucosamine Sulfate	Used in treating osteoarthritis to slow or reverse cartilage damage. Also helps to rejuvenate synovial fluid around the joints. May also decrease pain in osteoarthritic joints. Can take 4-8 weeks before any improvement is noticed.	Can cause stomach upset if taken on an empty stomach. Some side effects are nausea, heartburn and diarrhea. Can cause allergic reactions in patients allergic to shellfish. Can also interfere with the effect of warfarin (Coumadin) - an anticoagulant.
Chondroitin Sulfate	Used in osteoarthritis to decrease pain symptoms. Most often taken in conjunction with glucosamine sulfate. May also be used in eye drops to relieve dry eyes and also to treat interstitial cystitis.	Can cause allergic reactions in patients allergic to shellfish. Hives, rashes and sensitivity to the sun can be reported. For patients with prostate cancer, avoid use- it may encourage spread of cancer or recurrence.
Methylsulfonylmethane (MSM)	May be useful in decreasing joint pain and increasing range of motion in joints with osteoarthritis. Not as well researched as Glucosamine. In supplement form it is often combined with glucosamine and/or chondroitin sulfate.	Stomach pain and discomfort, diarrhea and headache.
SAMe	Used for many conditions: decreasing pain in osteoarthritis (anti-inflammatory and analgesic properties), treating depression, fibromyalgia, cholestasis and liver disease	Side effects can include diarrhea, constipation, insomnia, nervousness, sweating. Patients with bipolar disorder and Parkinson's should not take SAMe. It may lower blood glucose levels, so care should be taken with a diabetic patient taking SAMe. SAMe does cross the placenta, so should not be taken in the first trimester of pregnancy.

DIGESTIVE SUPPORT SUPPLEMENTS

This chart contains a few examples of supplements used to help improve digestive effectiveness and efficiency or will decrease unwanted symptoms of some digestive conditions.

Digestive Support Supplement	Proposed Health Benefits	Proposed Health Risks
Probiotics *For example: Lactobacillus acidophilus, Bifidobacterum longum, Saccharomyces boulardii*	To treat diarrhea (especially after antibiotic usage), to relieve symptoms of IBS, treat vaginal yeast infections, treat UTI's, and improve overall immune health	Not many reported
Prebiotics	Are used as a food and energy source for the probiotics. Helps to improve colony health of the probiotics in the body	Not many reported
Fiber Supplements *For example: Inulin, Psyllium (Metamucil), Methylcellulose (Citrucel)*	Used to improve bowel movement regularity, soften fecal material, and relieve constipation. Other uses may be to lower cholesterol, control diabetes/blood sugar levels	Abdominal bloating, cramping, gas. Can decrease absorption of medications (aspirin, warfarin, lithium). Can also decrease blood sugar levels, which may need to be monitored in a diabetic patient.
Licorice (DGL)	Used to relieve heartburn, acid reflux and indigestion	May increase blood pressure. Should not be taken in pregnancy
Papaya Enzymes	Used to relieve heartburn, acid reflux and indigestion	May interact with blood thinning medications (warfarin, aspirin). May cause a rash in some people. Individuals with a latex allergy should avoid papaya enzymes.
Peppermint Oil	Used to relieve IBS, acid reflux, heartburn, nausea	Can cause heartburn, flushing, headaches
Ginger	Used to relieve IBS, acid reflux, heartburn, nausea, gas, bloating. It can also be helpful in relieving nausea in morning sickness, as a result of chemotherapy, or motion sickness	Gas, belching, stomach upset, nausea. Ginger may have interactions with anticoagulant medications. It may alter blood pressure or blood glucose levels, so patients taking medications for hypertension or diabetes should be aware.
Hydrochloric acid	Used to treat acid reflux/ heartburn, belching, bloating	May increase heartburn, stomach pain, nausea, and vomiting
Pancreatin	Treats indigestion, or to replace pancreatic enzymes in a patient with pancreatitis, pancreatic cancer, cystic fibrosis	Abdominal cramps, nausea, diarrhea can occur
Lactase	In lactose intolerant people, used to diminish pain, gas, bloating and diarrhea when consuming dairy	Few reported. Possibly rash and swelling

HORMONE SUPPLEMENTS

This chart contains a few examples of supplements used when working with hormone related conditions or issues.

Hormonal Supplement	Proposed Health Benefits	Proposed Health Risks
Melatonin	Used for insomnia and sleep issues. Taken by people with jet-lag, people working swing shifts, children with ADHD or autism. May be useful for patients suffering from anxiety.	Daytime sleepiness, headache, depression, dizziness, irritability
Wild yams	Contains a chemical which can be made (in a laboratory setting) into estrogen or dehydroepiandrosterone (DHEA). Used as a natural estrogen replacement therapy (usually for menopause) or DHEA replacement therapy.	Might cause nausea, could worsen hormone related conditions (endometriosis, uterine fibroids) and cancer (breast, uterine, ovarian)
DHEA	May be taken for: slowing aging, reducing confusion and dementia, lessening effects of Alzheimer's, increasing sex drive, treating depression, weight loss	In women, changes in menses, headaches, growth of facial hair and deepening of voice may be seen. Men may see gynecomastia, increased blood pressure, increased aggression
Progesterone creams	Beware- OTC creams (not regulated by FDA) may not carry the amount of progesterone claimed on label. Prescription forms (regulated by FDA) are also available. Used to increase fertility, decrease miscarriages, PMS, regulate irregular menses, menopausal symptoms, headaches	Weight gain, fluid retention, fatigue, insomnia, rashes, depression
Human Chorionic Gonadotropin (HCG)	Weight loss	Combined with the calorie restriction guidelines in the HCG diet can lead to: gallstones, irregular heartbeat, electrolyte imbalances
Leptin	Weight loss and appetite suppressant. OTC supplements sold do not actually contain leptin, but may try to stimulate it in the body.	If leptin is injected, injection site reactions may occur (swelling, redness)
Human Growth Hormone (HGH)	Used for: anti-aging, muscle building, improvement of athletic performance	Edema, nerve and muscle pain, numbness and tingling in the skin. Can increase cholesterol and can increase risk of diabetes.

MOOD SUPPORT SUPPLEMENTS

Mood Support Supplement	Proposed Health Benefits	Proposed Health Risks
SAMe	See earlier discussion in this chapter	
St John's Wort	For treatment of mild to moderate depression	Can cause psychoses, photosensitivity, dry mouth, dizziness, confusion. Can have adverse drug reactions if patient is also taking other antidepressants, anticoagulants, NSAIDs, antiplatelet medications, digoxin, antiseizure medications, antiretrovirals, oral contraceptives and some chemotherapy medications.
5-Hydroxytryptophan (5-HTP)	For treatment of depression, fibromyalgia, sleep disorders, migraine headaches, appetite suppressant	In the past, some people taking 5-HTP have developed eosinophilia myalgia syndrome (due to supplement contamination- prior to regulation standards in 2007). Can also cause heartburn, nausea, vomiting, diarrhea. Can have interactions with prescription antidepressants and anti-Parkinson's medications
Valerian	For treatment of anxiety and insomnia	Can cause headaches, excitability, and sluggishness. May interfere with antiseizure medications. If taking valerian long term, withdrawal symptoms may be seen when discontinuing use.
Kava Kava	For treatment of anxiety, stress and insomnia. It can also reduce withdrawal symptoms in patients tapering off of benzodiazepine use.	Liver damage (jaundice, liver failure, death) has been seen with only short term usage. It may also make a person unsafe to be operating machinery and driving a car. (Do not drive after consuming kava). May interfere with oral contraceptives, diuretics and some chemotherapy medications
Gamma-Aminobutyric Acid (GABA)	For treatment of anxiety, depression, relieving PMS symptoms, and treatment for ADHD	Has not been studied enough to determine adverse effects
Passionflower	Used for treatment of anxiety and insomnia	Dizziness, confusion, poor muscle coordination. May have negative interactions with anticoagulant medications

OTHER COMMONLY USED WESTERN HERBS AND SUPPLEMENTS

Herb and/or Supplement	Proposed Health Benefits	Proposed Health Risks
Saw Palmetto	Used for treating Benign Prostatic Hypertrophy (BPH)	May cause headache and diarrhea. May have interactions with anticoagulants, NSAIDs, antiplatelet medications
Milk Thistle	Used for treating liver disease (cirrhosis, jaundice, hepatitis) and type 2 diabetes	Nausea, diarrhea, bloating, gas, upset stomach. May mimic estrogen and should not be taken by women with breast, ovarian or uterine cancers. It may alter medications which are normally processed by the liver.
Goldenseal	Can act as an antiseptic, used in preventing colds and flu. Can be used as an ointment on skin wounds to stimulate healing and minimize infection. Has been used to try to mask illegal drugs in urine tests (however, not very effective in this)	Should not be taken by pregnant women- may trigger uterine contractions. Should not be used by people with high blood pressure or people with heart conditions. May cause nausea and digestive issues.
Hawthorn	Used in treating angina, CHF, atherosclerosis, high blood pressure, arrhythmias	May cause abdominal pain, nausea, headaches, dizziness, palpitations, insomnia
Black Cohosh	Used in treating menopause symptoms, painful menses, PMS	Weight gain, headaches, abdominal pain, abdominal cramping, vaginal spotting or bleeding. May cause liver damage. Should not be taken during early pregnancy as it may increase the risk of miscarriage. Atorvastatin (Lipitor) may interact with Black Cohosh.
Evening Primrose	Used in treating osteoarthritis, PMS, cardiovascular disease, eczema and ADHD in children	May cause stomach upset, diarrhea, nausea, headaches. May interact with NSAIDs, aspirin, anticoagulants and antiplatelet medications.
Echinacea	Strengthens immune system (preventing colds and flu)	Fatigue, dizziness, headache, nausea, stomach discomfort. May cause an allergic reaction in people allergic to ragweed. Echinacea may interact with caffeine and immunosuppressant drugs.
Feverfew	Used in treating migraine headaches, menstrual cramps	May cause stomach upset, nausea, diarrhea, constipation, dizziness, sleep disturbances. Should be avoided by pregnant women as it may trigger uterine contractions and possibly a miscarriage. May cause an allergic reaction in people allergic to ragweed. May interact with NSAIDs, anticoagulants and antiplatelet medications.

OTHER COMMONLY USED WESTERN HERBS AND SUPPLEMENTS (CONTINUED)

Herb and/or Supplement	Proposed Health Benefits	Proposed Health Risks
Garlic	Used in treating high cholesterol, high triglycerides, atherosclerosis. Boosts immune system	Nausea, halitosis, increased body odor. May also cause burning sensation in the mouth, throat and stomach. May have interactions with anticoagulants, NSAIDs, antiplatelet medications, hypoglycemic medications, anti-retrovirals
Gingko	Used as an anti-aging treatment. Increases blood flow to the brain to improve memory	May cause heartburn, acid indigestion, nausea, headache and heart palpitations. May have interactions with anticoagulants, NSAIDs, antiplatelet medications, hypoglycemic medications, antiseizure medications, diuretics
Ginseng	Used to elevate energy levels, and improve stress resistance.	May cause rash, blood pressure changes, headache. May have interactions with anticoagulants, NSAIDs, antiplatelet medications, hypoglycemic medications, digoxin, diuretics, anti-retrovirals, and some chemotherapy medications
Cranberry	Treats and prevents urinary tract infections	Stomach upset, nausea, diarrhea. May have interactions with anticoagulants, NSAIDs, antiplatelet medications, hypoglycemic medications, diuretics, anti-retroviral medications, and some chemotherapy medications. May cause an allergic reaction in people allergic to aspirin. High levels of supplement may increase risk of kidney stones.

Practice Study and Test Questions:

1) Beriberi may be seen with a deficiency of
   A) Vitamin B1
   B) Vitamin B3
   C) Vitamin B9
   D) Vitamin B12

2) Excessive levels of _____ can lead to mottling of teeth.
   A) Iron
   B) Selenium
   C) Vitamin D
   D) Fluorine

3) Which vitamin is needed for proper clotting of the blood?
    A) Vitamin A
    B) Vitamin K
    C) Vitamin B7
    D) Vitamin B3

4) Which of the following supplements is often taken for benign prostatic hypertrophy?
    A) Evening primrose
    B) Passionflower
    C) Milk thistle
    D) Saw Palmetto

5) Proposed health risks for a woman who is taking DHEA are
    A) changes in menses, headaches, growth of facial hair, and deepening of voice
    B) abdominal cramps, nausea, or diarrhea
    C) gallstones and irregular heartbeat
    D) sweating, low blood pressure and a fishy body odor

6) Pellagra may be seen with a deficiency of
    A) Folic Acid
    B) Vitamin C
    C) Thiamin
    D) Niacin

7) Which of the following minerals is the main cation in intracellular fluid and is needed in the body for proper fluid balance, nerve and muscle function?
    A) Sodium
    B) Potassium
    C) Chloride
    D) Calcium

8) Which of the following supplements may be taken to improve bone and joint health?
    A) papaya enzymes
    B) glucosamine
    C) riboflavin
    D) iodine

9) Which of the following substances might be taken by a patient for depression or decreasing pain from osteoarthritis?
    A) HCG
    B) Valerian
    C) SAMe
    D) Ginseng

10) Which of the following supplements might be helpful for a patient who suffers from migraines?
    A) Coenzyme Q10
    B) Feverfew
    C) Lycopene
    D) both A and B

11) A BMI of 31 is
    A) normal
    B) overweight
    C) obese
    D) severely obese

12) Which supplements may be helpful in treating high cholesterol?
   A) Psyllium
   B) Garlic
   C) Selenium
   D) Plant sterols and stanols
   E) All of the above

13) Which of the following conditions could cause a person to be underweight?
   A) anorexia nervosa
   B) bulimia nervosa
   C) Crohn's disease
   D) all of the above
   E) only A and B

14) Liver damage is a proposed health risk when taking
   A) Peppermint oil
   B) Kava Kava
   C) Melatonin
   D) Lycopene

15) Which supplement might support eye health?
   A) Lutein
   B) Vitamin C
   C) SAMe
   D) Echinacea

16) Lactobacillus, Acidophilus, and Bifidobacterium longum are examples of
   A) Hormone supplements
   B) Antioxidants
   C) Mood support supplements
   D) Probiotics

17) Which of the following may be taken to relieve heartburn and acid reflux?
   A) DHEA
   B) Ginger
   C) Papaya enzymes
   D) both B and C

18) Which nutrient contains 4 kilocalories/gram?
   A) Carbohydrates
   B) Proteins
   C) Fats (Lipids)
   D) Both A and B

Answers: 1) A 2) D 3) B 4) D 5) A 6) D 7) B 8) B 9) C 10) D 11) C 12) E 13) D 14) B 15) A 16) D 17) D 18) D

CHAPTER 18: SAFETY PRACTICES

OSHA (Occupational Safety/ Health Act)

OSHA helps to establish the Universal Precautions we follow to ensure a safe environment in our clinics.

Here are <u>some</u> topics related to OSHA guidelines. Refer to your CNT booklet and any OSHA guidelines you follow in student clinic for more protocols you should follow when in practice.

Exposure Control Plan: OSHA requires that an acupuncturist has an **"Exposure Control Plan"** created and in placed in the office. For more information on what an Exposure Control Plan is and how to create one, please visit OSHA's document on this at: **http://www.osha.gov/Publications/osha3186.pdf.**

The Exposure Control Plan should be updated:
- annually
- whenever there is a new procedure added
- if a new staff position is created.

Blood-Borne Pathogen Training – must be done YEARLY for every at-risk *employee*. This does NOT apply to self-employed people in solo practice; it only applies if there are employees in the acupuncturist's office.

Vaccinations: *Hepatitis B vaccine-* OSHA requires employers to make Hepatitis B vaccines available for health care workers and also requires that employees are taught the benefits and risks of the vaccine. The Hepatitis B vaccine should be administered within 10 days of initial employment for health care workers. If an employee declines the vaccination, the acupuncturist MUST obtain a signed declination form from the employee. If the employee chooses later to obtain the vaccination, the acupuncturist must make the vaccine available, at no cost, to the employee. For more information, OSHA has a fact sheet and other resources available. The Hepatitis B Vaccination Fact Sheet can be accessed at: **https://www.osha.gov/OshDoc/data_BloodborneFacts/bbfact05.pdf**

Universal Precautions and CNT

The following information is a summary from the *Clean Needle Technique Manual for Acupuncturists, 6th edition, by the National Acupuncture Foundation*. Please refer to this text for additional information.

The main goal of Universal Precautions is the prevention of disease if exposure occurs. According to the concept of Universal Precautions, all human blood and certain human body fluids are treated as if known to be infectious for Human Immunodeficiency Virus, Hepatitis B Virus, and other blood-borne pathogens. Universal precautions must be used in the care of all patients.

Definitions:

Contamination – the transmission of pathogens to a sterile object. Sources for contamination in the clinic can be: fluid from open lesions/ blood/ saliva/ vaginal secretions/ fecal contamination. Tap water is not a usual source of contamination.

Sterilization – a procedure that destroys ALL microbial life, (bacteria, fungi, viruses, etc.).

Antiseptic – a substance that kills and reduces the number of pathogens on the skin. 70% Isopropyl alcohol – is the most effective antiseptic (allow to dry and avoid cross contamination with cotton swab). Use a different cotton swab for each area of the body. Do not use an alcohol concentration of greater than 70%, the antiseptic ability actually decreases with a concentration higher than 70%.

Disinfectant – a substance that reduces the number of pathogens on inanimate objects.

Basic elements of CNT and the Universal Precautions (not all inclusive, refer to the Clean Needle Technique Manual for more information):

✓ Risk control – assume that ALL patients have HBV and/or HIV
✓ For Immunocompromised Patients – (ex. HIV, or patients undergoing chemotherapy or dialysis) use antimicrobial products, alcohol-based disinfectants and germicidal soap
✓ Any material (towel, sheet, gown) applied or one that comes in contact with patient skin should NOT be re-used for another person. Blood-soiled gowns – should be put into laundry identified as such in the Exposure Control Plan.
✓ If blood or bodily fluids are present, gloves must be utilized. Protective clothing and eyewear must also be used if there is potential for splattering of bodily fluids into face or onto clothing. Gloves should not be re-used and should be disposed properly. Protective clothing must be cleaned or disposed of properly to avoid contamination. Hands should be immediately washed after encountering blood or bodily fluids.
✓ Universal precautions apply to the following bodily fluids: blood, serum/plasma, semen, vaginal secretions, cerebrospinal fluid, synovial fluid, fluid oozing out of wounds, tears, saliva, sputum, nasal secretions, feces, urine, vomit, and breast milk.
✓ Gloves or finger cots should be used if the acupuncturist has any cuts, lesions, damaged cuticles on their hand.
✓ A health care provider with weeping or oozing lesions should refrain from patient contact or handling equipment

✓ **Acupuncture Needles and Other Devices:**
  • Ensure needles are sterile, packaging is not damaged, needles are transported in protective equipment,
  • Dispose of needles in properly marked containers. And then dispose of container contents in the manner directed by state and local statutes.
  • Do not try to re-cap needles
  • Biohazard Needle containers should not be overfilled- dispose of contents when fill line has been reached (or earlier) - preferably 2/3 to 3/4 full.
  • Biohazard needle containers should be: Wall Mounted (if possible), "Biohazard" labeled, be RED in color, and have positive closures
  • The acupuncturist is legally accountable for EVERY acupuncture needle in their office until the contaminated ones are transferred to a licensed medical waste disposal company.

✓ **Hand washing:**
  • Have access to sink with hot and cold water, liquid soap, and disposable (single use) towels for drying hands.
  • Observe proper hand washing technique for health care providers (Wash entire hand – between fingers, under nails, and up to above the wrist).
  • The CDC recommends washing hands after removing gloves.
  • Wash hands before performing acupuncture procedure. Avoid re-contaminating hands before beginning treatment (answering phone, picking up pen/chart notes, etc.). Hands should be washed again after contacting patient. Hands should be washed also between every patient visit

✓ **Disinfecting in the Office:**
  - Disinfect non porous surfaces that were in contact with patient
  - Disinfectants are recommended for use on non-porous surfaces. Be sure to check expiration labels on disinfectants to ensure potency.
  - A Bleach dilution of 1:100 can be used to disinfect smooth surfaces. A bleach solution of 1:10 should be used for disinfecting porous surfaces. These solutions must be discarded after 24 hours and re-made if needed. The bottle of bleach solution should be labeled appropriately.
  - Over the counter hydrogen peroxide (usually sold as 3%) is not strong enough to act as an antiseptic or disinfectant. For sterilization, a concentration of 6%-25% must be used.
  - Treatment tabletops, and all work surfaces need to be cleaned with disinfectant at least once a day.

The prior information was a summary of information from the *Clean Needle Technique Manual for Acupuncturists, 6th edition, by the National Acupuncture Foundation*. Please refer to this text for additional information.

Methods of Communicable/Infectious Disease Transmission:

Infectious pathogens can be spread through many methods:
  - **Droplet contact**: through aerosolized droplets spread by sneezing, coughing, talking.
  - **Airborne**: smaller particulates (than in droplet contact) spread in the air. Pathogens can survive longer in the air without drying out (chickenpox, tuberculosis)
  - **Oral-fecal:** fecal material comes in contact with something that is ingested orally (food, water)
  - **Bodily fluids**: Coming in contact with bodily fluids that harbor the pathogen (semen, vaginal secretions, blood, lymph, saliva, sweat)
  - **Vector**: another organism carries the pathogen. It may be mechanical or biological. *Mechanical vector*- where the vector carries the pathogen on the outside of its body and transmits it. *Biological vector*- the pathogen enters the vector and then is spread by the vector usually through a bite (for example: a mosquito spreading West Nile Virus)
  - **Indirect contact**: touching a contaminated surface (door knob, table surface, computer keypad, telephone)

To read more about communicable disease and infectious pathogens, please refer to Chapter 10.

Federal Requirements / FDA (US Food and Drug Administration)

The FDA classifies medical devices into different classes. This allows for different rules and regulations for the different classes of devices to help improve safety when using these devices. Device classification is dependent on the intended use of the device and the indications for the use of the device.

Classification of Medical Devices Used in Acupuncture:

Class II Medical Devices:
FDA considers Acupuncture needles to be a CLASS II Medical device. For this reason, it is possible to simply verbally talk about the risks involved before the procedure, and not obtain written consent. However, obtaining written consent is a better method to utilize in your practice (it is proof that the discussion of the use of needles in the treatment did indeed occur).

CPR:

CPR stands for Cardiopulmonary Resuscitation. Upon arriving at a scene with a victim or victims, the rescuer should first determine that the scene is safe. If safe, the rescuer should see if the victim is responsive (tap and shout "Are you OK?"). If no response, call 911 (or instruct another bystander to do so). Check for a pulse for no more than 10 seconds. If no pulse, begin CPR.

When performing CPR, remember C-A-B. **C-A-B** stands for **C**= Compressions, **A**= Airway, **B**= Breathing. *Compressions* should be done in the center of the chest, contacting the lower half of the sternum (avoiding the xiphoid process) on an adult or child. The compressions should be performed at a fast rate – at about **100 per minute** (the beat to "Stayin' Alive"). *Airway* should be opened by performing a head tilt- chin lift maneuver. *Breathing*- each rescue breath should last about **1 second** and make the chest rise and fall. Once CPR is intitiated, CPR (compressions and rescue breaths) should continue until the scene becomes unsafe, another trained responder arrives and can take over, an AED (Automated external defibrillator) becomes available, or the rescuer becomes too exhausted to continue.

- **Adult victim**= anyone post-puberty. Single rescuer and 2-rescuers: 30 compressions followed by 2 rescue breaths. Chest compressions should be 2 inches deep using 2 hands
- **Child victim**= Age 1- puberty. Single rescuer and 2 rescuers: 30 compressions followed by 2 rescue breaths. Compressions should be 2 inches deep using one or two hands (depending on child size).
- **Infant**= less than one year of age. Single rescuer: 30 compressions followed by 2 rescue breaths. 2-rescuer CPR should have 15 compressions followed by 2 rescue breaths. Compressions should be performed just below the nipple line (using only 1 or 2 fingers), compressing to a depth of 1.5 inches.

Choking: If an *adult or child victim* cannot breathe, speak or make a sound, perform **abdominal thrusts** until object is expelled. If they CAN cough or make sounds, do not give abdominal thrusts- offer encouragement and stand by to help more, if needed. For an *infant*, perform **5 back blows and 5 chest compressions** (continue until object is removed from airway). If victim becomes unresponsive, begin CPR.

Basic First Aid

When performing basic first aid, please keep the following recommendations in mind:

- **Seizure:** Do not put anything in victim's mouth. Move any objects away from them that they might accidently strike. Assist in lowering them to the floor (so they do not fall down) and place some sort of a cushion behind their head. Do not try to physically restrain the victim during the seizure.
- **Fainting:** If no back or neck injury is suspected, raise legs 6-12 inches off of the floor. If victim feels nauseated when regaining consciousness, place in side lying recovery position.
- **Bleeding:** Wear gloves before contacting victim. Apply pressure over wound with sterile dressing. Wrap wound with gauze roller from first aid kit. Apply pressure over wound. If victim bleeds through wrap, do not remove it. Add more absorbent material over top (another dressing), secure it with another gauze roller, and apply pressure. Repeat if necessary. Watch for signs of shock. Tourniquets or pressure points to control bleeding are not advised.
- **Hypothermia:** Get victim out of cold environment and wet clothes (if present). Warm the body slowly by wrapping in blankets. Do not put them in a hot shower or hot tub. Give small amounts of warm fluid (not alcohol) to drink. Watch consciousness levels. For severe cases, call 911.
- **Hyperthermia:** Get victim out of sun/hot environment. Place cool damp towels over head and chest. Fan victim to assist in cooling. Give small amounts of fluid to drink (not alcohol). Watch consciousness levels. For **heat stroke** call 911.
- **Anaphylaxis:** Call 911. If patient has a prescribed auto-injector, help the victim self-administer the epinephrine. If victim is unable, the responder should administer the epinephrine *if they have been trained (and <u>state law allows</u>)*.

Please see your CPR and First Aid materials for more detailed information.

Practice Study and Test Questions:

1) If a mosquito harboring West Nile virus bites a human, the virus may be transmitted through the bite. This is an example of what type of infectious disease transmission?
      A) biological vector
      B) mechanical vector
      C) bodily fluid
      D) indirect contact

2) A bleach solution of _____ should be used to disinfect smooth surfaces and a bleach solution of _____should be used for porous surfaces.
      A) 1:100; 1:10
      B) 1:10; 1:100
      C) 1:50; 1:2
      D) 1:10; 1:2

3) The bleach solution discussed in Question #2 should be discarded after _____ and re-made, if needed.
      A) 12 hours
      B) 24 hours
      C) 6 hours
      D) 1 hour

4) Which of the following is not a blood-borne pathogen?
      A) Human immunodeficiency virus
      B) hepatitis A
      C) hepatitis B
      D) hepatitis C

5) The FDA considers acupuncture needles to be a
      A) unclassified medical device
      B) class III medical device
      C) class I medical device
      D) class II medical device

6) A sheet that was used to cover one patient during treatment may be re-used to cover the next patient- as long as there is no blood on it.
      A) True
      B) False

7) During CPR, depth of chest compressions on an adult victim should be
      A) 0.5 inches deep
      B) 1 inch deep
      C) 2 inches deep
      D) 3 inches deep

8) The acupuncturist should wash hands
      A) only when they arrive in the office first thing in the morning
      B) before performing an acupuncture procedure
      C) after contacting patient
      D) both B and C

9) Universal precautions apply to which bodily fluids?
> A) breast milk
> B) blood
> C) semen
> D) all of the above

10) Which of the following procedures destroys all microbial life?
> A) sterilization
> B) disinfecting
> C) vacuuming
> D) dusting

11) A patient is having a seizure in your office. You should not
> A) move objects away from the patient that they could strike while having the seizure
> B) assist them off of the treatment table or chair and onto the floor
> C) put a wallet or spoon in their mouth to prevent them from swallowing their tongue
> D) place a cushion or something soft under their head

12) OSHA requires that employers make the _____ vaccine available for health care workers.
> A) Hepatitis A
> B) Hepatitis B
> C) Hepatitis C
> D) all of the above

13) For a victim of hypothermia, a first-aid responder should not
> A) get the victim out of any wet clothing
> B) wrap the victim in blankets to gradually warm the body
> C) put the victim in a hot shower or tub to warm up their body
> D) give small amounts of warm fluids to drink

14) During a treatment, finger cots or gloves should be worn by the acupuncturist if the acupuncturist has any cuts or lesions on their hands/fingers.
> A) True
> B) False

15) CPR on an adult victim should have a ratio of ___ compressions and ___ rescue breaths
> A) 30:2
> B) 30:1
> C) 15:2
> D) 1:1

16) Biohazard containers should follow all of the following protocols, except
> A) they should be wall mounted (if possible)
> B) they should be labeled "Biohazard"
> C) they should be green in color
> D) they should have positive closures

17) An Exposure Control Plan is required by
> A) FDA
> B) OSHA
> C) Department of Homeland Security
> D) USDA

Answers: 1) A 2) A 3) B 4) B 5) D 6) B 7) C 8) D 9) D 10) A 11) C 12) B 13) C 14) A 15) A 16) C 17) B

CHAPTER 19: PRACTICE MANAGEMENT

For this section of materials, please reference any experiences in Clinic on charting and record maintenance, the CNT booklet, materials from HIPAA trainings, NCCAOM Code of Conduct and NCCAOM Rules and Regulations (found on their website) and discussions on how to establish a business.

But, here are a few links that may provide you with some information, or some quick definitions of terms that you may find helpful. The state guidelines mentioned here will vary from state to state. This text uses Washington State as its sample state for rules and regulations. If you are planning on practicing in a different state, check with that particular states rules and regulations pertaining to maintaining an acupuncture practice. Another state may have different (or in some cases, similar) guidelines as Washington State.

Charting and Record Keeping:

On every visit, documentation must be made. On the patient's first visit, a detailed history should be taken. This may include a thorough intake form (filled out by the patient) as well as notes taken during the consultation and examination. (See review notes on the Physical Examination the earlier chapter). Also refer to and think about the protocols you have been taught at school and in student clinic. The state you practice in (not the NCCAOM) determines how long you must retain patient records.

One common method of documenting a visit is SOAP charting/notes. These notes should be completed after you have finished the treatment.
- **S = Subjective**. This includes information that the patient tells you about how they are feeling and/or doing.
- **O = Objective**. This is where you detail things that you observed about the patient during any examination you have performed (pulses, palpation, etc.).
- **A = Assessment**. This is where any "diagnosis" of condition would be documented. Can summarize the S and O section here.
- **P= Plan.** It is here that you document the therapeutic intervention you performed during the visit. Also includes follow up treatment schedule, anything prescribed for home care (exercises, dietary changes, herbs, supplements, medications), and referrals or recommendations.

Some other things about medical records that should be kept in mind:
- A medical practice must respond to a patient's request to amend a record within 60 days. The maximum time allowed to comply with a medical records release order is 90 days
- If the provider notices a wrong entry in the medical records: Draw a line through the entry. Make sure that the inaccurate information is still legible. **Write "error"** by the incorrect entry and state the reason for the error in the margin or above the note if room. **Sign and date** the entry. **Document the correct information**. If the error is in a narrative note, it may be necessary to enter the correct information on the next available line, documenting the current date and time and referring back to the incorrect entry. **Never obliterate or otherwise alter the original entry** by blacking out with marker, using whiteout, or writing over an entry.
- Medical notes can ONLY be signed by the provider (not by any other staff members).
- Medical records belong to the health care provider, but the patient has access to them and can ask to view and/or amend them.
- If a patient misses or cancels an appointment, it should be documented in BOTH the appointment book AND the medical record
- Appointment logs should be kept just beyond the Statute of Limitations (this is determined by the state in which you practice)
- If the acupuncturist refers a patient out and there is a request for their records to be transferred, there must be written permission from the patient. Make a note in the patient's chart: **What** was

sent, **when** it was sent and **to whom** the records were provided. **Make a copy** of the records given to the health care provider to keep for your own record.

- Medical records are not primarily a legal document, however, they can serve as a legal document in court representing quality of care (in the case of a malpractice suit) or in the case of an injury court case (auto accident, etc.).
- From a legal perspective, if an action is not charted, it is assumed not to have happened.

HIPAA:

The Health Insurance Portability and Accountability Act of 1996. HIPAA is designed to help protect a patient's **Personal Health Information (PHI).** Here are some regulatory points about the HIPAA policies.

- A **Notice of Privacy Practices (NOPP)** must be given to every patient on their first visit to the office. It should detail how the patients PHI will be used and who it would be disclosed to (please take a look at the one distributed in student clinic to be familiar with what information the NOPP should contain). This NOPP also must be provided to non-patients who request to view it. It also should be prominently posted in a place available for viewing in the clinic.
- A patient must sign a consent form after reading the NOPP for permission to disclose PHI to the parties mentioned in the NOPP (insurance companies, law enforcement, etc.). This consent form only needs to be signed once.
- Office procedures should also make sure that PHI cannot be compromised.
  - Files should be locked and secure when not in use.
  - Computers should be password protected and computer screens not visible to others (for example- not facing the waiting room).
  - PHI should not be released to anyone (unless authorized in the NOPP), over the telephone or used for marketing purposes without written consent from the patient.
  - Transmission of PHI must be done in a secure manner (submitting insurance claims, referrals). Regular email should not be used to transmit PHI- encryption or other secure measures must be in place before email can be used.
  - ALL privacy breaches to PHI must be documented and followed up on.
  - Maintain records of all disclosures of PHI for 6 years (*"Disclosure"* is the release, transfer, provision of access to, or divulging of information outside of the original entity holding the information). Deceased patients signed PHI consent form never expires.
  - Penalties for leaving PHI information unsecured is $1000 per occurrence and criminal penalties for improperly disclosing PHI are $250,000 and up to 10 years in prison
  - Parents are allowed to have PHI of their children (who are still minors) released and discussed with them. A parent with a child (minor) will sign the NOPP consent form on behalf of their child. A minor can be viewed as having the legal capacity of an adult ("adult status") if they are any of the following: an emancipated minor, in the armed forces, married, or self-supporting and living on their own. Otherwise, legally a minor is anyone age seventeen (17) and below.
- Employees should be trained in HIPAA protocols, but no follow up CEU's are required after initial training. One employee should be named as the Information Security Officer and should be in charge of releasing any records and ensuring that protection of PHI is being done at all times.
- Business associates who have access to PHI must have contracts signed (associates in practice, billing companies you use to handle your insurance claim submissions, even housekeeping services) to assure security of PHI
- For more information Visit the Dept. of Health and Human Services website:
  - **http://www.hhs.gov/ocr/privacy/**

Referral Guidelines (in general)

Referrals to another health care provider (patient's primary care physician-PCP, a specialist, an urgent care facility, the emergency room, or contacting 911) may be needed, depending on what symptoms the patient presents with in the office. Following is a list of some conditions that should be referred out and the timeframe of when the patient should follow up with another health care provider. *This list is NOT all-inclusive!* It is here just to give some examples of situations when a referral is necessary. Each state may have specific laws and regulations detailing referral procedures for an acupuncturist. Please consult with the specific state rules and regulations that you may be practicing in for more information. Referral guidelines for acupuncturists practicing in Washington State will be listed later in this chapter, as an example of some state regulations.

Emergent referral (refer for immediate care)	Urgent referral (care should be obtained within 24-48 hours)	Routine referral (care should be obtained within 48 hours-7 days)
If you suspect the patient may have (or shows signs and symptoms of): • Myocardial infarction • Difficulty breathing (and not responding to medication) • Cerebrovascular accident (stroke) • Fever over 105° • Suspected fracture • Acute appendicitis • Acute pancreatitis • Pulmonary embolism • Severe pneumothorax • Suicidal depression • Anaphylaxis • Hypertensive crisis • Atrial fibrillation • Pyelonephritis (with high fever) • Ectopic pregnancy	*If you suspect the patient may have (or shows signs and symptoms of):* • Seizure (new onset) • Lung cancer • Breast cancer • Gastroenteritis • Otitis media • Pyelonephritis (with mild fever) • Malignant melanoma • Deep vein thrombosis • Neuropathy with high levels of pain, paresthesia, numbness	*If you suspect the patient may have (or shows signs and symptoms of):* • ADHD • Autism • Sleep apnea • Cancer- colorectal, bladder, uterine • Radiculopathy with mild pain and intermittent paresthesia • Myasthenia gravis • Rheumatoid arthritis • Temporomandibular joint disorder (TMJD) • Heartburn not responding to acupuncture treatment • Narcolepsy • Basal Cell Carcinoma • Erectile dysfunction • Cataracts

Mandated Reportable Conditions:

- Abuse, neglect, or endangerment of a child or elderly person must be reported to the authorities (for example: failure to provide a child with food, shelter, or clothing is considered neglect). Communicable and other diseases may need to be reported to the health department.
- **Child abuse** can involve physical and/or sexual abuse, emotional abuse, neglect or endangerment. Child abuse should be reported to the state Child Protective Services. If that resource is not available in the state, a practitioner can call 911 and ask for the appropriate referral agency to contact or ask for immediate police help.
- **Elder abuse** can involve physical abuse, emotional abuse, financial abuse (misusing the elderly person's assets), endangerment and neglect. In some states there is an Adult Protective Services that can be called to report the condition. If you are unsure who to call, you can call 911 and ask for the appropriate agency to contact or ask for immediate police help.
- **Communicable diseases** (and a few other diseases) must be reported to the health department. In most states there is a local health department and a state health department. In some states, certain conditions may need to be reported to the *local* health department and some may need to be reported to the *state* health department. Please see the state guidelines for the state you are practicing in to know which department to call and which conditions are reportable.
- For an example of state regulation of reporting a communicable disease, please see the section below. This is the WAC regarding Communicable Diseases which must be reported in Washington State:

WAC 246-101-101
Notifiable conditions and the health care provider

This section describes the conditions that Washington's health care providers must notify public health authorities of on a statewide basis. The board finds that the conditions in Table HC-1 of this section are notifiable for the prevention and control of communicable and noninfectious diseases and conditions in Washington.

(1) Principal health care providers shall notify public health authorities of the conditions identified in Table HC-1 of this section as individual case reports following the requirements in WAC 246-101-105, 246-101-110, 246-101-115, and 246-101-120.

*(2) **Other health care providers in attendance, other than the principal health care provider, shall notify public health authorities of the conditions identified in Table HC-1 of this section <u>unless the condition notification has already been made</u>.***

(3) Local health officers may require additional conditions to be notifiable within the local health officer's jurisdiction.

Some sample notifiable conditions from Table HC-1 are:
- **Conditions Notifiable to Local Health Department Immediately**: Anthrax, Animal bites where rabies is suspected, Diphtheria, Measles, Small Pox, Tuberculosis
- **Conditions Notifiable to Local Health Department Within 3 Business Days**: AIDS, chlamydia, gonorrhea, hepatitis C, Lyme disease, syphilis, tetanus, giardia, malaria
- **Conditions Notifiable to the State Health Department Monthly**: Asthma (occupational), autism spectrum disorder, cerebral palsy, alcohol related birth defects

**The table (Table HC-1) referenced in this WAC is many pages long, so it will not be posted here. Should you be interested in viewing the entire table (along with the information on this WAC that is listed above), please visit:
- **http://apps.leg.wa.gov/wac/default.aspx?cite=246-101-101**.

Coding for Treatment and Billing:

CPT Codes:

CPT codes- Current Procedural Terminology Codes. These are the codes the practitioner uses to describe what procedures and services were performed on the patient. For example:

- **97810:** Acupuncture, one or more needles; without electrical stimulation; initial 15 minutes.
- **97813**: Acupuncture, with electrical stimulation; initial 15 minutes

E&M Codes:

E&M codes- Evaluation and Management codes. These codes are based on the CPT codes and are used for office visits where a consultation or examination is performed. There are four levels of E&M codes: Problem Focused, Expanded Problem Focused, Detailed, and Comprehensive. These different levels reflect the depth in which the health care provider performed the health history intake and the examination. Different fees can be charged based on the level of complexity of the office visit.

ICD Codes:

ICD Codes- International Statistical Classification of Diseases and Related Health Problems Codes. These codes are the codes used to describe the condition the health care provider is treating or the "diagnosis" given the patient (will be provided by a referring MD, ND, DO, etc.). Following are some examples of ICD-9 and ICD-10 codes.

ICD-9 Code	ICD-10 Code	Diagnosis
724.2	M54.5	Low back pain
723.1	M54.2	Cervicalgia (Neck Pain)
530.11	K21.0	Reflux esophagitis
493.81	J45.990	Exercise induced bronchospasm (asthma)
346.10	G43.009	Migraine without aura, not intractable, without status migrainosus

Insurance:

Malpractice insurance: Malpractice insurance is purchased by health care professionals to financially cover them in the event they are sued for malpractice. Malpractice is the act of causing damage or injury to a person or persons as a result of negligently performing a professional duty or intentional wrongdoing. This type of injury is sometimes called an *iatrogenic injury* (an inadvertent adverse effect or complication resulting from medical treatment or advice). Malpractice insurance is sometimes called Personal Liability Insurance.

General Liability Insurance: sometimes also called "slip and fall" insurance. This is purchased to protect the practitioner from lawsuits should someone be injured on the business premises, but not as a result of the medical treatment. Some companies include general liability coverage in their malpractice policies. Other insurance companies do not; therefore the practitioner would have to purchase a separate policy. Landlords may require that the practitioner has this type of insurance in place before leasing office space.

Communication Issues

Medical Records Release: If a patient wants their medical records released, standard release forms must contain:
- ✓ Patient's dated signature and authorization for release.
- ✓ Address of the acupuncturist and include the ID of the patient (if known)
- ✓ What information is to be released (dates of service of needed, progress reports, etc.)
- ✓ Who will be receiving the records

Termination of a Patient: This is unfortunate, but occasionally will happen. If a practitioner is unilaterally terminating the care of a patient, the practitioner does not need to say WHY, but the practitioner needs to follow appropriate guidelines. The practitioner must notify the patient of termination of care in writing at least 30 days prior to termination. In that communication, these points must be stated
- the last day care will be provided, assuring the patient at least 15 days of emergency treatment and prescriptions before discontinuing service;
- alternative sources of medical care; for example: referral to another health care provider, the patient's insurer (for a provider list), or the local county's medical society; and
- how the patient can obtain their medical records from the practitioner.

Patient referral – If a patient comes via a referral, find out the purpose of the referral: Examine, Evaluate and Treat for that purpose. Send a report back to the referring physician about the services provided and document this report in the patient's chart.

Cost of Treatment – should be communicated to all new patients at the time of their initial appointment

Relationships with patients- It is best to keep interactions with patients on a strictly professional level. However, if an acupuncturist chooses to have an intimate relationship with a patient, the patient must be terminated from care (and referred to another acupuncturist for treatment, if necessary). The relationship must wait until 6 months after the last treatment (per NCCAOM guidelines in their "Code of Ethics").

Licensure Requirements:

TCM colleges must be accredited by the ACAOM (The Accreditation Commission for Acupuncture and Oriental Medicine).

Licensure:

Licensure is the process in which a governmental unit (state or local) grants an individual permission to pursue an occupation or carry out a business. This occupation or business is subject to regulation under the government's regulatory policies. Each practitioner should familiarize themselves with the licensure process in the <u>city</u> and <u>state</u> in which they will be practicing. In Washington State, for example, the practitioner's license must be renewed (and renewal fee paid) every year on the practitioner's birthday. And, the state (not NCCAOM) determines the title/identifier used by a health care practitioner. In Washington State, for example, these are the following titles which may be used in practice:
- ✓ **East Asian Medicine Practitioner**
- ✓ **EAMP**
- ✓ **Acupuncturist**
- ✓ **Licensed Acupuncturist**
- ✓ **L.Ac**

Certification:

Certification, a form of self-regulation, is a voluntary program by a private nonprofit organization (for example, the NCCAOM). The certification process is used to evaluate practitioners in a particular profession or business. Certification is usually granted for a limited period of time and must be renewed. The NCCAOM requires the practitioner to complete 60 CEU's every four years. The practitioner is responsible for notifying them of the CEU's that they have taken prior to the expiration of the certification each four years. CEU's are also referred to as PDA's (Professional Development Activities) by the NCCAOM.

NCCAOM certification- For students wishing to receive certification by the NCCAOM, it is HIGHLY recommended that the student be well familiarized with the NCCAOM's "Code of Ethics". The Code of Ethics and other documents (such as: Grounds for Professional Discipline, Ethics Complaint Form, and Procedures for Upholding Professional Conduct) can be found at the NCCAOM's website: **www.NCCAOM.org**. This website has great information on the certification and examination process, renewal process, and other helpful topics pertaining to the NCCAOM certification and to the practice of acupuncture in general.

Scope of Practice and Qualifications

Scope of practice is determined by each state. In Washington State, for example, the law requires each East Asian Medicine Practitioner / Acupuncturist to inform a patient of the practitioner's qualifications and scope of practice. The patient must be notified in writing of these criteria on their initial visit. In the following section in this chapter we will review the specific scope of practice regulations for Washington State (as an example of state regulation of this topic). Please check the regulations for any state you wish to practice in, as they may be similar or different from our sample state example (Washington State).

Laws That Govern the Profession in the State of Washington:

Revised Code of Washington (RCW's)

A *statute* or **Revised Code of Washington (RCW)** is written by the Washington State Legislature. Once legislation is signed by the Governor, it becomes law. Use the following link to guide you to RCW's that apply to abuse reporting, medical records disclosure, etc...

> **http://apps.leg.wa.gov/RCW/default.aspx?cite=18.06**

Washington Administrative Code (WAC)

A *rule* or **Washington Administrative Code (WAC)** is written to provide interpretive support for the individuals to whom the rule applies. Department of Health rules are written and adopted by a Board, Commission or the Secretary of the Department of Health. Rules or WACs carry the full force of the law.

In 2011, the name "Acupuncturist" in the WAC's was replaced with the name "**East Asian Medicine Practitioner**". The WAC's that apply to East Asian Medicine Practitioners (Acupuncture) are found in Chapter 246-803 WAC. Items included in the WAC's include topics such as: referral to health care providers, examination guidelines, patient informed consent, documentation requirements, etc. and can be found at:

- **http://apps.leg.wa.gov/wac/default.aspx?cite=246-803**

Referral Guidelines for East Asian Medicine Practitioner / Acupuncturists in Washington State

When needing to refer a patient out, document the referral in the chart note. If possible, offer the name of a few health care providers to refer the patient to. This allows patients options for selecting their provider.

Referral to Primary Health Care Providers

Approved primary health care providers for referral in Washington State include: *medical physician, physician assistant, osteopathic physician, osteopathic physician assistant, naturopathic physician, or advanced registered nurse practitioners*. Here is the WAC for when an East Asian Medicine Practitioner/Acupuncturist should refer to a Primary Health Care Provider.

WAC 246-803-310
Referral to Primary Health Care provider.

(1) *When an East Asian medicine practitioner sees a patient with a potentially serious disorder, the East Asian medicine practitioner shall immediately request a consultation or written diagnosis from a primary health care provider.*

(2) *Potentially serious disorders include, but are not limited to:*
    (a) Cardiac conditions including uncontrolled hypertension;
    (b) Acute abdominal symptoms;
    (c) Acute undiagnosed neurological changes;
    (d) Unexplained weight loss or gain in excess of fifteen percent body weight within a 3 month period;
    (e) Suspected fracture or dislocation;

(f) Suspected systemic infection;

(g) Any serious undiagnosed hemorrhagic disorder; and

(h) Acute respiratory distress without previous history or diagnosis.

(3) In the event a patient with a potentially serious disorder refuses to authorize such consultation or provide a recent diagnosis from a primary health care provider, East Asian medical treatments, including acupuncture, may only continue after the patient signs a written waiver acknowledging the risks associated with the failure to pursue treatment from a primary health care provider.

(4) The written waiver must include:

(a) A statement acknowledging that failure by the patient to pursue treatment from a primary health care provider may involve risks that such a condition can worsen without further warning and even become life threatening;

(b) An explanation of an East Asian medicine practitioner's scope of practice, to include the services and techniques East Asian medicine practitioners are authorized to provide; and

(c) A statement that the services and techniques that an East Asian medicine practitioner is authorized to provide will not resolve the patient's underlying potentially serious disorder.

[Statutory Authority: Chapter 18.06 RCW and 2010 c 286. WSR 11-17-105, § 246-803-310, filed 8/22/11, effective 9/22/11.]

(The above WAC can be found at **http://apps.leg.wa.gov/wac/default.aspx?cite=246-803-310**)

Emergency Transfer and Referral

The East Asian Medicine Practitioner /Acupuncturist must have a plan in place in an emergency situation. Here is the WAC pertaining to this topic

WAC 246-803-330
Plan for consultation, emergency transfer and referral.

Every East Asian medicine practitioner shall develop a written plan for consultation, emergency transfer, and referral. The written consultation plan must be submitted to the department after initial licensure but prior to treating any patients, and annually with the license renewal fee. The written plan for consultation, emergency transfer and referral must include:

(1) The name, license number and telephone numbers of two consulting primary health care providers.

(2) A statement attesting that in an emergency, the East Asian medicine practitioner will:

(a) Initiate the emergency medical system (EMS) by dialing 911;

(b) Request an ambulance; and

(c) Provide patient support until emergency response arrives.

(3) Confirmation from the primary health care providers listed as to their agreement to consult with and accept referred patients from the applicant.

[Statutory Authority: Chapter 18.06 RCW and 2010 c 286. WSR 11-17-105, § 246-803-330, filed 8/22/11, effective 9/22/11.]

(The above WAC can be found at: **http://apps.leg.wa.gov/wac/default.aspx?cite=246-803-330**)

Scope of Practice and Qualifications in Washington State

Scope of practice is determined by each state. In Washington State, for example, the law requires each East Asian Medicine Practitioner / Acupuncturist to inform a patient of the practitioner's qualifications and scope of practice. The patient must be notified in writing of these criteria on their initial visit. **(WAC 246-803-300).**

The following is a sample document from the Washington State Department of Health.

SAMPLE-- Patient Notification of Qualifications and Scope of Practice

East Asian medicine means a health care service using East Asian medicine diagnosis and treatment to promote health and treat organic or functional disorders.

1. *My qualifications include the following education and license information:*
(a) _____
(b) _____
(c) _____
(d) _____

2. *The scope of practice for an East Asian medicine practitioner in the state of Washington includes the following:*
     (a)Acupuncture, including the use of acupuncture needles or lancets to directly or indirectly stimulate acupuncture points and meridians;
     (b)Use of electrical, mechanical, or magnetic devices to stimulate acupuncture points and meridians;
     (c)Moxibustion;
     (d)Acupressure;
     (e)Cupping;
     (f)Dermal friction technique;
     (g)Infra-red;
     (h)Sonopuncture;
     (i)Laserpuncture;
     (j)Point injection therapy (aquapuncture); and
     (k)Dietary advice and health education based on East Asian medical theory, including the recommendation and sale of herbs, vitamins, minerals, and dietary and nutritional supplements;
     (l)Breathing, relaxation, and East Asian exercise techniques;
     (m)Qi gong;
     (n)East Asian massage and Tui na, which is a method of East Asian bodywork, characterized by the kneading, pressing, rolling, shaking, and stretching of the body and does not include spinal manipulation;
     (o)Superficial heat and cold therapies.

3. *Side effects may include, but are not limited to:*
     (a)Pain following treatment;
     (b)Minor bruising;
     (c)Infection;
     (d)Needle sickness; and
     (e)Broken needle.

4. *The patient must inform the East Asian medicine practitioner if the patient has a severe bleeding disorder or pace maker prior to any treatment.*

(The above sample form can be found at:
http://www.doh.wa.gov/LicensesPermitsandCertificates/ProfessionsNewReneworUpdate/EastAsianMedicine
Practitioner/FrequentlyAskedQuestions.aspx#1)

Practice Study and Test Questions:

1) You find an error in one of your chart notes. You should
    A) use white-out to cover the error and write over it
    B) take notes in pencil so that you can erase any errors
    C) draw a single line through the error, and initial it. Then write the correct information on the next line available.
    D) use a dark marker to completely cover the error, and then write the correct information

2) HIPAA stands for
    A) Health Insurance Portability and Accountability Act
    B) Health Information Privacy and Accountability Act
    C) Health Information Practices and Adjustment Act
    D) Health Intelligence Procedures And Assessments

3) You suspect a patient is experiencing a cerebrovascular accident in your office. This condition warrants a
    A) Emergent referral (immediate care)
    B) Urgent referral (care should be obtained within 24-48 hours)
    C) Routine referral

4) Mr. And Mrs. Jones are both patients of yours. Do the HIPAA regulations allow you to speak with Mr. Jones' wife about his condition during one of her treatments?
    A) Yes
    B) No
    C) It would depend if Mr. Jones has authorized (in writing) that you may do so.

5) PHI stands for
    A) Personal Health Information
    B) Private Health Information
    C) Notice of Privacy Practices
    D) Both A and B

6) Housekeeping, janitorial, and billing services which may have access to the PHI in your office should have a business associate contract signed, to assure security of PHI.
    A) True
    B) False

7) A patient describes that she wakes up consistently at 3:00 am and then has a hard time falling back asleep. This should be recorded in which portion of the SOAP chart?
    A) S- Subjective
    B) O-Objective
    C) A- Assessment
    D) P-Plan

8) You suspect a 10 year old patient may be suffering from ADHD. This condition warrants a
    A) Emergent referral (immediate care)
    B) Urgent referral (care should be obtained within 24-48 hours)
    C) Routine referral

9) Mrs. Smith calls your office very irate. Her 25 year old daughter, Sally, has been coming for treatment in your office. Mrs. Smith demands to know why her daughter has been seeking care. Are you allowed to discuss this with Sally's mother?
        A) Yes, of course. She is her mother!
        B) No, not without written consent from Sally.

10) Mandated reportable conditions can include
        A) Child abuse
        B) Elder abuse
        C) Certain communicable diseases (if specified by the state or local law in the area you are practicing in)
        D) All of the above

11) Which codes does an acupuncturist use to describe the condition for which the patient is being treated?
        A) DPT codes
        B) E and M codes
        C) CPT codes
        D) ICD codes

12) What code is used to indicate the procedure performed during the visit (not an examination or consultation).
        A) DPT codes
        B) E and M codes
        C) CPT codes
        D) ICD codes

13) A patient trips over one of the chairs in your waiting room and falls, breaking her wrist. Which insurance of yours will pay for the medical care as a result of her accident?
        A) Malpractice Insurance
        B) General Liability Insurance
        C) Personal Injury Protection Insurance
        D) Both A and B

14) The title under which you will be able to practice (ex: LAc, Licensed Acupuncturist, EAMP) is determined
        A) by the ACAOM
        B) by the local or state governmental regulations in the area you practice
        C) by the NCCAOM
        D) by yourself- you can decide which title you'd like to use.

15) 97810 is an example of a
        A) ICD-9 code
        B) ICD-10 code
        C) CPT code

16) An acupuncturist would document their pulse findings in which part of the SOAP chart?
        A) S-subjective
        B) O-objective
        C) A-Assessment
        D) P-Plan

Answers: 1) C 2) A 3) A 4) C 5) A 6) A 7) A 8) C 9) B 10) D 11) D 12) C 13) B 14) B 15) C 16) B

CHAPTER 20: MEDICAL TERMINOLOGY

Following is a list of terms which can be used in forming many of the biomedical words.

A "**prefix**" is a term found at the beginning of a word. A medical term may or may not have a prefix present.
A "**word root**" makes up the main body of the word.
A "**suffix**" is the word ending.

Here are a few examples of biomedical terms and how they can be broken down into their roots, prefixes and suffixes.

Osteoporosis- can be broken down into
- **"Osteo"-** word root meaning "bone"
- **"-porosis"-** suffix meaning "condition of pores (spaces or holes)"
- Note: there is no prefix present in this example.

Hyperthyroidism- can be broken down into
- **"Hyper-"** prefix meaning "excessive or increased"
- **"thyroid"** word root meaning "thyroid gland"
- **"-ism"** is a suffix meaning "a process or condition"

a- *(at beginning of word)*	not, without, no, away from
a- / an- *(at beginning of word)*	without/ not/ no
ab-	away from
-ac	pertaining to
Acr/o	extremities (hands and feet), top, extreme point
ad-	toward
Aden/o-	gland
Adren/o	adrenal glands
Af-	toward, to
Agglutin/o	clumping, stick together
-al	pertaining to
-algia	pain
Aliment/o	to nourish
An-	without
Ana-	apart, backward, excessive
Andr/o	relationship to male
Ankyl/o	crooked/bent/stiff
Anter/o-	front
Anti-	against
-ar	pertaining to
Arachn/o	spider web, spider
Arter/o, arteri/o	artery
Arthr/o	joint
-ary	pertaining to
Asmat/o	gasping/ choking
-asthenia	weakness/ lack of strength
Astr/o	star, star-shaped
Ather/o	plaque, fatty paste
Auscult/o	listen

Auto-	self, own
Bio-	life
-blast	to build, immature,
Brachi/o	arm
Brady-	slow
Bronch/o	bronchial tube, bronchiole
Bronchi/o	bronchus
Bronchiol/o	small bronchus
Burs/o	bursae
Calc/o	calcium
Calci/o	calcium
Carb/o-	carbon
Carcin/o	cancerous/ cancer
Cardi/o	heart
Catabol/o-	breaking down
Caud/o	lower part of body, tail
Cephal/o-	head
Cerebr/o	cerebrum, brain
Chem/o	drug, chemical
Chol/e	bile
Chondr/o	cartilage
Chore/o	dance
Chrom/o-	color
Cirrh/o	orange/yellow, tawny
-clast	to destroy
Co-	together/ with
Coagul/o	clotting
Cochle/o	spiral, snail, snail shell
Colon/o	large intestine
Concuss/o	shaken together, violently agitated
-constriction	narrowing
Conten/o-	keep in, contain, hold back
Contus/o	bruise
Cort-	covering
Cost/o	ribs
Crani/o	cranium/skull bones
-crit	to separate
Cutane/o	skin
Cyan/o	blue
Cyst-	urinary bladder / fluid filled sac
Cyt/o-	cell
-cyte	cell
De-	down, lack of, from, not, removed
Defecat/o	free from waste, clear
Dendr/o	branching, resembling a tree
Derm/o	skin
di-	twice, twofold, double
Dia-	complete/ through
-dilation	widening, stretching, expanding
Dis-	negative/ apart/ absence of
Dist/o-	far/distant
Diur/o, diuret/o	tending to increase urine output
Dors/i, dors/o	back of body
Duct/o	to lead, carry
-dypsia	thirst

Dys-	bad, difficult, painful
-ectomy	surgical removal, cutting out, excision
Edem/o	swelling, fluid
-edema	swelling
Ef-	out
Ejaculato-	throw or hurl out
Electr/o-	electricity
Embol/o	something inserted in or thrown in
-emesis	vomiting
-emia	blood, blood condition
Encephal/o	brain
Endo-	in, within, inside
Endo-	in/ within
Endocrin/o	secrete within
Epi-	above, upon, on
Epiglott/o	epiglottis
Equin/o	pertaining to a horse
Erythem/o	redness
Erythr/o	red
Estro-	female
Eu-	good, normal, well, easy
Ex-	out of, outside, away from
Exo-	out of, outside, away from
Fasci/o	fascia, fascial
Fer/o	bear, carrying
-ferent	carrying
Fibr/o	fiber
Fimbrio-	fringe
Gastr/o	stomach
Gemin/o	twin, double
-gen	producing, forming
-genesis	creation, reproduction, the beginning of
Gest/o	bear, carry young offspring
Gigant/o	giant, very large
-gli/o, -gli/a	neurologic tissue, support tissue of nervous system
-globin	protein
-globulin	protein
Glomerul/o-	glomerulus portion of kidney
Gloss/o	tongue
Glyc/o	sugar
Glyc/o-	glucose, sugar
Gonad/o	gonad, sex glands
Gyr/o-	turning, folding
Hem/o Hemat/o-	blood
Hepa	liver
Hiat/o	opening
Hist/o-	tissue
Home/o-	sameness/unchanging/ constant
Hydr/o- ; Hydr/a-	relating to water
Hyper-	excessive, above, increased
Hypo-	deficient, decreased, below
-ia	abnormal condition
-iferous	bearing/ carrying/ producing
Immun/o-	immune/ protection/ safe
In-	into/in/not

-ine	pertaining to
Infarct/o	filled in, stuffed
Insipid/o	tasteless
Integument	covering
Inter-	between, among
-ion	action, process, state or condition
Isch/o	to hold back
-ism	process/condition
-itis	inflammation
-ium	tissue
Jaund/o	yellow
Juxta-	beside, near, nearby
Kerat/o	hard/ horny/ cornea
Kinesi/o	movement
Kyph/o	kyphotic/ humpback
Lact/o, lact-	milk
Laryng/o	larynx/ voice box
Later/o-	side
Leuk/o	white
Ligament/o	ligament
Lingu/o	tongue
-lithiasis	presence of stones
Loc/o	place
Lord/o	bent backwards
Lun/o	moon
Lux/o	to slide
Lymph/o	lymph
-lysis	breakdown/separation/loosening
-lytic	to reduce, destroy
Macro-	large
Mal-	bad
-malacia	softening
Mandibul/o	mandible, lower jaw
Masticat/o	to chew
Medi/o-	middle
Medull/o-	inner section, middle, soft, marrow
-megaly	enlargement
Melan/o	black
Mellit/o	honey, honeyed
Men/o-	menstruation
Mening/o	membranes, meninges
Meta-	to change/ beyond
Metr/i, metri/o-	uterus
Micro-	small
Micturit/o- , Mictur/o-	urinate
mid-	middle
Mono-	one, single
Mot/o	movement, motion
Muscul/o	muscle
My/o, Myos/o	muscle
Myel/o	bone marrow/spinal cord
Myx/a	mucus
Nas/o	nose
Nephro-	nephron portion of kidney
Neur/o	nerve, neuron, nerve tissue

Noct-	night
Nom/o	control
Non-	no
Nor	chemical compound
Nucle/o-	nucleus
Occipit/o	back of skull
Ocul/o	eye
Olfact/o	smell, sense of smell
Olig/o	scanty, few
-oma	tumor/ mass
-one	hormone
Oo-	egg
-opsy	to view
Opthalm/o	eye, vision
-ory	pertaining to
-osis	condition, usually abnormal
Osseous	bony
Oste/o	bone
Ovulo-	egg
Oxy-	swift, sharp
Para-	beside, near, along side
Paralys/o, paralyt/o	disable
Parturit/o-	childbirth
Path/o	disease
-pathy	disease condition
-penia	deficiency, lack, too few
Peri-	surrounding, around
Peritone/o-	peritoneum
Phag/o-	eat, swallow
-phage	eat, swallow
-phagia	eating, swallowing
Pharyng/o	pharynx/ throat
-phil, -philia	attraction to, like, love
Phleb/o	vein
-phylactic	protective, preventative
Physi/o-	nature, function
-physis	to grow
Pir/o	breathing
-plegia	paralysis, stroke
-plegic	one affected with paralysis
Pleur/o	pleura
Plex/o	network
-pnea	breathing
Pneum/o; pneumon/o	air, lung
-poiesis	formation/ to make
Poly-	many
-porosis	condition of pores (spaces or holes)
Poster/o-	back/behind
Pro-	before, in, behalf of
Proxim/o-	nearest
Psor/i ; Psor/o	itching/ itch
Pulmon/o	lung
Pyelo-	renal pelvis
Pyr/o-	fever, fire
Quadr/i, quadr/o-	four

Re-	back, again
Renal	pertaining to kidney
Retro-	behind, backward, back of
Rheumat/o	watery flow (synovial fluid)
Rhin/o	nose
-rrhea	abnormal flow/ discharge
Scler/o	hard, white of eye
Scoli/o	crooked/bent
-scope	instrument to visually examine
Seb/o	sebum
Semi-	half
-sis	state of
Skelet/o	skeleton
Somat/o	body
Spermato-	sperm/spermatozoa
-sphyxia	pulse
Spin/o	spine, backbone
Spir/o	breathing
Splen/o	spleen
-stalsis	contraction, constriction
-stasis	control, maintenance of a constant level
Ster/o	solid structure
Sub-	below/ under/ less
Sudor/o	sweat
Symptomat/o	symptom, falling together
Tachy-	fast
Tax/o	coordination, order
Ten/o, Tend/o, Tendin/o	tendon
Tens/o	strain, stretch out
Test/o	testes, testicle
Thermo	temperature
Thorac/o	chest, thoracic spine
Thromb/o	clot
Thyroid, thyro	thyroid gland
-tocin	labor, birth
Ton/o	tension/ tone/ stretching
Tox/o	poison
tri-	three
Trochle/o	pulley
-trophy	nourishment/ development
Tropic	turning
Tubercul/o	little knot, swelling
-um/ -ium	structure/ tissue
Un-	not
Ureth-	urethra
-uria	urination
-us	thing
Vas/o-	ductus (Vas) deferens/ vessel
Ventilat/o	expose to air
Ventr/o	in front, belly side of body
Vestibul/o	entrance
Viscer/o	viscera/ internal organ

Practice Study and Test Questions:

1) This prefix means "against"
      A) Anti-
      B) Semi-
      C) Rhino-
      D) Oo-

2) The word root which means "cancer" is
      A) micturo
      B) ischo
      C) juxta
      D) carcino

3) "Ankylo" means
      A) crooked, bent, or stiff
      B) opening
      C) giant, very large
      D) stomach

4) Which word root means "cartilage"?
      A) chondro
      B) contuso
      C) integument
      D) epiglotto

5) The suffix _____ means "tumor or mass"?
      A) -oma
      B) -emia
      C) -ium
      D) both A and C

6) "Edemo" means
      A) presence of stones
      B) to destroy
      C) swelling or fluid
      D) covering

7) Which word root means "brain"?
      A) encephalo
      B) hemato
      C) cerebro
      D) both A and C

8) The suffix "-itis" means
      A) good, normal
      B) to hold back
      C) inflammation
      D) to cut

9) Which term means "white"?
      A) disto
      B) cutaneo
      C) leuko
      D) cyano

10) Which word root means "clotting"?
      A) pyelo
      B) viscero
      C) ovulo
      D) coagulo

11) "Defecato" means
      A) childbirth
      B) free from waste
      C) membrane
      D) spine

12) Which term means "black"?
      A) jaundo
      B) toxo
      C) melano
      D) contuso

13) "Infarcto" means
      A) turning/folding
      B) stomach
      C) filled in, stuffing
      D) covering

14) "Cyto" means
      A) tissue
      B) cell
      C) life
      D) skin

15) Which term means "red"?
      A) jaundo
      B) leuko
      C) estro
      D) erythro

16) Which word root means "eye"?
      A) oculo
      B) opthalmo
      C) mono
      D) both A and B

17) Which word root means "kidney"?
      A) hepato
      B) esophago
      C) renal
      D) spleno

18) Which word root means "joint"?
    A) kerato
    B) endocrino
    C) medullo
    D) arthro

19) Which word suffix means "pain"?
    A) -physis
    B) -pnea
    C) -algia
    D) -malacia

20) Which word root means "liver"?
    A) opthalmo
    B) hepa
    C) nephro
    D) musculo

21) "-asthenia" means
    A) weakness or lack of strength
    B) crooked/bent
    C) fever
    D) breathing

22) Which word rood means "bone"?
    A) osteo
    B) osseous
    C) sudoro
    D) both A and B

23) "Pulmono" means
    A) lung
    B) nose
    C) mandible
    D) pharynx/throat

24) Which prefix means "fast'
    A) brady
    B) nomo
    C) macro
    D) tachy

25) "-osis" means
    A) back of skull
    B) breathing
    C) a condition, usually abnormal
    D) paralysis

Answers: 1) A 2) D 3) A 4) A 5) A 6) C 7) D 8) C 9) C 10) D 11) B 12) C 13) C 14) B 15) D 16) D 17) C 18) D 19) C 20) B 21) A 22) D 23) A 24) D 25) C

PLEASE USE THIS PAGE FOR ANY ADDITIONAL NOTES YOU MIGHT WANT TO WRITE DOWN

PLEASE USE THIS PAGE FOR ANY ADDITIONAL NOTES YOU MIGHT WANT TO WRITE DOWN

Made in United States
Troutdale, OR
03/11/2024

18378768R00186